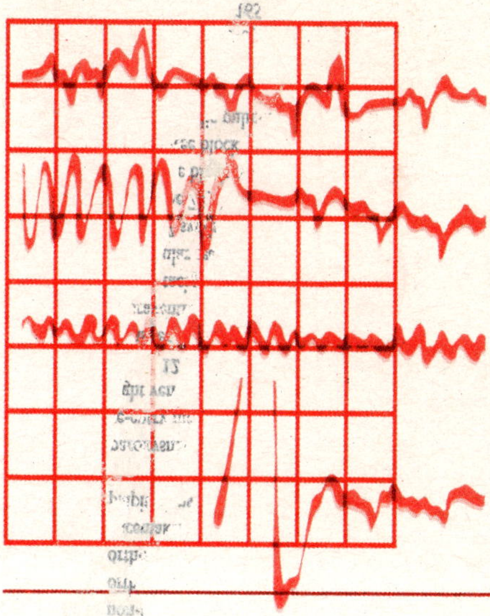

THE ECG IN PRACTICE

FIFTH EDITION

Commissioning Editor: Laurence Hunter
Development Editor: Hannah Kenner
Project Manager: Susan Stuart and Helius
Designer: Sarah Russell
Illustrator: Helius and Gecko Ltd
Illustration Manager: Bruce Hogarth

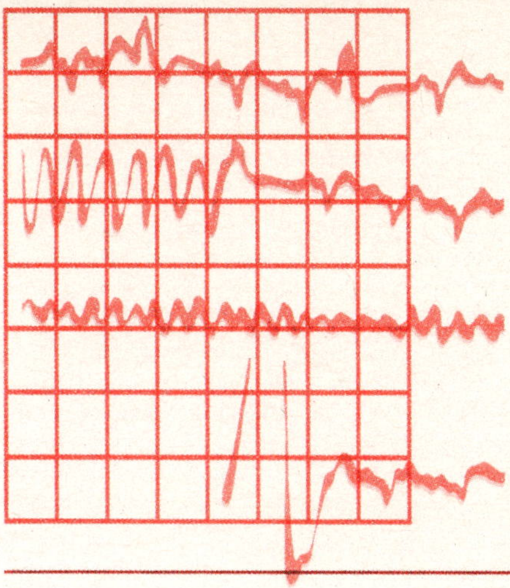

THE ECG IN PRACTICE

FIFTH EDITION

John R. Hampton

DM MA DPhil FRCP FFPM FESC

Emeritus Professor of Cardiology
University of Nottingham
Nottingham, UK

With a contribution by

David Adlam DPhil BA BM BCh MRCP DPhil

Specialist Registrar in Cardiology
and General (Internal) Medicine
Oxford, UK

CHURCHILL LIVINGSTONE
ELSEVIER

EDINBURGH LONDON NEW YORK OXFORD PHILADELPHIA ST LOUIS SYDNEY TORONTO 2008

CHURCHILL
LIVINGSTONE
ELSEVIER

First edition 1986
Second edition 1992
Third edition 1997
Fourth edition 2003
Fifth edition 2008

Standard edition ISBN: 978-0-443-06825-6
International edition ISBN: 978-0-443-06824-9

British Library Cataloguing in Publication Data
A catalogue record for this book is available from the British Library

Library of Congress Cataloguing in Publication Data
A catalogue record for this book is available from the Library of Congress

Printed in China

Note

Knowledge and best practice in this field are constantly changing. As new research and experience broaden our knowledge, changes in practice, treatment and drug therapy may become necessary or appropriate. Readers are advised to check the most current information provided (i) on procedures featured or (ii) by the manufacturer of each product to be administered, to verify the recommended dose or formula, the method and duration of administration, and contraindications. It is the responsibility of the practitioner, relying on their own experience and knowledge of the patient, to make diagnoses, to determine dosages and the best treatment for each individual patient, and to take all appropriate safety precautions. To the fullest extent of the law, neither the Publisher nor the Author assume any liability for any injury and/or damage to persons or property arising out or related to any use of the material contained in this book.

The Publisher

The publisher's policy is to use paper manufactured from sustainable forests

Preface

WHAT TO EXPECT OF THIS BOOK

I assume that the reader of this book will have the level of knowledge of the ECG that is contained in *The ECG Made Easy*, to which this is a companion volume. The ECG is indeed easy in principle, but the variations in pattern seen both in normal people and in patients with cardiac and other problems can make the ECG seem more complex than it really is. This book concentrates on these variations, and contains several examples of each abnormality. It is intended for anyone who understands the basics, but now wants to use the ECG to its maximum potential as a clinical tool.

The ECG is not an end in itself, but is an extension of the history and physical examination. Patients do not visit the doctor wanting an ECG, but come either for a health check or because they have symptoms. Therefore this book is organized according to clinical situations, and the chapters cover the ECG in healthy subjects and in patients with palpitations, syncope, chest pain, breathlessness or non-cardiac conditions. To emphasize that the ECG is part of the general assessment of a patient, each chapter begins with a brief section on history and examination and ends with a short account of what might be done once the ECG has been interpreted.

This fifth edition adopts the philosophy of its predecessors regarding the relative importance of the ECG and the individual from whom it was recorded. There is a series of changes in the text, with the introduction of more summaries and more tables of clinical conditions associated with ECG patterns. Most importantly, there is a completely new chapter on pacemakers, defibrillators and electrophysiology, all of which involve the ECG and are becoming increasingly important in patient treatment. The format of the book has been changed, to allow each 12-lead ECG to be printed across a single page.

WHAT TO EXPECT OF THE ECG

The ECG has its limitations. Remember that it provides a picture of the electrical activity of the heart, but gives only an indirect indication of the heart's structure and function. It is, however, invaluable for assessing patients whose symptoms may be due to electrical malfunction in the heart, including patients with conduction problems and those with arrhythmias.

In healthy people, finding the ECG to appear normal may be reassuring. Unfortunately the ECG can be totally normal in patients with severe coronary disease. Conversely, the range of normality is such that a healthy subject may quite wrongly be labelled as having heart disease on the basis of the ECG. Some ECG patterns that are undoubtedly abnormal (for example, right bundle branch block) are seen in perfectly healthy people. It is a good working principle that it is the individual's clinical state that matters, not the ECG.

When a patient complains of palpitations or syncope, the diagnosis of a cardiac cause is only certain if an ECG is recorded at the time of symptoms – but even when the patient is symptom-free, the ECG may provide a clue for the prepared mind. In patients with chest pain the ECG may indicate the diagnosis and treatment can be based upon it, but it is essential to remember that the ECG may remain normal for a few hours after the onset of a myocardial infarction. In breathless patients a totally normal ECG probably rules out heart failure, but it is not a good way of diagnosing lung disease or pulmonary embolism. Finally it must be remembered that the ECG can be quite abnormal in a patient with a variety of non-cardiac conditions, and one must not jump to the conclusion that an abnormal ECG indicates cardiac pathology.

ACKNOWLEDGEMENTS

This fifth edition of *The ECG in Practice* has been changed in many ways, and I have been helped by many people. In particular, I am grateful to David Adlam for contributing the chapter on devices and electrophysiology, which takes the book beyond the routine ECG into the realm of sophisticated diagnosis and electrical treatments – which are nevertheless based on an understanding of the ECG. I am also extremely grateful to my copy-editor, Alison Gale, for her enormous attention to detail that led to many improvements in the text. The new format of the book required a totally new layout compared with the previous edition, and this has been inroduced most expertly by Rich Cutler of Helius; this new edition could not have been produced without his help and patience. As before, I am grateful to many friends and colleagues who have helped me to find the wide range of examples of normal and abnormal ECGs that form the backbone of the book.

John Hampton
Nottingham, 2008

Contents

12-lead ECGs

1 The ECG in healthy people

For the purposes of this chapter, we shall assume that the subject from whom the ECG was recorded is asymptomatic, and that physical examination has revealed no abnormalities. We need to consider the range of normality of the ECG, but of course we cannot escape from the fact that not all disease causes symptoms or abnormal signs, and a subject who appears healthy may not be so and may therefore have an abnormal ECG. In particular, individuals who present for 'screening' may well have symptoms about which they have not consulted a doctor, so it cannot be assumed that an ECG obtained through a screening programme has come from a healthy subject.

The range of normality in the ECG is therefore debatable. We first have to consider the variations in the ECG that we can expect to find in completely healthy people, and then we can think about the significance of ECGs that are undoubtedly 'abnormal'.

THE NORMAL CARDIAC RHYTHM

Sinus rhythm is the only normal sustained rhythm. In young people the R–R interval is reduced (that is, the heart rate is increased) during inspiration, and this is called sinus arrhythmia (Fig. 1.1). When sinus arrhythmia is marked, it may mimic an atrial arrhythmia. However, in sinus arrhythmia each P–QRS–T complex is normal, and it is only the interval between them that changes.

Sinus arrhythmia becomes less marked with increasing age of the subject, and is lost in conditions such as diabetic autonomic neuropathy due to impairment of the vagus nerve function.

THE HEART RATE

There is no such thing as a normal heart rate, and the terms 'tachycardia' and 'bradycardia' should be used with care. There is no point at which a high

Fig. 1.1

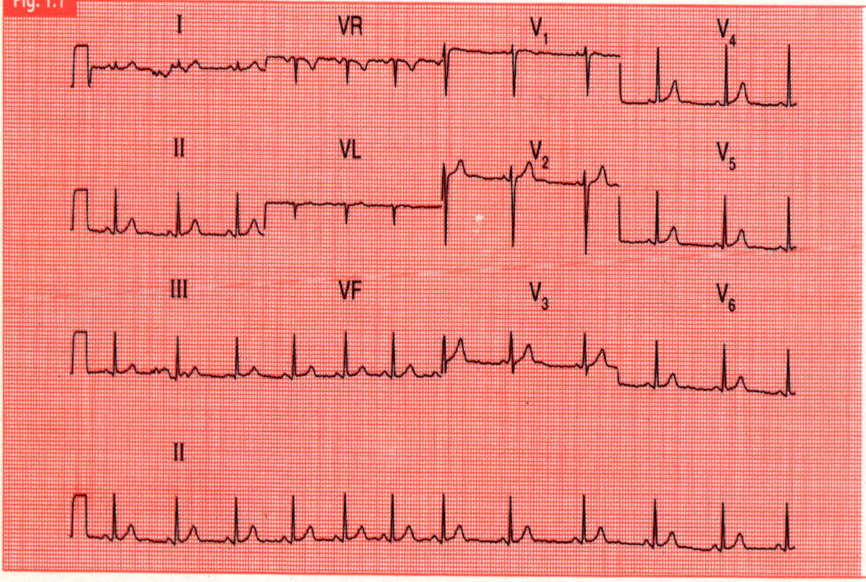

heart rate in sinus rhythm has to be called 'sinus tachycardia' and there is no upper limit for 'sinus bradycardia'. Nevertheless, unexpectedly fast or slow rates do need an explanation.

SINUS TACHYCARDIA

The ECG in Figure 1.2 was recorded from a young woman who complained of a fast heart rate. She had no other symptoms but was anxious. There were no other abnormalities on examination, and her blood count and thyroid function tests were normal.

Box 1.1 shows possible causes of sinus rhythm with a fast heart rate.

Sinus arrhythmia

Note

- Marked variation in R–R interval
- Constant PR interval
- Constant shape of P wave and QRS complex

Box 1.1 Possible causes of sinus rhythm with a fast heart rate

- Pain, fright, exercise
- Hypovolaemia
- Myocardial infarction
- Heart failure
- Pulmonary embolism
- Obesity
- Lack of physical fitness
- Pregnancy
- Thyrotoxicosis
- Anaemia
- Beri-beri
- CO_2 retention
- Autonomic neuropathy
- Drugs:
  — sympathomimetics
  — salbutamol (including by inhalation)
  — caffeine
  — atropine

Fig. 1.2

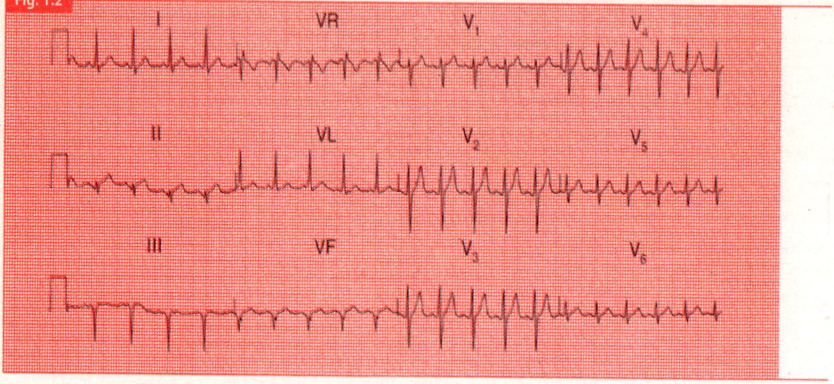
I
VR
V_1
V_4
II
VL
V_2
V_5
III
VF
V_3
V_6

Fig. 1.3

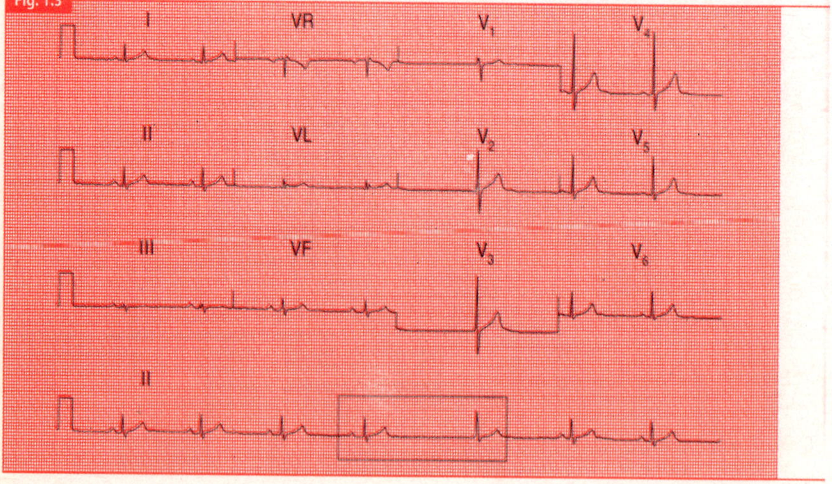
I
VR
V_1
V_4
II
VL
V_2
V_5
III
VF
V_3
V_6
II

Sinus tachycardia

Note

- Normal P–QRS–T waves
- R–R interval 500 ms
- Heart rate 120/min

SINUS BRADYCARDIA

The ECG in Figure 1.3 was recorded from a young professional footballer. His heart rate was 44/min, and at one point the sinus rate became so slow that a junctional escape beat appeared.

The possible causes of sinus rhythm with a slow heart rate are summarized in Box 1.2.

Sinus bradycardia

Note

- Sinus rhythm
- Rate 44/min
- One junctional escape beat

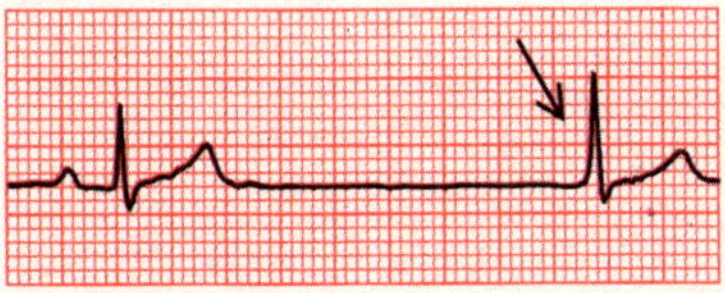

Junctional escape beat

Box 1.2 Possible causes of sinus rhythm with a slow heart rate

- Physical fitness
- Vasovagal attacks
- Sick sinus syndrome
- Acute myocardial infarction, especially inferior
- Hypothyroidism
- Hypothermia
- Obstructive jaundice
- Raised intracranial pressure
- Drugs:
  - — beta-blockers (including eye drops for glaucoma)
  - — verapamil
  - — digoxin

Fig. 1.4

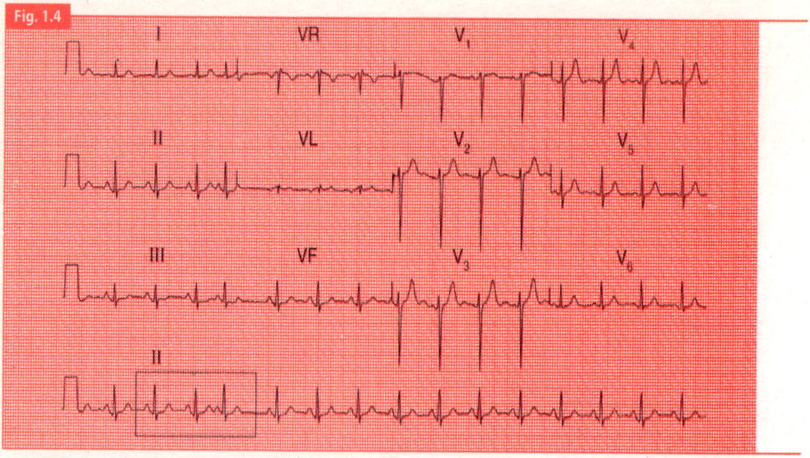
I
VR
V1
V4
II
VL
V2
V5
III
VF
V3
V6
II

Fig. 1.5

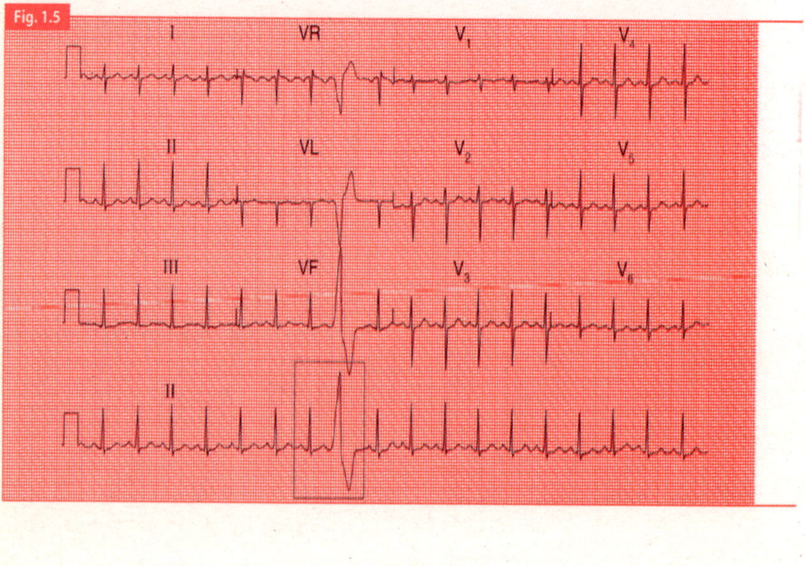
I
VR
V1
V4
II
VL
V2
V5
III
VF
V3
V6
II

Supraventricular extrasystole

Note

- In supraventricular extrasystoles the QRS complex and the T wave are the same as in the sinus beat
- The fourth beat has an abnormal P wave and therefore an atrial origin

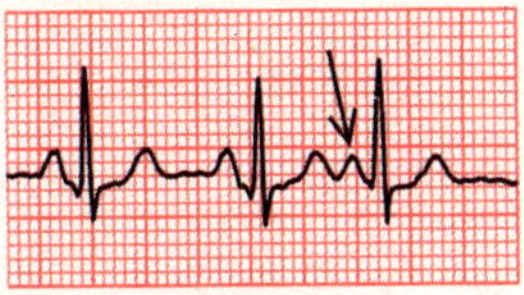

Early abnormal P wave

Ventricular extrasystole

Note

- Sinus rhythm, with one ventricular extrasystole
- Extrasystole has a wide and abnormal QRS complex and an abnormal T wave

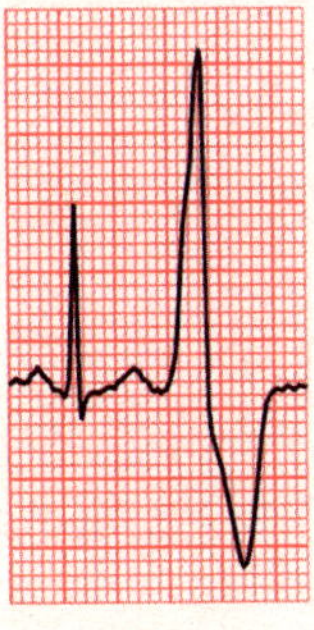

Ventricular extrasystole

EXTRASYSTOLES

Supraventricular extrasystoles, either atrial or junctional (AV nodal), occur commonly in normal people and are of no significance (Fig. 1.4). Atrial extrasystoles have an abnormal P wave; in junctional extrasystoles, either there is no P wave or the P wave may follow the QRS complex.

Ventricular extrasystoles are also commonly seen in normal ECGs (Fig. 1.5).

THE P WAVE

In sinus rhythm, the P wave is normally upright in all leads except VR. When the QRS complex is predominantly downward in lead VL, the P wave may also be inverted (Fig. 1.6).

A notched or bifid P wave is the hallmark of left atrial hypertrophy, and peaked P waves indicate right atrial hypertrophy – but bifid or peaked P waves can also be seen with normal hearts.

In patients with dextrocardia the P wave is inverted in lead I (Fig. 1.7). In practice this is more often seen if the limb leads have been wrongly attached, but dextrocardia can be recognized if leads V_5 and V_6, which normally 'look at' the left ventricle, show a predominantly downward QRS complex.

If the ECG of a patient with dextrocardia is repeated with the limb leads reversed, and the chest leads are placed on the right side of the chest instead of the left, in corresponding positions, the ECG becomes like that of a normal patient (Fig. 1.8).

Fig. 1.6

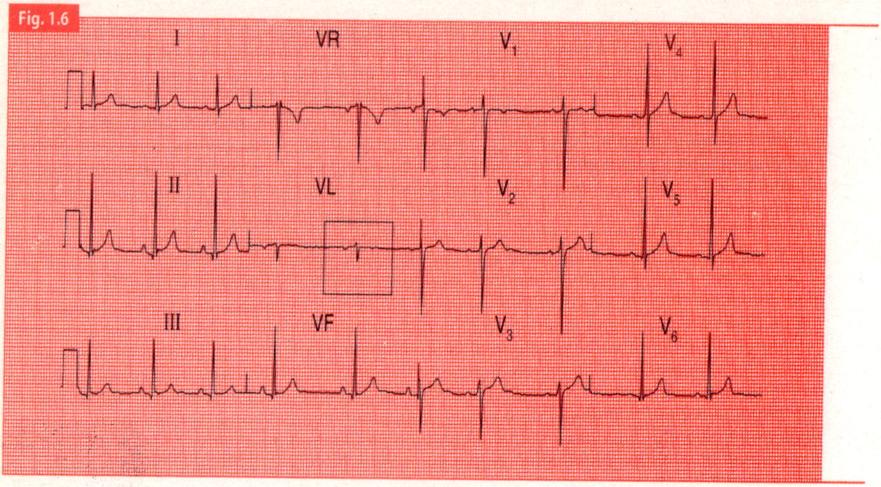

Fig. 1.7

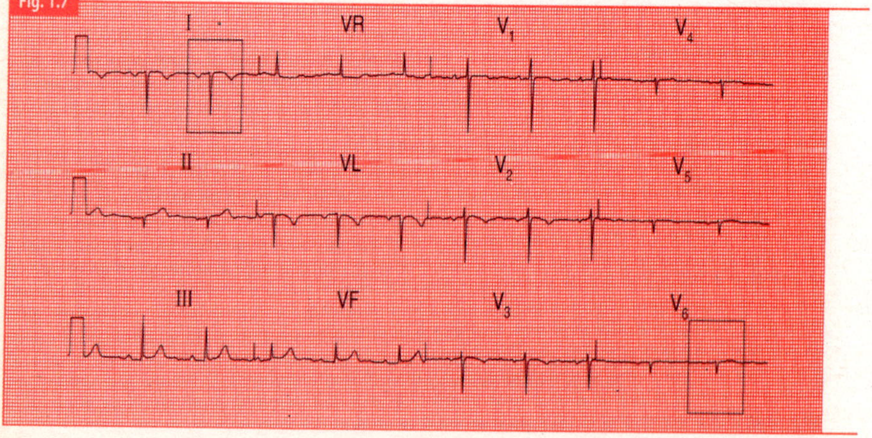

Normal ECG

Note

- In both leads VR and VL the P wave is inverted, and the QRS complex is predominantly downward

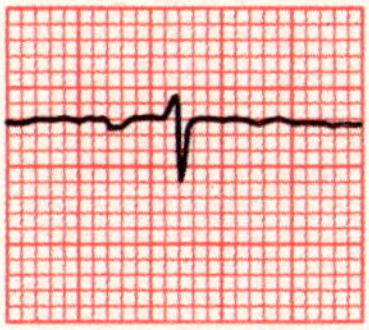

Inverted P wave in lead VL

Dextrocardia

Note

- Inverted P wave in lead I
- No left ventricular complexes seen in leads V_5–V_6

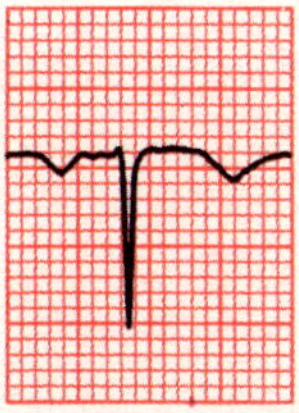

Inverted P wave and dominant S wave in lead I

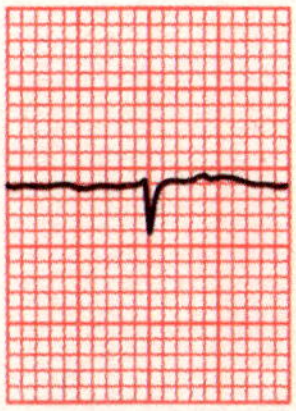

Persistent S wave in lead V_6

Fig. 1.8

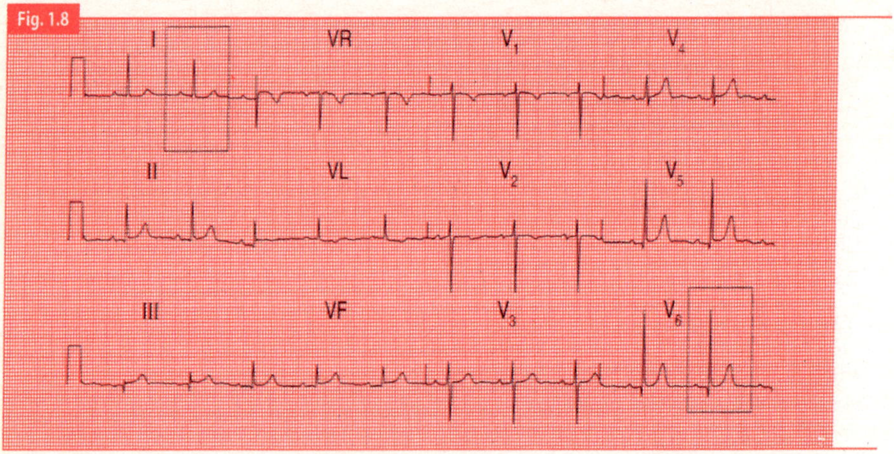

Fig. 1.9

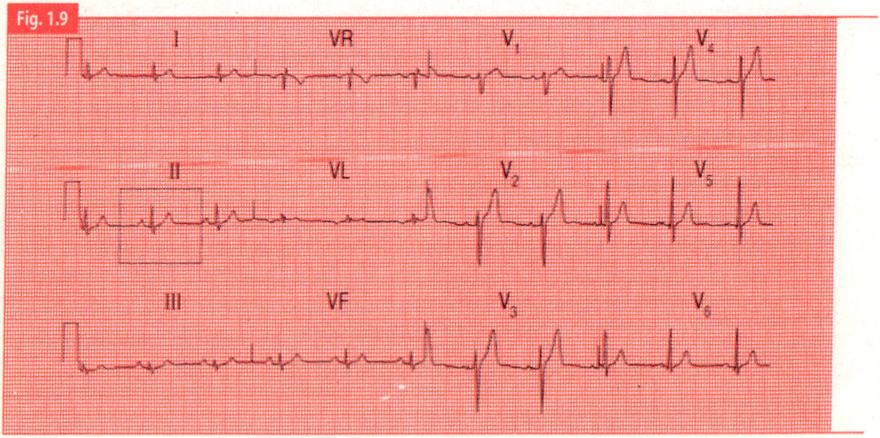

Dextrocardia, leads reversed

Note

- P wave in lead I upright
- QRS complex upright in lead I
- Typical left ventricular complex in lead V_6

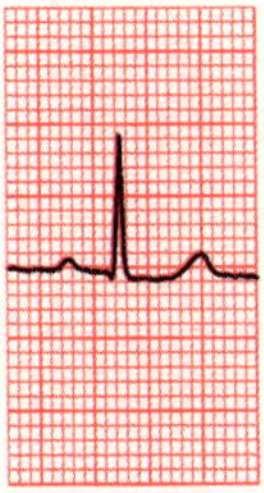

Upright P wave and QRS complex in lead I

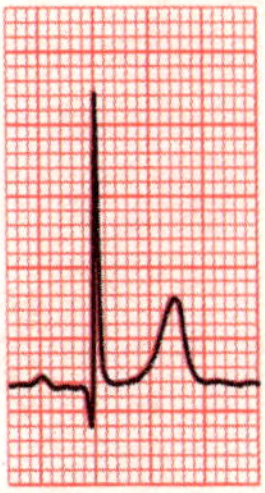

Normal QRS complex in lead V_6

Normal ECG

Note

- PR interval 170 ms
- PR interval constant in all leads
- Notched P wave in lead V_5 is often normal

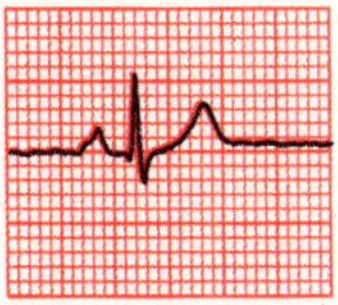

PR interval 170 ms

THE PR INTERVAL

In sinus rhythm, the PR interval is constant and the normal range is 120–200 ms (3–5 small squares of ECG paper) (Fig. 1.9).

A PR interval of less than 120 ms suggests pre-excitation, and a PR interval of longer than 200 ms is due to first degree block. Both of these 'abnormalities' are seen in normal people, and will be discussed further in Chapter 2.

Fig. 1.10

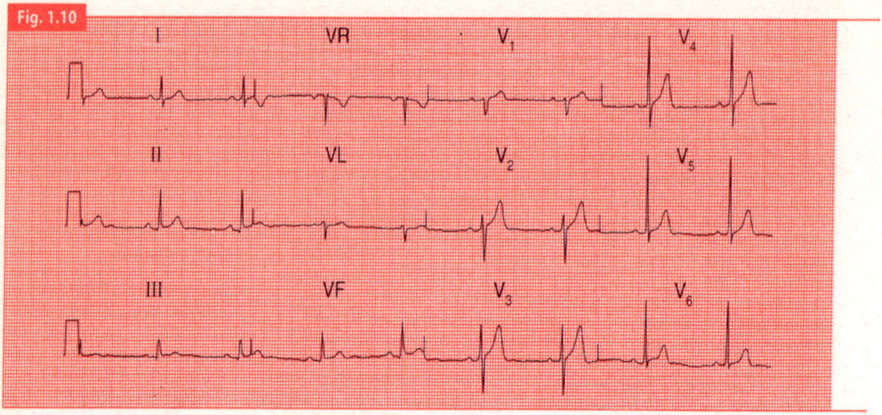

Fig. 1.11

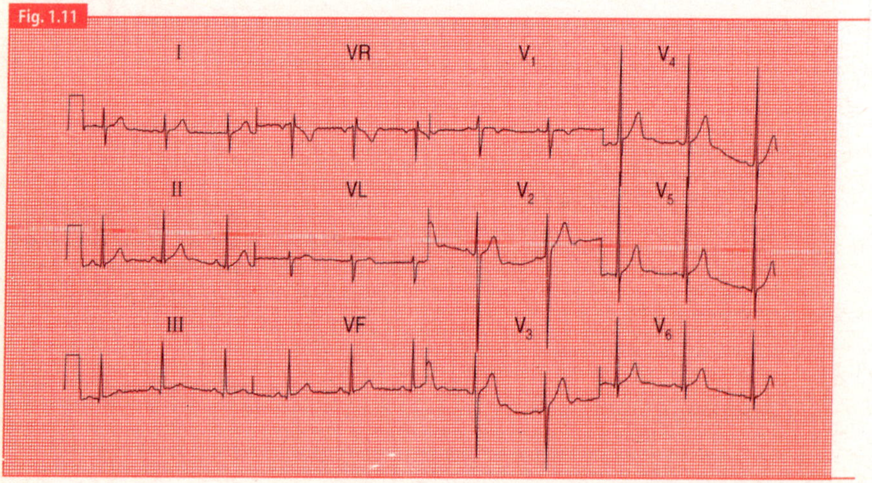

Normal ECG

Note

- QRS complex upright in leads I–III
- R wave tallest in lead II

Normal ECG

Note

- This record shows the 'rightward' limit of normality of the cardiac axis
- R and S waves equal in lead I

THE QRS COMPLEX

THE CARDIAC AXIS

There is a fairly wide range of normality in the direction of the cardiac axis. In most people the QRS complex is tallest in lead II, but in leads I and III the QRS complex is also predominantly upright (i.e. the R wave is greater than the S wave) (Fig. 1.10).

The cardiac axis is still perfectly normal when the R wave and S wave are equal in lead I: this is common in tall people (Fig. 1.11).

When the S wave is greater than the R wave in lead I, right axis deviation is present. However, this is very common in perfectly normal people. The ECG in Figure 1.12 is from a professional footballer.

It is common for the S wave to be greater than the R wave in lead III, and the cardiac axis can still be considered normal when the S wave equals the R wave in lead II. These patterns are common in fat people and during pregnancy (Fig. 1.13).

When the depth of the S wave exceeds the height of the R wave in lead II, left axis deviation is present (see Fig. 2.26).

Fig. 1.12

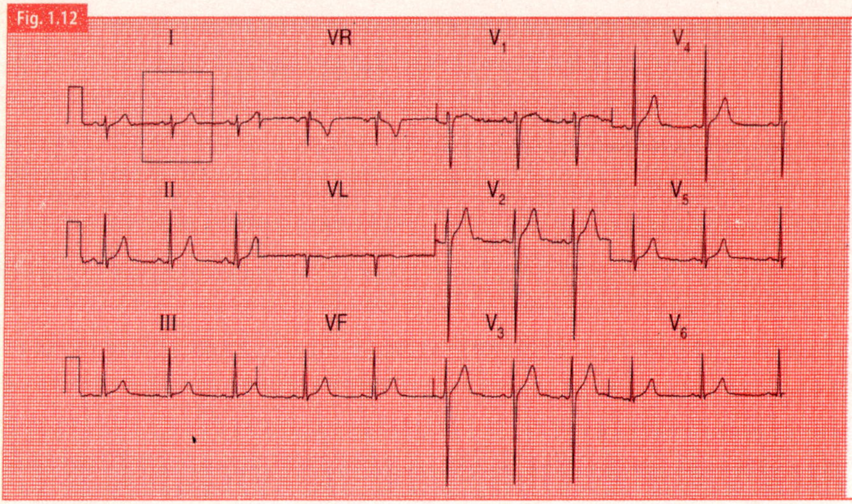

Fig. 1.13

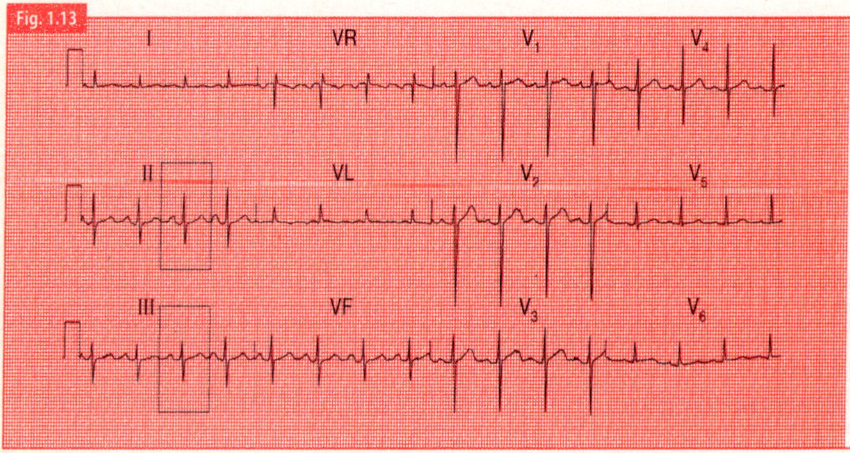

?Normal ECG

Note

- Right axis deviation: S wave greater than R wave in lead I
- Upright QRS complexes in leads II–III

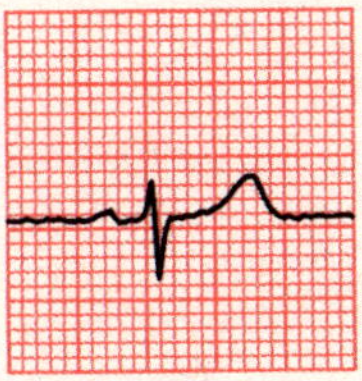

Dominant S wave in lead I

Normal ECG

Note

- This shows the 'leftward' limit of normality of the cardiac axis
- S wave equals R wave in lead II
- S wave greater than R wave in lead III

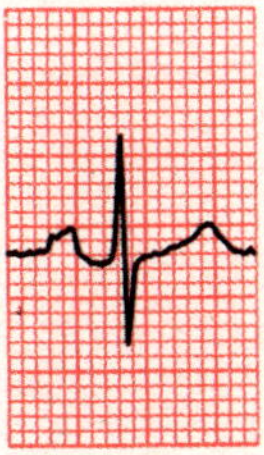

S wave = R wave in lead II

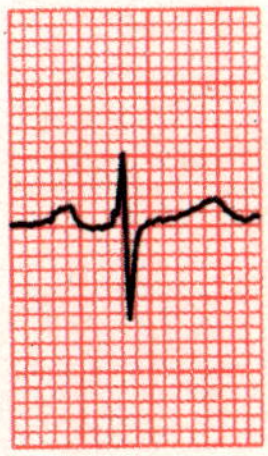

S wave > R wave in lead III

Fig. 1.14

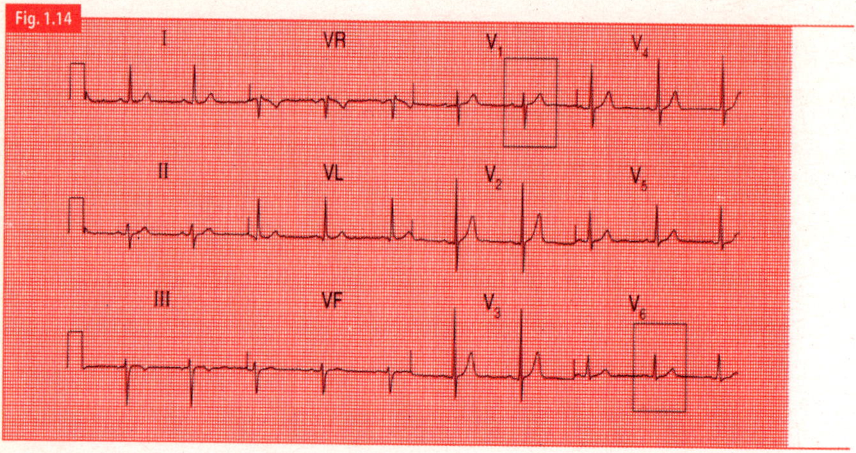

Fig. 1.15

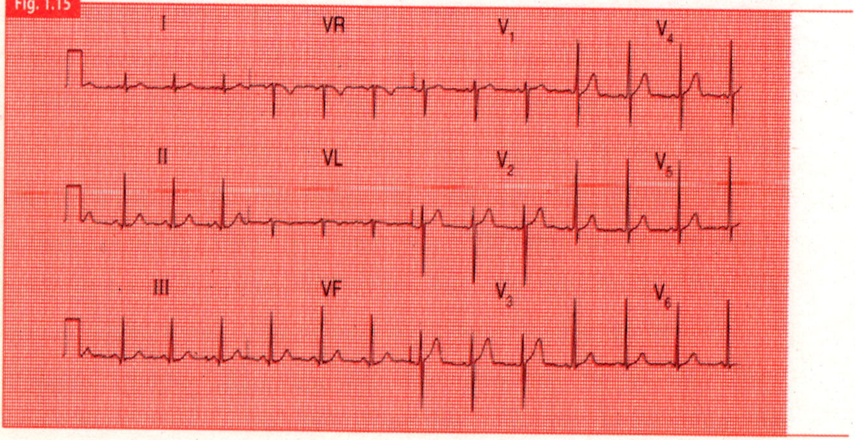

Normal ECG

Note

- Lead V_1 shows a predominantly downward complex, with the S wave greater than the R wave
- Lead V_6 shows an upright complex, with a dominant R wave and a tiny S wave

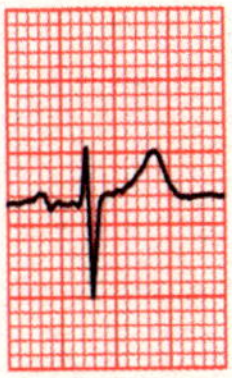

S wave > R wave in lead V_1

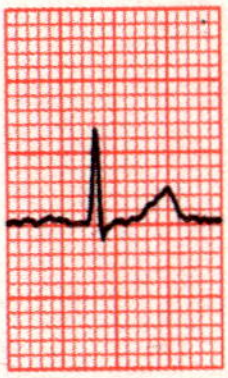

Dominant R wave in lead V_6

Normal ECG

Note

- In lead V_3 there is a dominant S wave
- In lead V_4 there is a dominant R wave
- The transition point is between leads V_3 and V_4

THE SIZE OF R AND S WAVES IN THE CHEST LEADS

In lead V_1 there should be a small R wave and a deep S wave, and the balance between the two should change progressively from V_1–V_6. In lead V_6 there should be a tall R wave and no S wave (Fig. 1.14).

Typically the 'transition point', when the R and S waves are equal, is seen in lead V_3 or V_4 but there is quite a lot of variation. Figure 1.15 shows an ECG in which the transition point is somewhere between leads V_3 and V_4.

Fig. 1.16

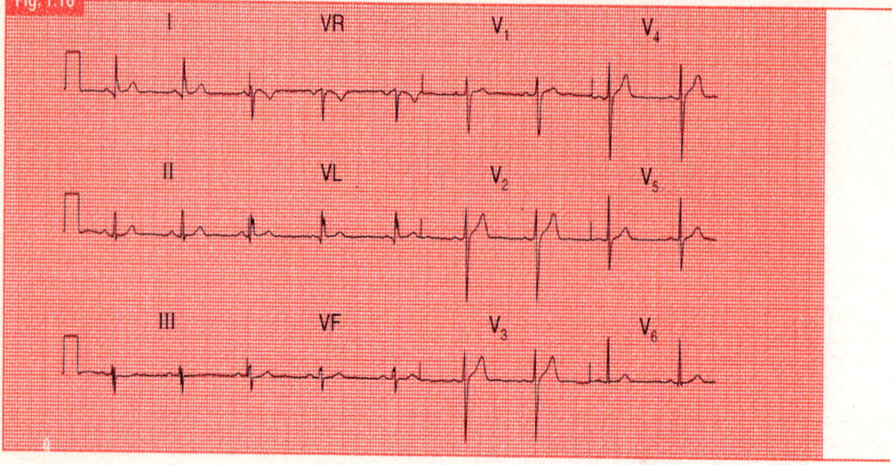

Fig. 1.17

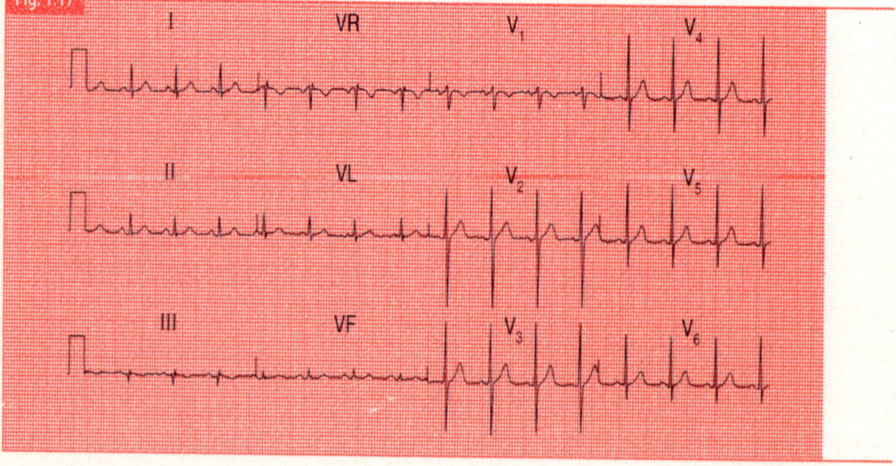

Normal ECG

Note

- Dominant S wave in lead V_4
- R wave just bigger than S wave in lead V_5

Normal ECG

Note

- Dominant S wave in lead V_2
- Dominant R wave in lead V_3
- The transition point is between leads V_2 and V_3

Figure 1.16 shows an ECG with a transition point between leads V_4 and V_5.

Figure 1.17 shows an ECG with a transition point between leads V_2 and V_3.

The transition point is typically seen in lead V_5 or even V_6 in patients with chronic lung disease (see Ch. 4), and this is called 'clockwise rotation'. In extreme cases, the chest lead needs to be placed in the posterior axillary line, or even further round to the back (leads V_7–V_9) before the transition point is demonstrated. A similar ECG pattern may be seen in patients with an abnormal chest shape, particularly when depression of the sternum shifts the mediastinum to the left, although in this case the term 'clockwise rotation' is not used. The patient from whom the ECG in Figure 1.18 was recorded had mediastinal shift.

Occasionally the ECG of a totally normal subject will show a 'dominant' R wave (i.e. the height of the R wave exceeds the depth of the S wave) in lead V_1. There will thus, effectively, be no transition point, and this is called 'counterclockwise rotation'. The ECG in Figure 1.19 was recorded from a healthy footballer with a normal heart. However, a dominant R wave in lead V_1 is usually due to either right ventricular hypertrophy (see Ch. 4) or a true posterior infarction (see Ch. 3).

Fig. 1.18

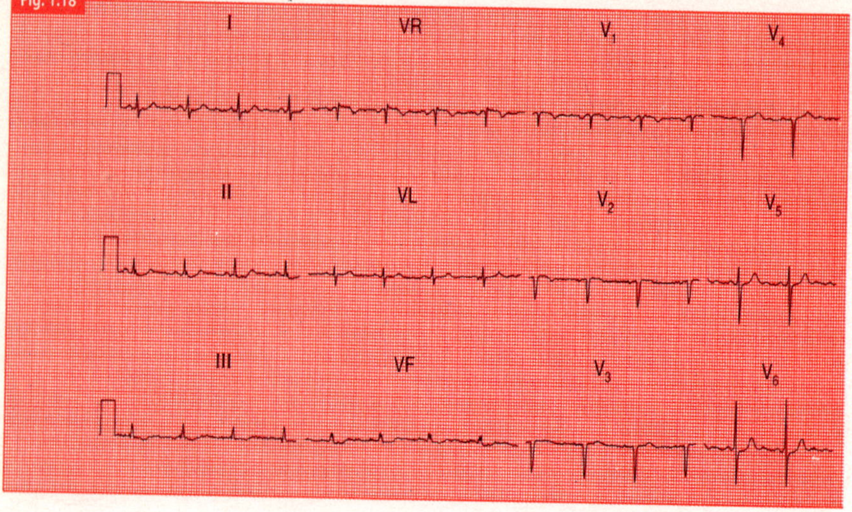

Fig. 1.19

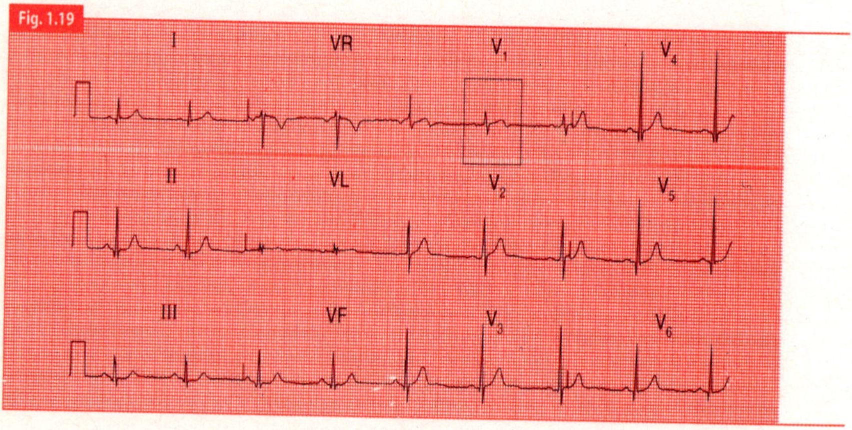

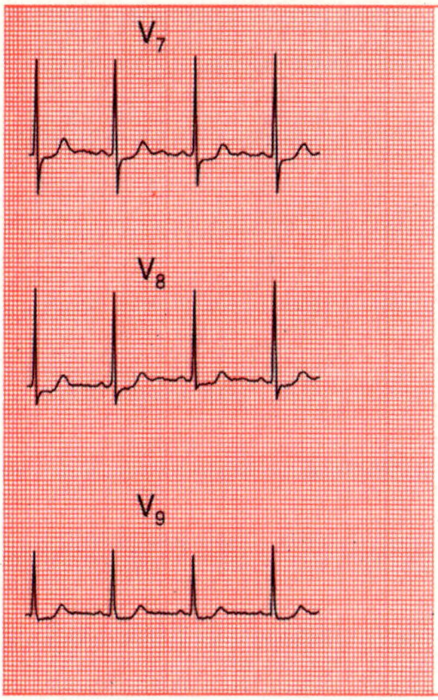

Mediastinal shift

Note

- 'Abnormal' ECG, but a normal heart
- Shift of the mediastinum means the transition point is under lead V_6
- Ventricular complexes are shown in leads round the left side of the chest, in positions V_7–V_9

Normal ECG

Note

- Dominant R waves in lead V_1

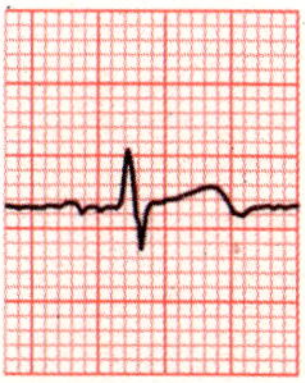

Dominant R wave in lead V_1

Fig. 1.20

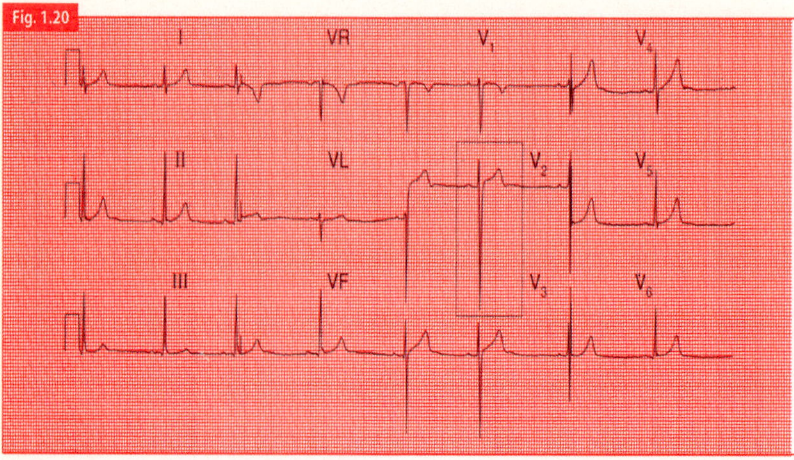

Fig. 1.21

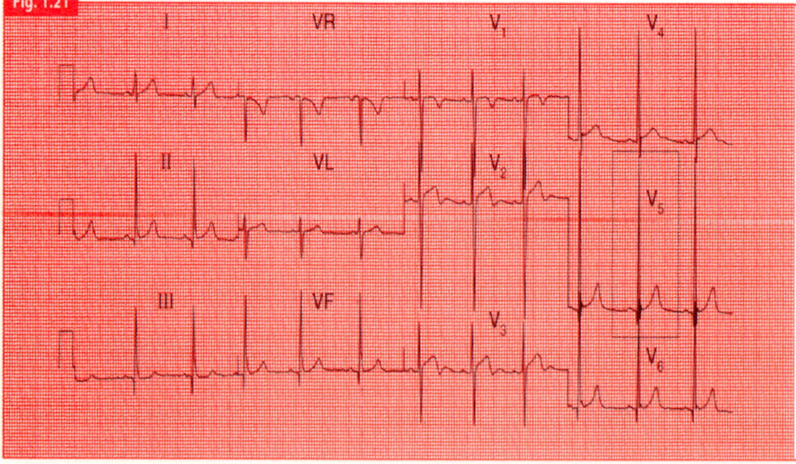

Normal ECG

Note

- S wave in lead V_2 is 36 mm

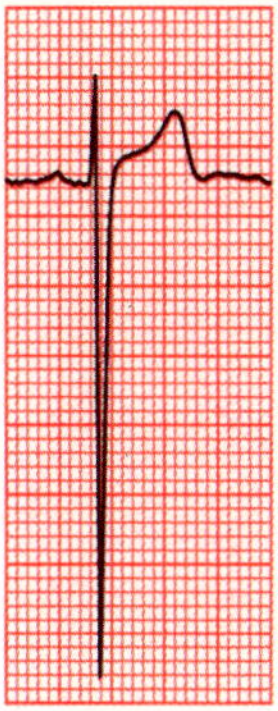

S wave > 25 mm in lead V_2

Normal ECG

Note

- R wave in lead V_5 is 42 mm

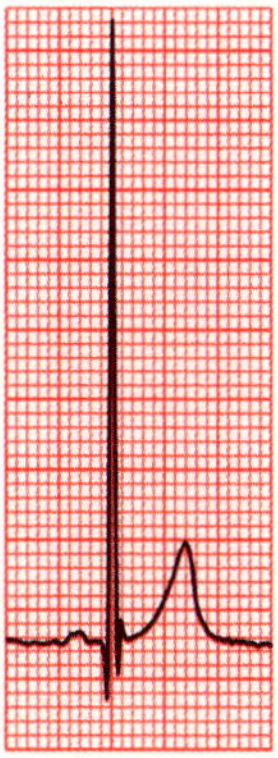

R wave > 25 mm in lead V_5

Although the balance between the height of the R wave and the depth of the S wave is significant for the identification of cardiac axis deviation, or right ventricular hypertrophy, the absolute height of the R wave provides little useful information. Provided that the ECG is properly calibrated (1 mV causes 1 cm of vertical deflection on the ECG), the limits for the sizes of the R and S waves in normal subjects are usually said to be:

- 25 mm for the R wave in lead V_5 or V_6
- 25 mm for the S wave in lead V_1 or V_2
- Sum of R wave in lead V_5 or V_6 plus S wave in lead V_1 or V_2 should be less than 35 mm.

However, R waves taller than 25 mm are commonly seen in leads V_5–V_6 in fit and thin young people, and are perfectly normal. Thus, these 'limits' are not helpful. The ECGs in Figures 1.20 and 1.21 were both recorded from fit young men with normal hearts.

THE WIDTH OF THE QRS COMPLEX

The QRS complex should be less than 120 ms in duration (i.e. less than 3 small squares) in all leads. If it is longer than this, then either the ventricles have been depolarized from a ventricular rather than a supraventricular focus (i.e. a ventricular rhythm is present), or there is an abnormality of conduction within the ventricles. The latter is most commonly due to bundle branch block. An RSR^1 pattern, resembling that of right bundle branch block (RBBB) but with a narrow QRS complex, is sometimes called 'partial right bundle branch block' and is a normal variant (Fig. 1.22). An RSR^1S^1 pattern is also a normal variant (Fig. 1.23), and is sometimes called a 'splintered' complex.

Fig. 1.22

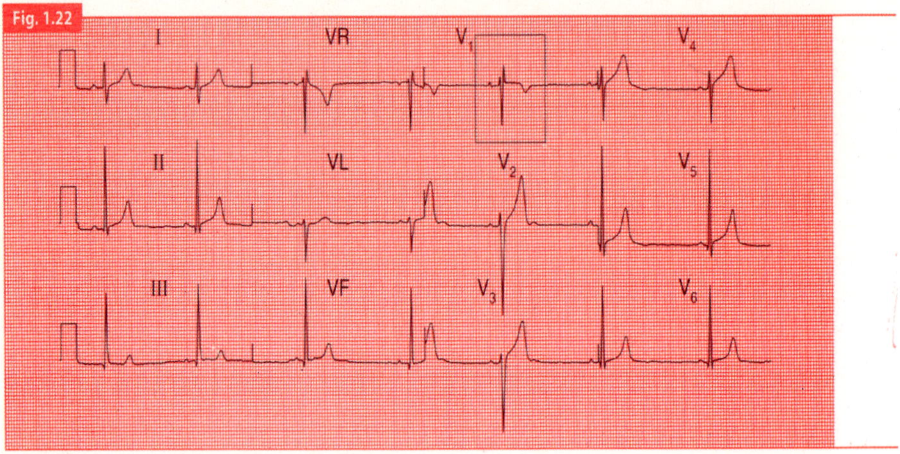

Fig. 1.23

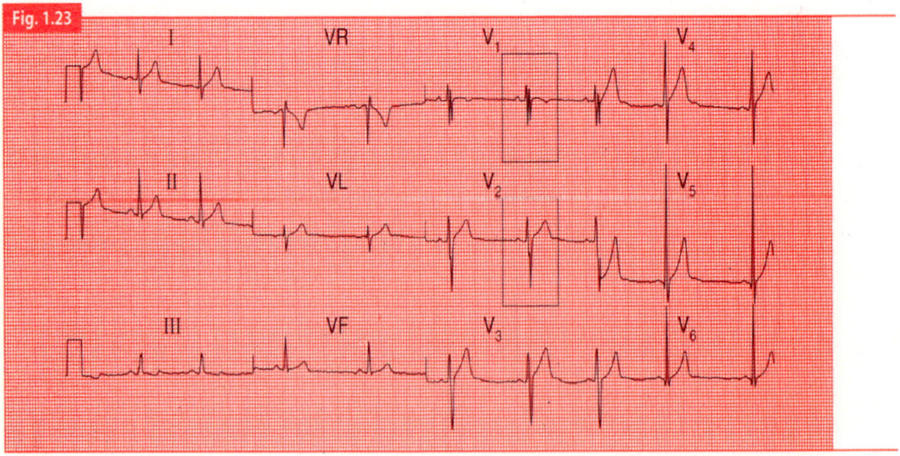

Normal ECG

Note

- RSR^1 pattern in lead V_2
- QRS complex duration 100 ms
- Partial RBBB pattern

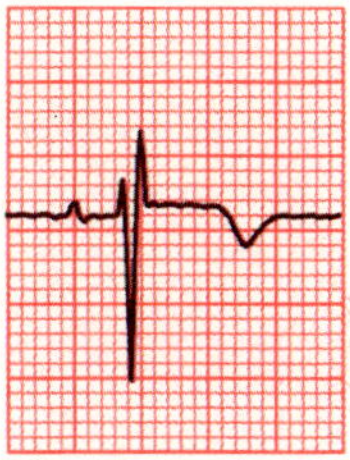

RSR^1 pattern and QRS complex 100 ms in lead V_1

Normal ECG

Note

- RSR^1S^1 pattern in lead V_1
- Notched S wave in lead V_2
- QRS complex duration 100 ms
- Partial RBBB pattern

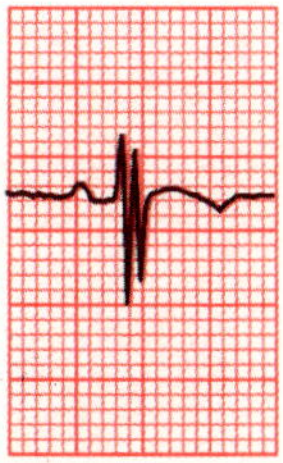

RSR^1S^1 pattern in lead V_1

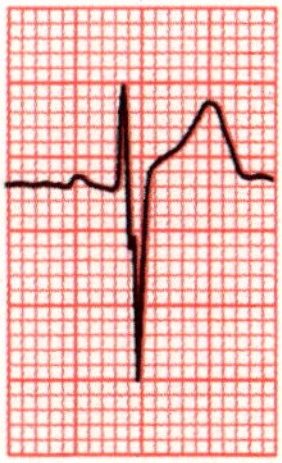

Notched S wave in lead V_2

Fig. 1.24

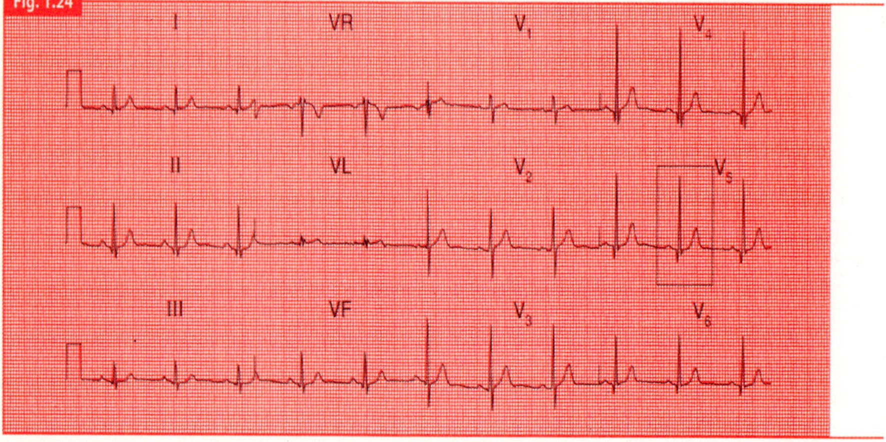

Fig. 1.25

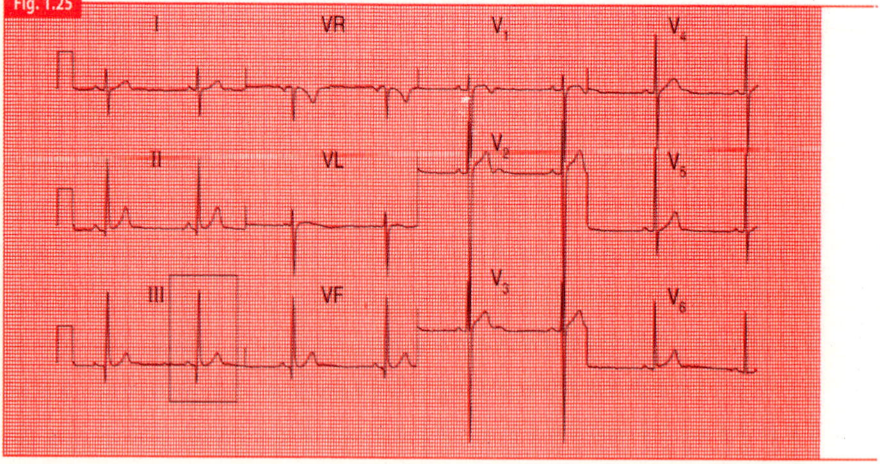

Normal ECG

Note

- Septal Q waves in leads I, II, V_4–V_6

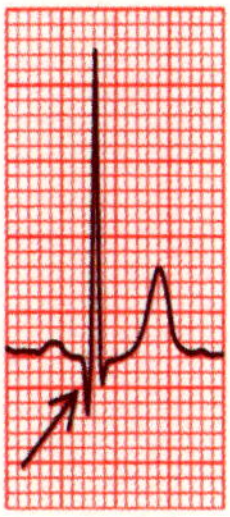

Septal Q wave in lead V_5

Q WAVES

The normal depolarization of the interventricular septum from left to right causes a small 'septal' Q wave in any of leads II, VL, or V_5–V_6. Septal Q waves are usually less than 3 mm deep and less than 1 mm across (Fig. 1.24).

A small Q wave is also common in lead III in normal people, in which case it is always narrow but can be more than 3 mm deep. Occasionally there will be a similar Q wave in lead VF (Fig. 1.25). These 'normal' Q waves become much less deep, and may disappear altogether, on deep inspiration (see Fig. 1.33).

Normal ECG

Note

- Narrow but quite deep Q wave in lead III
- Smaller Q wave in lead VF

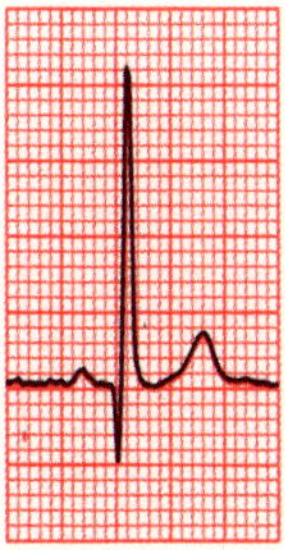

Narrow Q wave in lead III

Fig. 1.26

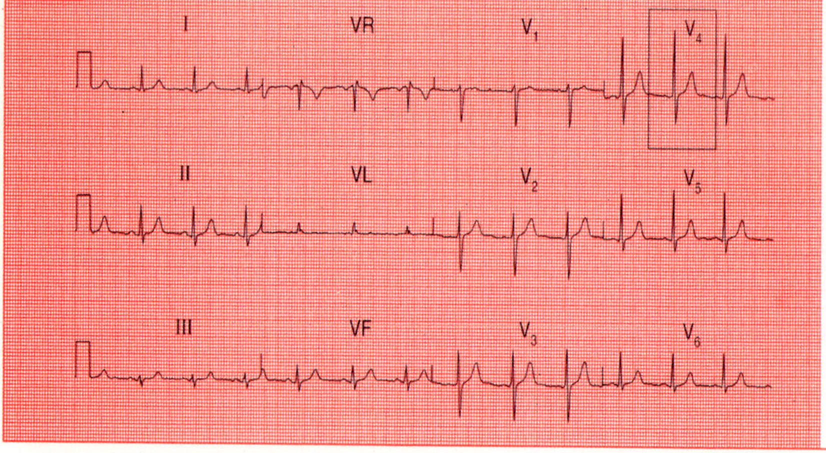

Fig. 1.27

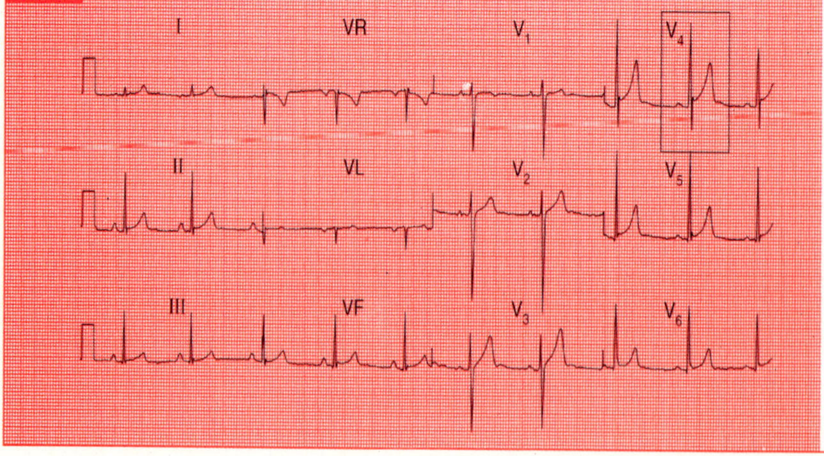

Normal ECG

Note

- ST segment is isoelectric but slopes upwards in leads V_2–V_5

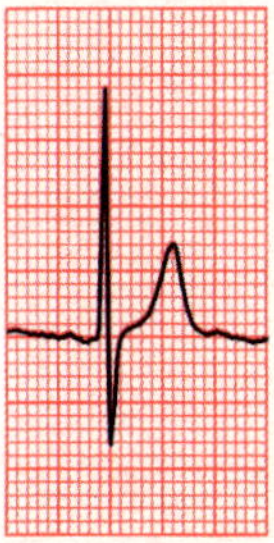

Upward-sloping ST segment in lead V_4

Normal ECG

Note

- In lead V_4 there is an S wave followed by a raised ST segment. This is a 'high take-off' ST segment

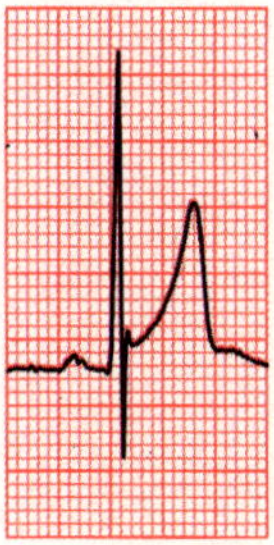

High take-off ST segment in lead V_4

THE ST SEGMENT

The ST segment (the part of the ECG between the S wave and the T wave) should be horizontal and 'isoelectric', which means that it should be at the same level as the baseline of the record between the end of the T wave and the next P wave. However, in the chest leads the ST segment often slopes upwards and is not easy to define (Fig. 1.26).

An elevation of the ST segment is the hallmark of an acute myocardial infarction (see Ch. 3), and depression of the ST segment can indicate ischaemia or the effect of digoxin. However, it is perfectly normal for the ST segment to be elevated following an S wave in leads V_2–V_5. This is sometimes called a 'high take-off ST segment'. The ECGs in Figures 1.27 and 1.28 were recorded from perfectly healthy young men.

Depression of the ST segment is not uncommon in normal people, and is then called 'nonspecific'. ST segment depression in lead III but not VF is likely to be nonspecific (Fig. 1.29). Nonspecific ST segment depression should not be more than 2 mm (Fig. 1.30), and the segment often slopes upwards. Horizontal ST segment depression of more than 2 mm indicates ischaemia (see Ch. 3).

Fig. 1.28

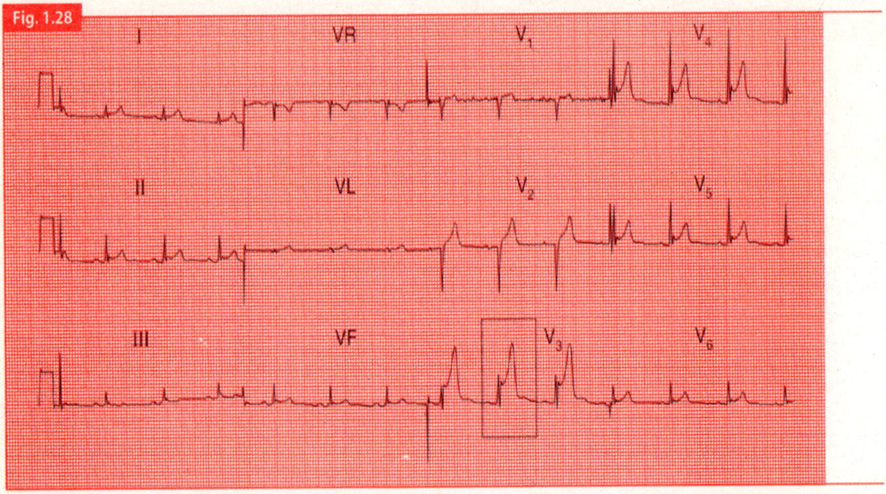

Fig. 1.29

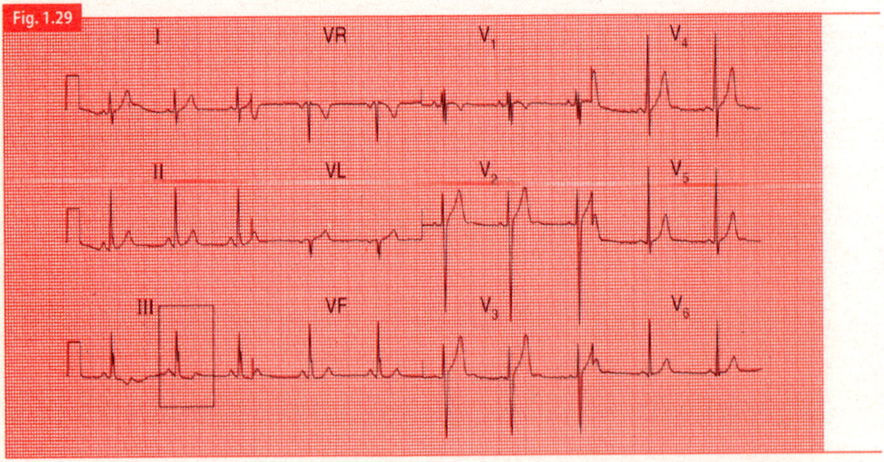

Normal ECG

Note

- Marked ST segment elevation in lead V_3 follows an S wave

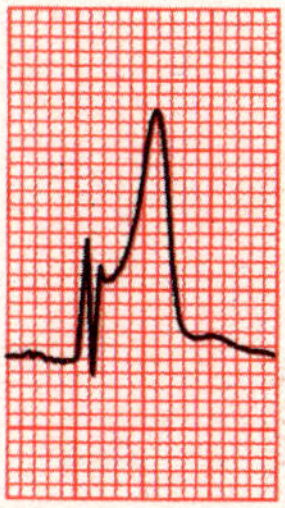

High take-off ST segment in lead V_3

Normal ECG

Note

- ST segment depression in lead III but not VF
- Biphasic T wave (i.e. initially inverted but then upright) in lead III but not VF
- Partial right bundle branch block pattern

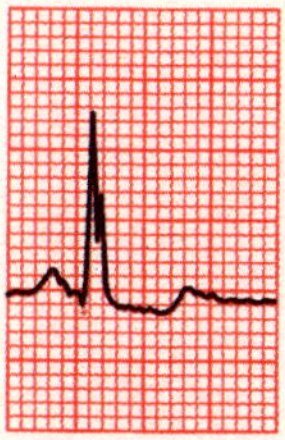

ST segment depression and biphasic T wave in lead III

Fig. 1.30

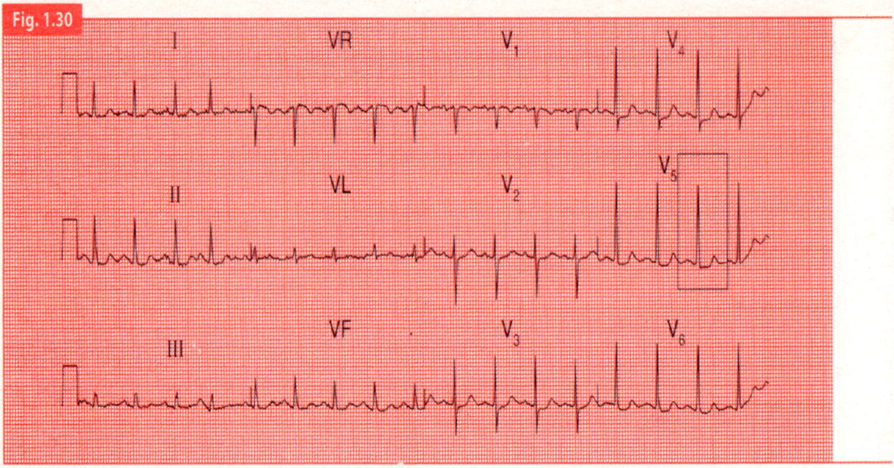

Fig. 1.31

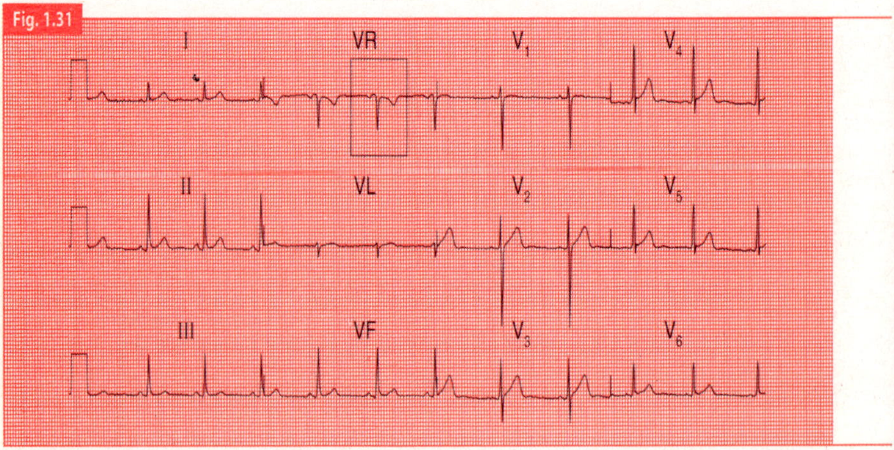

Possibly normal ECG

Note

- ST segment depression of 1 mm in leads V_3–V_6
- In a patient with chest pain this would raise suspicions of ischaemia but, particularly in women, such changes can be nonspecific

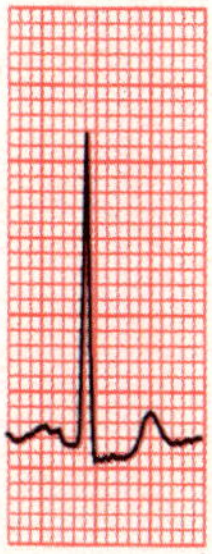

Nonspecific ST segment depression in lead V_5

Normal ECG

Note

- T wave is inverted in VR but is upright in all other leads

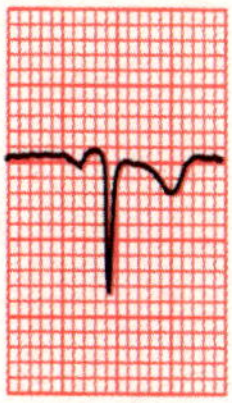

Inverted T wave in lead VR

THE T WAVE

In a normal ECG the T wave is always inverted in lead VR, and often in lead V_1, but is usually upright in all the other leads (Fig. 1.31).

The T wave is also often inverted in lead III but not VF. However, its inversion in lead III may be reversed on deep inspiration (Figs 1.32 and 1.33).

Fig. 1.32

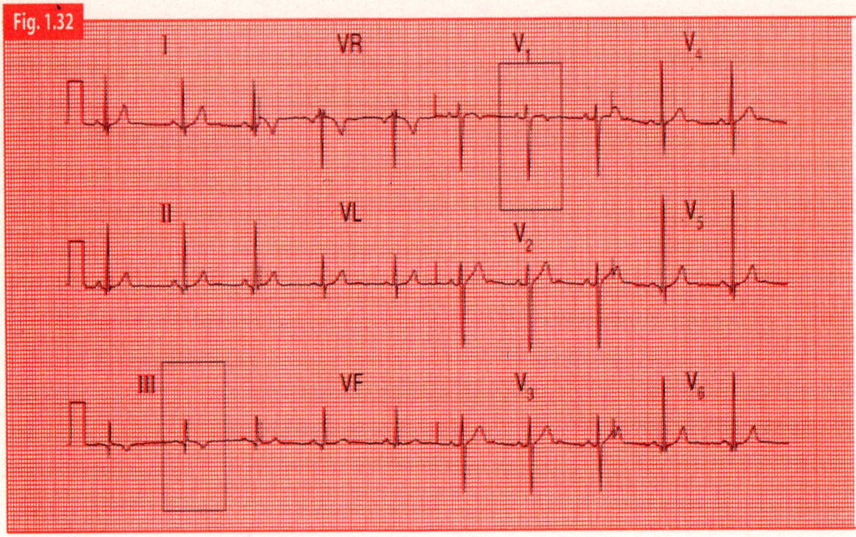

Fig. 1.33

Normal ECG during inspiration

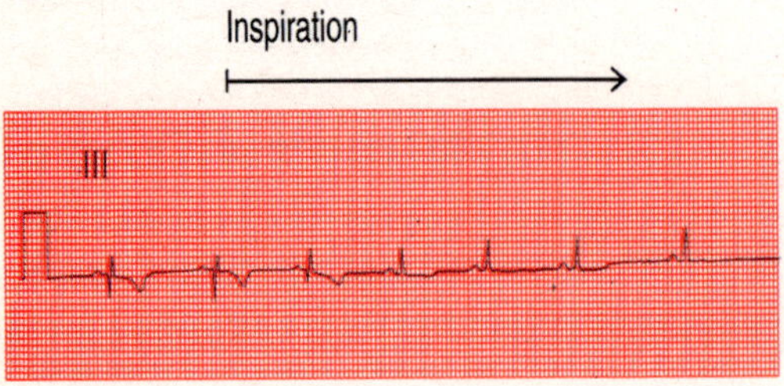

Note

- ECG recorded from same patient as in Figure 1.32, but during deep inspiration
- Q wave in lead III disappears
- T wave becomes upright

Normal ECG

Note

- Small Q wave in lead III but not VF
- Inverted T wave in lead III but upright T wave in VF
- Inverted T wave in lead V_1

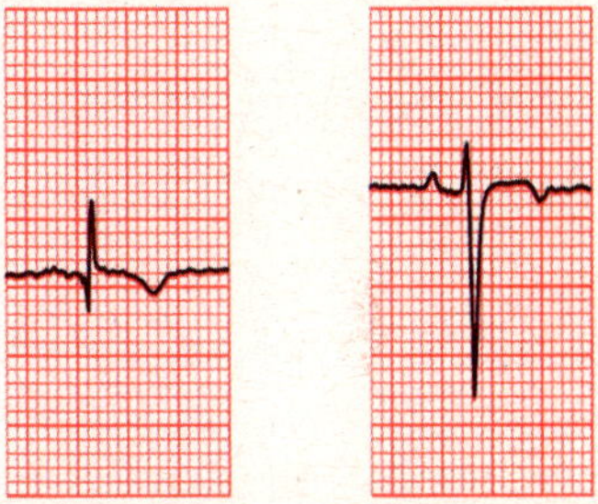

Q wave and inverted T wave in lead III

Inverted T wave in lead V_1

T wave inversion in lead VL as well as in VR can be normal, particularly if the P wave in lead VL is inverted. The ECG in Figure 1.34 was recorded from a completely healthy young woman.

T wave inversion in leads V_2–V_3 as well as in V_1 occurs in pulmonary embolism and in right ventricular hypertrophy (see Chs 3 and 4) but it can be a normal variant. This is particularly true in black people. The ECG in Figure 1.35 was recorded from a healthy young white man, and that shown in Figure 1.36 from a young black professional footballer. The ECG in Figure 1.37 was recorded from a middle-aged black woman with rather non-specific chest pain, whose coronary arteries and left ventricle were shown to be entirely normal on catheterization.

Generalized flattening of the T waves with a normal QT interval is best described as 'non-specific'. In a patient without symptoms and whose heart is clinically normal, the finding has little prognostic significance. This was the case with the patient whose ECG is shown in Figure 1.38. In patients with symptoms suggestive of cardiovascular disease, however, such an ECG would require further investigation.

Peaked T waves are one of the features of hyperkalaemia, but they can also be very prominent in healthy people (Fig. 1.39).

The T wave is the most variable part of the ECG. It may become inverted in some leads simply by hyperventilation associated with anxiety.

Fig. 1.34

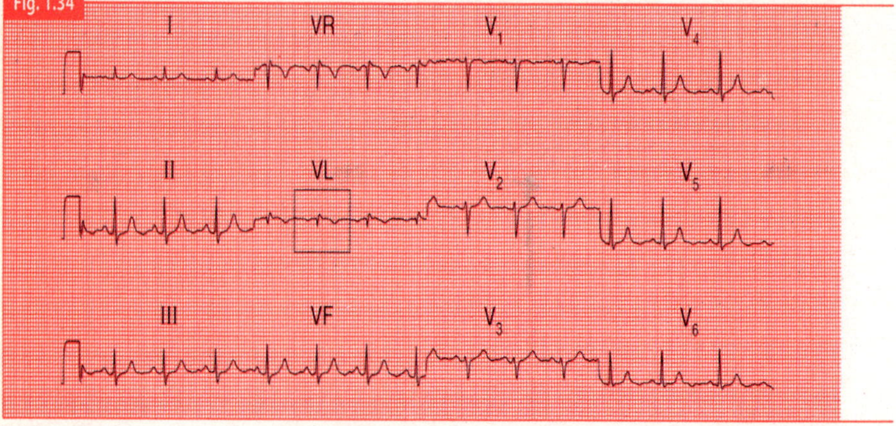

Fig. 1.35

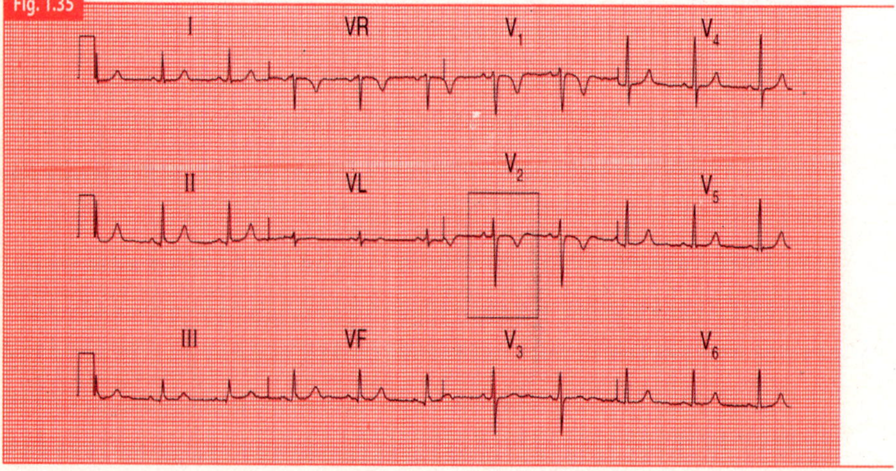

Normal ECG

Note

- Inverted T waves in leads VR, VL
- Inverted P waves in leads VR, VL

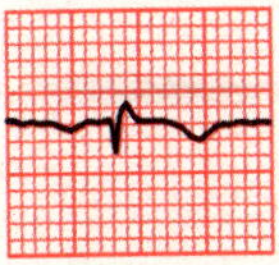

Inverted P and T waves in lead VL

Normal ECG

Note

- T wave inversion in leads VR, V_1–V_2
- Biphasic T wave in lead V_3

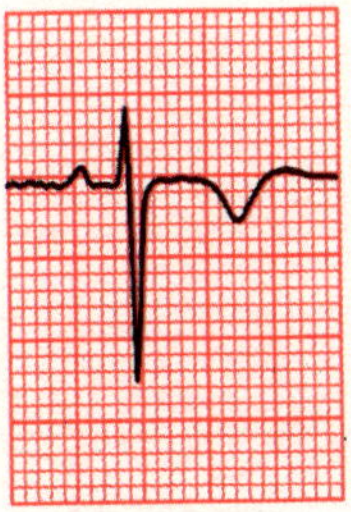

Inverted T wave in lead V_2

Fig. 1.36

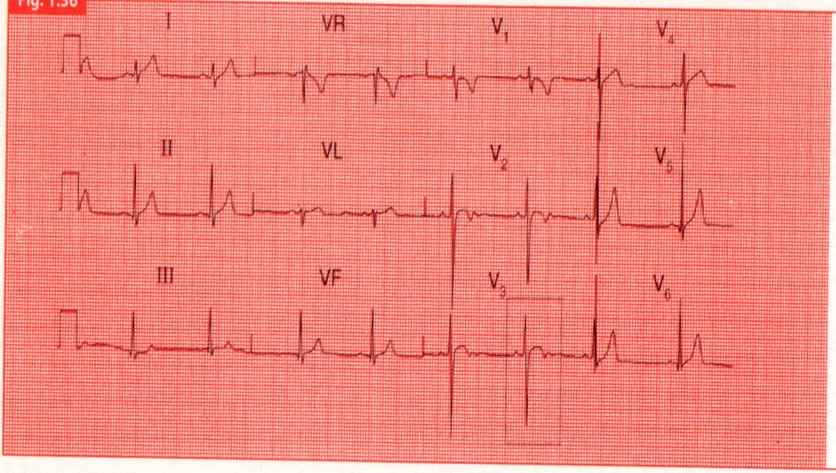

Fig. 1.37

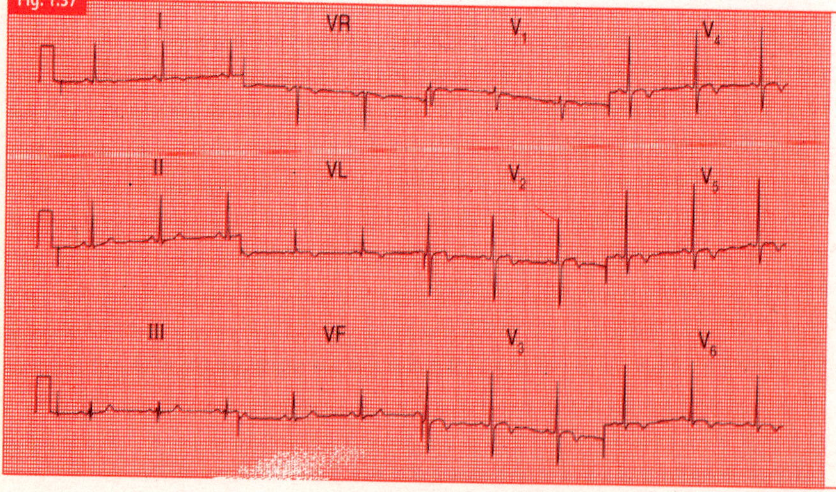

Normal ECG, from a black man

Note

- T wave inversion in leads VR, V_1–V_3

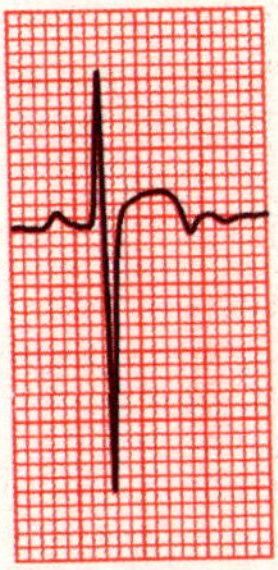

Inverted T wave in lead V_3

Normal ECG, from a black woman

Note

- Sinus rhythm
- T wave inversion in lead VL and all chest leads
- Presumably a normal variant: coronary angiography and echocardiography were normal

Fig. 1.38

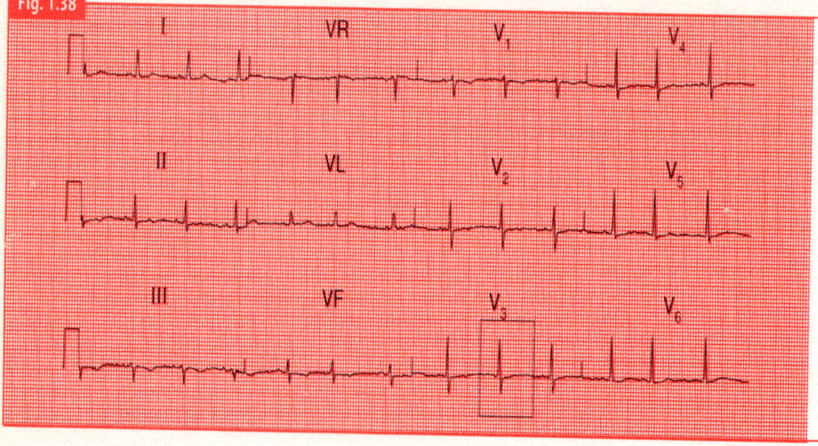

Fig. 1.39

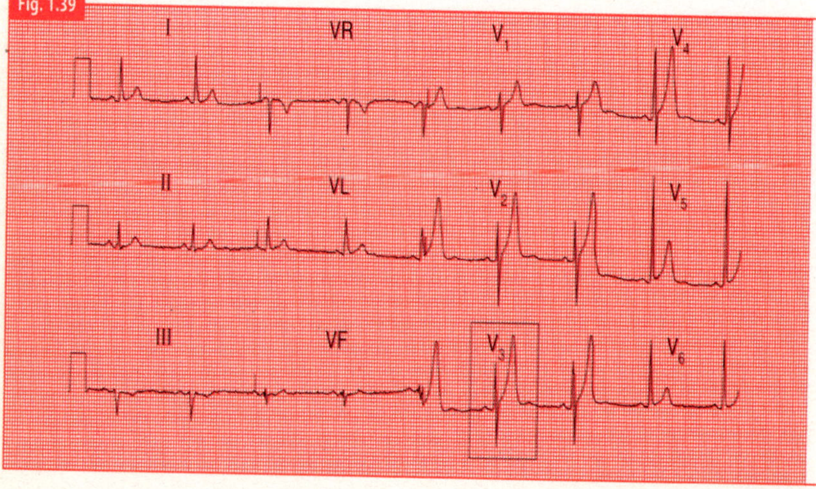

Possibly normal ECG

Note

- Sinus rhythm
- Normal axis
- Normal QRS complexes
- T wave flattening in all chest leads
- T wave inversion in leads III, VF
- In an asymptomatic patient, these changes are not necessarily significant

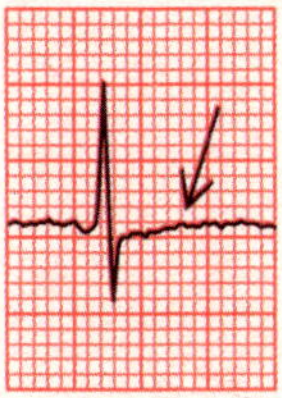

Flattened T wave in lead V_3

Normal ECG

Note

- Sinus rhythm
- Normal axis
- Normal QRS complexes
- Very tall and peaked T waves

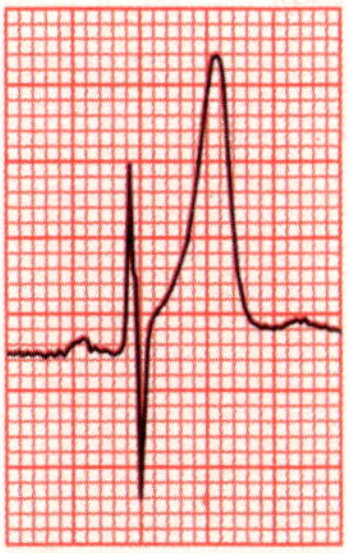

Tall peaked T wave in lead V_3

Fig. 1.40

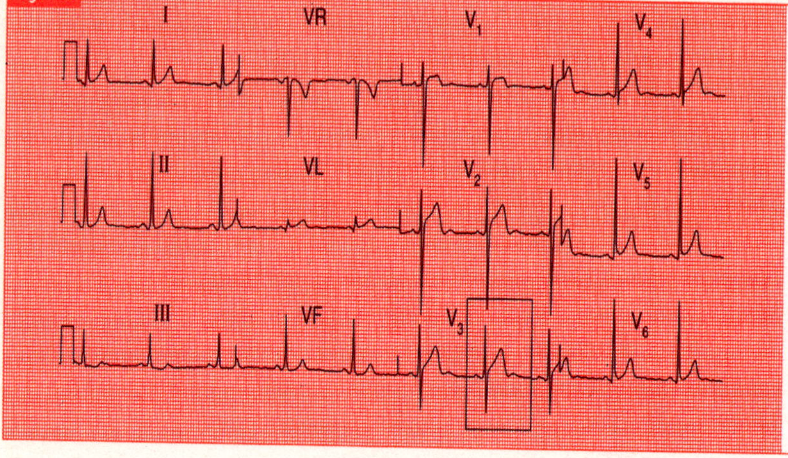

An extra hump on the end of the T wave, a 'U' wave, is characteristic of hypokalaemia. However, U waves are commonly seen in the anterior chest leads of normal ECGs (Fig. 1.40). It is thought that they represent repolarization of the papillary muscles. A U wave is probably only important if it follows a flat T wave.

THE QT INTERVAL

The QT interval (from the Q wave to the end of the T wave) varies with the heart rate, gender and time of day. There are several different ways of correcting for heart rate, but the simplest is Bazett's formula. In this, the corrected QT interval (QT_c) is calculated by:

$$QT_c = \frac{QT}{\sqrt{(\text{R–R interval})}}$$

An alternative is Fridericia's correction, in which QT_c is the QT interval divided by the cube root of the R–R interval. It is uncertain which of the corrections is clinically more important.

The upper limit of the normal QT_c interval is longer in women than in men, and increases with age. Its precise limit is uncertain, but is usually taken

Normal ECG

Note

- Prominent U waves following normal T waves in leads V_2–V_4

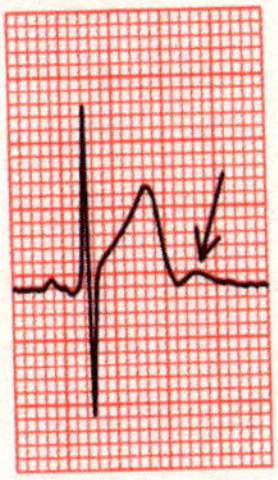

U wave in lead V_3

(following Bazett's correction) as 450 ms for adult men and 470 ms for adult women.

THE ECG IN ATHLETES

Any of the normal variations discussed above can be found in athletes. There can be changes in rhythm and/or ECG pattern, and the ECGs of athletes may also show some features that might be considered abnormal in non-athletic subjects, but are normal in athletes (see Box 1.3).

The ECGs in Figures 1.41, 1.42 and 1.43 were all recorded during the screening examinations of healthy young footballers.

Box 1.3 Possible ECG features of healthy athletes

Variations in rhythm
- Sinus bradycardia.
- Marked sinus arrhythmia
- Junctional rhythm
- 'Wandering' atrial pacemaker
- First degree block
- Wenckebach phenomenon
- Second degree block

Variations in ECG pattern
- Tall P waves
- Tall R waves and deep S waves
- Prominent septal Q waves
- Counterclockwise rotation
- Slight ST segment elevation
- Tall symmetrical T waves
- T wave inversion, especially in lateral leads
- Biphasic T waves
- Prominent U waves

Fig 1.41

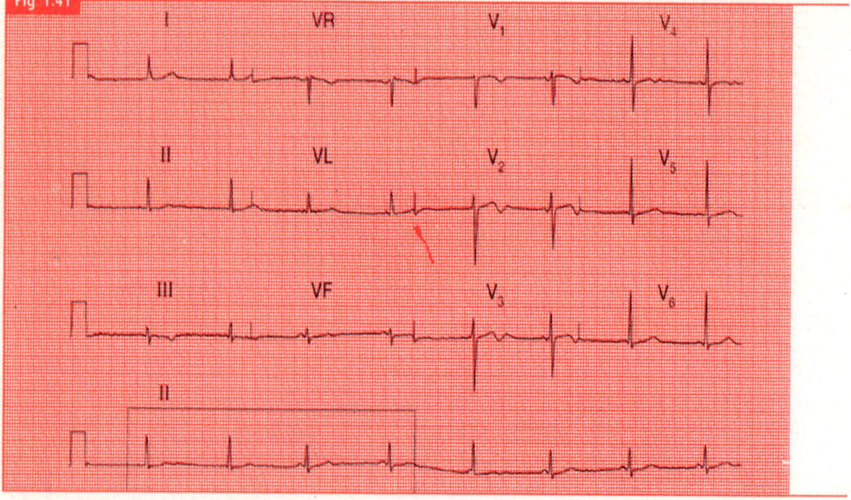

Fig 1.42

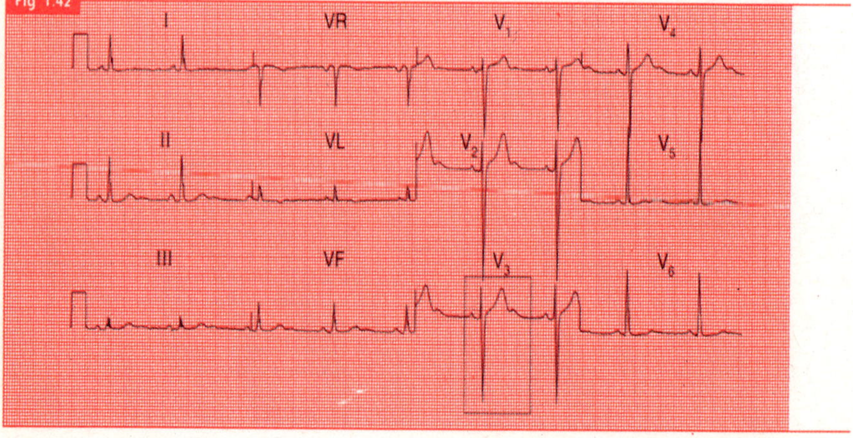

Normal ECG

Note

- Heart rate 49/min
- Accelerated idionodal rhythm ('wandering pacemaker')
- Biphasic T wave in lead V_3
- Prominent U waves

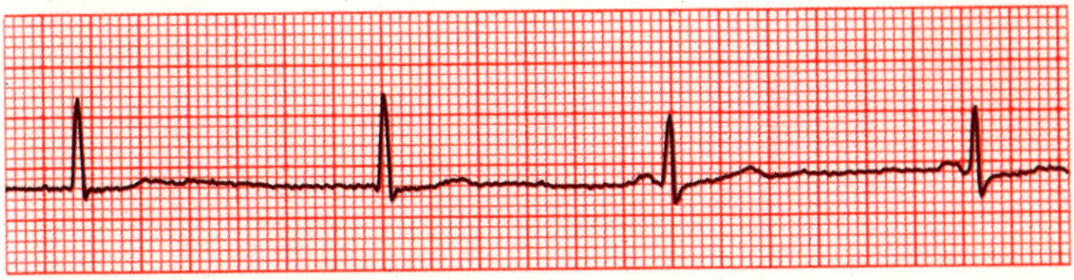

Accelerated idionodal rhythm

Normal ECG

Note

- Heart rate 53/min
- Sinus rhythm
- Prominent U waves in leads V_2–V_5
- Inverted T waves in lead VL

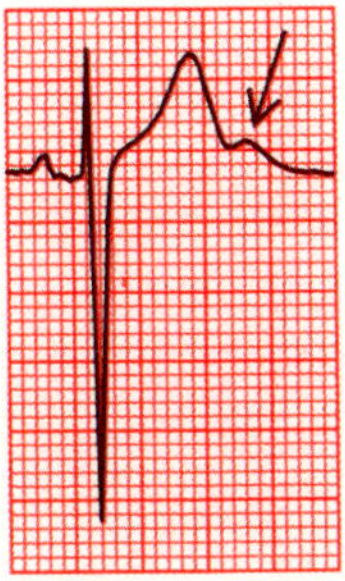

U wave in lead V_3

Fig. 1.43

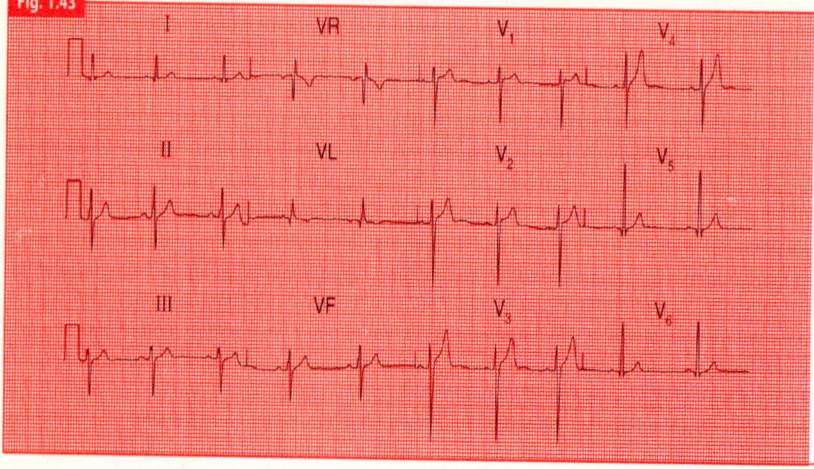

Fig. 1.44

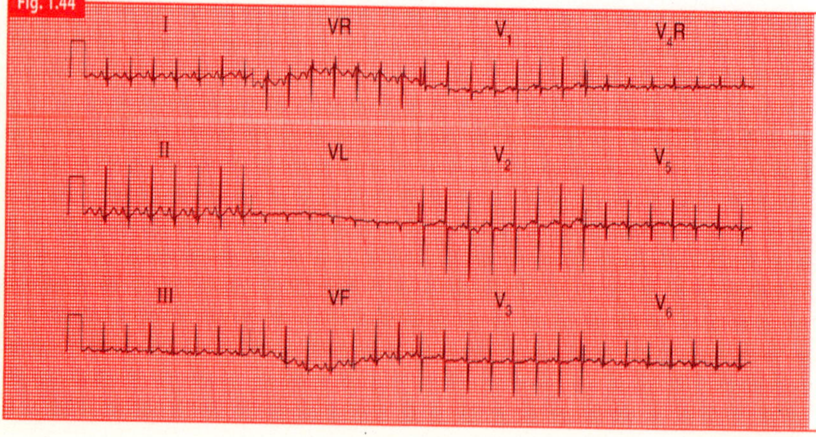

Normal ECG

Note

- Sinus rhythm
- Left axis deviation
- Septal Q waves in leads V_5–V_6

Normal ECG, from a child 1 month old

Note

- Heart rate 170/min
- Sinus rhythm
- Normal axis
- Dominant R waves in lead V_1
- Inverted T waves in leads V_1–V_2
- Biphasic T waves in lead V_3
- Lead V_4R (a position on the chest equivalent to V_4, but on the right side) has been recorded instead of V_4

THE ECG IN PREGNANCY

Minor changes in the ECG are commonly seen in pregnancy (see Box 1.4). Ventricular extrasystoles are almost universal.

Box 1.4 Possible ECG features in pregnancy

- Sinus tachycardia
- Supraventricular and ventricular extrasystoles
- Nonspecific ST segment/T wave changes

THE ECG IN CHILDREN

The normal heart rate in the first year of life is 140–160/min, falling slowly to about 80/min by puberty. Sinus arrhythmia is usually quite marked in children.

At birth, the muscle of the right ventricle is as thick as that of the left ventricle. The ECG of a normal child in the first year of life has a pattern that would indicate right ventricular hypertrophy in an adult. The ECG in Figure 1.44 was recorded from a normal child aged 1 month.

The changes suggestive of right ventricular hypertrophy disappear during the first few years of life. All the features other than the inverted T waves in leads V_1 and V_2 should have disappeared by the age of 2 years, and the adult pattern of the ECG should have developed by the age of 10 years. In general, if the infant ECG pattern persists beyond the age of 2 years, then right ventricular hypertrophy is indeed present. If the normal adult pattern is present in the first year of life, then left ventricular hypertrophy is present.

Box 1.5 The ECG in normal children

At birth
- Sinus tachycardia
- Right axis deviation
- Dominant R waves in lead V_1
- Deep S waves in lead V_6
- Inverted T waves in leads V_1–V_4

At 1 year of age
- Sinus tachycardia
- Right axis deviation
- Dominant R waves in lead V_1
- Inverted T waves in leads V_1–V_2

At 2 years of age
- Normal axis
- S waves exceed R waves in lead V_1
- T waves inverted in leads V_1–V_2

At 5 years of age
- Normal QRS complexes
- T waves still inverted in leads V_1–V_2

At 10 years of age
- Adult pattern

The ECG changes associated with childhood are summarized in Box 1.5.

FREQUENCY OF ECG ABNORMALITIES IN HEALTHY PEOPLE

The ECG findings we have discussed so far can all be considered to be within the normal range. Certain findings are undoubtedly abnormal as far as the ECG is concerned, yet do occur in apparently healthy people.

The frequency with which abnormalities are detected depends on the population studied: most abnormalities are found least often in healthy young people recruited to the armed services, and become progressively more common in populations of increasing age. An exception to this rule is that frequent ventricular extrasystoles are very common in pregnancy. The frequency of right and left bundle branch block has been found to be 0.3% and 0.1% respectively in populations of young recruits to the services, but in older working populations these abnor-

Table 1.1 Prevalence of the more common ECG abnormalities in 18 000 civil servants (after Rose et al 1978 British Heart Journal 40: 636-643)

ECG abnormality	Rate of abnormality per 1000 individuals in age range		
	40–49 years	50–59 years	60–64 years
Frequent ventricular extrasystoles	8	14	26
Atrial fibrillation	2	4	11
Left axis deviation	23	32	49
First degree block	18	26	33
Left bundle branch block	9	16	31
Abnormal T wave inversion	9	54	76
Wolff–Parkinson–White syndrome	0.3	0.2	0

malities have been detected in 2% and 0.7% respectively of apparently healthy people.

Table 1.1 shows the frequency with which the more common ECG abnormalities were encountered in a large survey of civil servants. All the abnormalities, except the Wolff–Parkinson–White syndrome, which is congenital, were found more frequently with increasing age. Some individuals had symptoms of heart disease and of course these were more common in the older age group. These findings suggest that the various abnormalities are all indicators of heart disease. This sort of survey shows how difficult it is to define the precise range of 'normality' in the ECG.

WHAT TO DO

When an apparently healthy subject has an ECG record that appears abnormal, the most important thing is not to cause unnecessary alarm. There are four questions to ask:

1. Does the ECG really come from that individual? If so, is he or she really asymptomatic and are the findings of the physical examination really normal?
2. Is the ECG really abnormal or is it within the normal range?
3. If the ECG is indeed abnormal, what are the implications for the patient?
4. What further investigations are needed?

THE RANGE OF NORMALITY

Normal variations in the P waves, QRS complexes and T waves have been described in detail. T wave changes usually give the most trouble in terms of ECG interpretation, because changes in repolarization occur in many different circumstances, and in any individual, variations in T wave morphology can occur from day to day.

Box 1.6 lists some of the ECG patterns that can be accepted as normal in healthy patients, and some that must be regarded with suspicion.

Box 1.6 Variations in the normal ECG in adults

Rhythm
- Marked sinus arrhythmia, with escape beats
- Lack of sinus arrhythmia (normal with increasing age)
- Supraventricular extrasystoles
- Ventricular extrasystoles

P wave
- Normally inverted in lead VR
- May be inverted in lead VL

Cardiac axis
- Minor right axis deviation in tall people
- Minor left axis deviation in fat people and in pregnancy

QRS complexes in the chest leads
- Slight dominance of R wave in lead V_1, provided there is no other evidence of right ventricular hypertrophy or posterior infarction
- The R wave in the lateral chest leads may exceed 25 mm in thin fit young people
- Partial right bundle branch block (RSR^1 pattern, with QRS complexes less than 120 ms)
- Septal Q waves in leads III, VL, V_5–V_6

ST segment
- Raised in anterior leads following an S wave (high take-off ST segment)
- Depressed in pregnancy
- Nonspecific upward-sloping depression

T wave
- Inverted in lead VR and often in V_1
- Inverted in leads V_2–V_3, or even V_4 in black people
- May invert with hyperventilation
- Peaked, especially if the T waves are tall

U wave
- Normal in anterior leads when the T wave is not flattened

THE PROGNOSIS OF PATIENTS WITH AN ABNORMAL ECG

In general, the prognosis is related to the patient's clinical history and to the findings on physical examination, rather than to the ECG. An abnormal ECG is much more significant in a patient with symptoms and signs of heart disease than it is in a truly healthy subject. In the absence of any other evidence of heart disease, the prognosis of an individual with one of the more common ECG abnormalities is as follows.

Conduction defects

First degree block (especially when the PR interval is only slightly prolonged) has little effect on prognosis. Second and third degree block indicate heart disease and the prognosis is worse, though the congenital form of complete block is less serious than the acquired form in adults.

Left anterior hemiblock has a good prognosis, as does right bundle branch block. The presence of left bundle branch block (LBBB) in the absence of other manifestations of cardiac disease is associated with about a 30% increase in the risk of death compared with that of individuals with a normal ECG. The risk of death doubles if a subject known to have a normal ECG suddenly develops LBBB, even if there are no symptoms – the ECG change presumably indicates progressive cardiac disease, probably most often ischaemia. Bifascicular block seldom progresses to complete block, but is always an indication of underlying heart disease – the prognosis is therefore relatively poor compared to that of patients with LBBB alone.

Arrhythmias

Supraventricular extrasystoles are of no importance whatsoever. Ventricular extrasystoles are almost universal, but when frequent or multiform they indicate populations with a statistically increased risk of death, presumably because in a proportion of people they indicate subclinical heart disease. The increased risk to an individual is, however, minimal and there is no evidence that treating ventricular extrasystoles prolongs survival.

Atrial fibrillation is frequently the result of rheumatic or ischaemic heart disease or cardiomyopathy, and the prognosis is then relatively poor. In about one third of individuals with atrial fibrillation no cardiac disease can be demonstrated. However, even in these people the risk of death is increased by three or four times, and the risk of stroke is increased perhaps tenfold, compared with people of the same age whose hearts are in sinus rhythm.

FURTHER INVESTIGATIONS

Complex and expensive investigations are seldom justified in asymptomatic patients whose hearts are clinically normal, but who have been found to have an abnormal ECG.

An echocardiogram should be recorded in all patients with bundle branch block, to assess the size and function of the individual heart chambers.

Patients with LBBB may have a dilated cardiomyopathy, and the echocardiogram will then show a dilated left ventricle which contracts poorly. Alternatively they may have ischaemia, and the echocardiogram will show some segments of the left ventricle failing to contract or contracting poorly. Patients with LBBB may also have unsuspected aortic stenosis.

Patients with RBBB may have an atrial septal defect or pulmonary hypertension, but quite frequently the echocardiogram shows no abnormality.

Echocardiography may also be helpful to establish the cause of T wave inversion, which might be due to ischaemia, ventricular hypertrophy or cardiomyopathy.

Patients with frequent ventricular extrasystoles seldom need detailed investigation, but if there is any question of underlying heart disease an echocardiogram may help to exclude the possibility of a cardiomyopathy. It is also worth checking their blood haemoglobin level.

In patients with atrial fibrillation, an echocardiogram is useful for defining or excluding structural abnormalities, and for studying left ventricular function. An echocardiogram is indicated if there is anything that might suggest rheumatic heart disease. Since atrial fibrillation can be the only manifestation of thyrotoxicosis, thyroid function must be checked. Atrial fibrillation may also be the result of alcoholism and this may be denied by the patient, so it may be fair to check liver function.

Table 1.2 shows investigations that should be considered in the case of various cardiac rhythms and indicates which underlying diseases may be present.

TREATMENT OF ASYMPTOMATIC ECG ABNORMALITIES

It is always the patient who should be treated, not the ECG. The prognosis of patients with complete heart block is improved by permanent pacing, but that of patients with other degrees of block is not. Ventricular extrasystoles should not be treated because of the risk of the pro-arrhythmic effects of antiarrhythmic drugs. Atrial fibrillation need not be treated if the ventricular rate is reasonable, but anticoagulation must be considered in all cases. In the case of patients with valve disease and atrial fibrillation, however, anticoagulant treatment is essential.

Table 1.2 Investigations in apparently healthy people with an abnormal ECG

ECG appearance	Investigation	Diagnosis to be excluded
Sinus tachycardia	Thyroid function Haemoglobin Echocardiogram	Thyrotoxicosis Anaemia Changes in heart size Heart failure Systolic dysfunction
Sinus bradycardia	Thyroid function	Myxoedema
Frequent ventricular extrasystoles	Echocardiogram Haemoglobin	Left ventricular dysfunction Anaemia
Right bundle branch block	Echocardiogram	Heart size Lung disease Atrial septal defect
Left bundle branch block	Echocardiogram	Heart size Aortic stenosis Cardiomyopathy Ischaemia
T wave abnormalities	Electrolytes Echocardiogram Exercise test	High or low potassium or calcium Ventricular systolic dysfunction Hypertrophic cardiomyopathy Ischaemia
Atrial fibrillation	Thyroid function Liver function Echocardiogram	Thyrotoxicosis Alcoholism Valve disease, ventricular and left atrial dimensions Myxoma

The ECG in patients with palpitations and syncope

2

The ECG is of paramount importance for the diagnosis of arrhythmias. Many arrhythmias are not noticed by the patient, but sometimes they cause symptoms. These symptoms are often transient, and the patient may be completely well at the time he or she consults a doctor. Obtaining an ECG during a symptomatic episode is then the only certain way of making a diagnosis, but as always the history and physical examination are also extremely important. The main purpose of the history and examination is to help decide whether a patient's symptoms could be the result of an arrhythmia, and whether the patient has a cardiac or other disease that may cause an arrhythmia.

THE CLINICAL HISTORY AND PHYSICAL EXAMINATION

PALPITATIONS

'Palpitations' mean different things to different patients, but a general definition would be 'an awareness of the heartbeat'. Arrhythmias, fast or slow, can cause poor organ perfusion and so lead to syncope (a word used to describe all sorts of collapse), breathlessness and angina. Some rhythms can be recognized from a patient's description, such as:

- A patient recognizes sinus tachycardia because it feels like the palpitations that he or she associates with anxiety or exercise.
- Extrasystoles are described as the heart 'jumping' or 'missing a beat'. It is not possible to distinguish between supraventricular and ventricular extrasystoles from a patient's description.
- A paroxysmal tachycardia begins suddenly and sometimes stops suddenly. The heart rate is often 'too fast to count'. Severe attacks are associated with dizziness, breathlessness and chest pain.

Table 2.1 compares the symptoms associated with sinus tachycardia and a paroxysmal tachycardia, and shows how a diagnosis can be made from the history. Note that a heart rate between 140/min and 160/min may be associated with either sinus or paroxysmal tachycardia.

DIZZINESS AND SYNCOPE

These symptoms may have a cardiovascular or a neurological cause. Remember that cerebral hypoxia, however caused, may lead to a seizure and that can make the differentiation between cardiac and neurological syncope very difficult. Syncope is defined as 'a transient loss of consciousness characterized by unresponsiveness and loss of postural tone, with spontaneous recovery and not requiring specific resuscitative intervention'.

Some causes of syncope are summarized in Box 2.1.

Table 2.1 Diagnosis of sinus tachycardia or paroxysmal tachycardia from a patient's symptoms

Symptoms	Sinus tachycardia	Paroxysmal tachycardia
Timing of initial attack	Attacks probably began recently	Attacks probably began in teens or early adult life
Associations of attack	Exercise, anxiety	Usually no associations, but occasionally exercise-induced
Rate of start of palpitations	Slow build-up	Sudden onset
Rate of end of palpitations	'Die away'	Classically sudden, but often 'die away'
Heart rate	< 140/min	> 160/min
Associated symptoms	Paraesthesia due to hyperventilation	Chest pain Breathlessness Dizziness Syncope
Ways of terminating attacks	Relaxation	Breath holding Valsalva's manoeuvre

Box 2.1 Cardiovascular causes of syncope

Obstructed blood flow in heart or lungs
- Aortic stenosis
- Pulmonary embolus
- Pulmonary hypertension
- Hypertrophic cardiomyopathy
- Pericardial tamponade
- Atrial myxoma

Arrhythmias
- Tachycardias: patient is usually aware of a fast heartbeat before becoming dizzy
- Bradycardias: slow heart rates are often not appreciated. A classical cause of syncope is a Stokes–Adams attack, due to a very slow ventricular rate in patients with complete heart block. A Stokes–Adams attack can be recognized because the patient is initially pale but flushes red on recovery

Postural hypotension, occurring immediately on standing

Seen with:
- Loss of blood volume
- Autonomic nervous system disease (e.g. diabetes, Shy–Drager syndrome, amyloid neuropathy)
- Patients being treated with antihypertensive drugs

Neurally-mediated reflex syncopal syndromes
- Vasovagal (neurocardiogenic) (simple faints)
- Situational (e.g. after coughing, sneezing, gastrointestinal stimulation of various sorts, post-micturition)
- Carotid sinus hypersensitivity

Table 2.2 **Diagnosis of causes of syncope**

Symptoms and signs	Possible diagnosis
Family history of sudden death	Long QT syndrome, Brugada syndrome, hypertrophic cardiomyopathy
Caused by unpleasant stimuli, prolonged standing, hot places (situational syncope)	Vasovagal syncope
Occurs within seconds or minutes of standing	Orthostatic hypotension
Temporal relation to medication	Orthostatic hypotension
Occurs during exertion	Obstruction to blood flow (e.g. aortic stenosis, pulmonary hypertension)
Occurs with head rotation or pressure on neck	Carotid sinus hypersensitivity
Confusion for more than 5 min afterwards	Seizure
Tonic-clonic movements, automatism	Seizure
Frequent attacks, usually unobserved, with somatic symptoms	Psychiatric illness
Symptoms or signs suggesting cardiac disease	Cardiac disease

Table 2.2 shows some clinical features of syncope, and possible causes.

PHYSICAL EXAMINATION

If the patient has symptoms at the time of examination, the physical signs shown in Table 2.3 may point towards the nature of an arrhythmia.

If the patient has no symptoms at the time of the examination, look for:

- Evidence of any heart disease that might cause an arrhythmia
- Evidence of non-cardiac disease that might cause an arrhythmia
- Evidence of cardiovascular disease that might cause syncope without an arrhythmia
- Evidence (from history or examination) of neurological disease.

Box 2.2 lists some of the rhythms and conditions associated with syncope, and Box 2.3 gives the rhythms and underlying disease associated with palpitations.

Table 2.3 **Physical signs and arrhythmias**

Pulse	Heart rate (beats/min)	Possible nature of any arrhythmia
Arterial		
Regular	< 50	Sinus bradycardia Second or third degree block Atrial flutter with 3:1 or 4:1 block Idionodal rhythm (junctional escape), with or without sick sinus syndrome
	60–140	Probable sinus rhythm
	140–160	Sinus tachycardia or an arrhythmia
	150	Probable atrial flutter with 2:1 block
	140–170	Atrial tachycardia Nodal tachycardia Ventricular tachycardia
	> 180	Probable ventricular tachycardia
	300	Atrial flutter with 1:1 conduction
Irregular		Marked sinus arrhythmia Extrasystoles (supraventricular or ventricular) Atrial fibrillation Atrial flutter with variable block Rhythm varying between sinus rhythm and any arrhythmia or conduction defect
Jugular venous pulse		
More pulsations visible than heart rate		Second or third degree block Cannon waves – third degree block

Box 2.2 Causes of syncope associated with various cardiac rhythms

Sinus rhythm
- Neurological diseases, including epilepsy
- Vagal overactivity:
  - simple faint
  - carotid sinus hypersensitivity
  - acute myocardial infarction
- Postural hypotension:
  - blood loss
  - hypotensive drugs
  - Addison's disease
  - autonomic dysfunction
- Circulatory obstruction:
  - aortic or pulmonary stenosis
  - hypertrophic cardiomyopathy
  - pericardial tamponade
  - pulmonary embolus
  - pulmonary hypertension
  - atrial myxoma
- Drugs, including beta-blockers

Atrial fibrillation with slow ventricular rate
- Rheumatic heart disease
- Ischaemic heart disease
- Cardiomyopathies
- Drugs:
  - digoxin
  - beta-blockers
  - verapamil
  - amiodarone

'Sick sinus' disease
- Congenital
- Familial
- Idiopathic
- Ischaemic heart disease
- Rheumatic heart disease
- Cardiomyopathy
- Amyloidosis
- Collagen diseases
- Myocarditis
- Drugs, e.g. lithium

Second or third degree block
- Idiopathic (fibrosis)
- Congenital
- Ischaemia
- Aortic valve calcification
- Surgery or trauma
- Tumours in the His bundle
- Drugs:
  - digoxin
  - beta-blockers

Box 2.3 Causes of palpitations associated with various cardiac rhythms

Extrasystoles
- Normal heart
- Any cardiac disease
- Anaemia

Sinus tachycardia
- Normal heart
- Anxiety
- Anaemia
- Acute blood loss
- Thyrotoxicosis
- Pregnancy
- Lung disease
- CO_2 retention
- Pulmonary embolus
- Phaeochromocytoma
- Sympathomimetic drugs, including inhalers and caffeine

Atrial fibrillation
- Rheumatic heart disease
- Thyrotoxicosis
- Ischaemic heart disease
- Cardiomyopathy
- Alcoholism
- Apparently normal heart with 'lone atrial fibrillation'

Supraventricular tachycardia
- Pre-excitation syndromes
- Apparently normal heart

Ventricular tachycardia
- Acute myocardial infarction
- Ischaemic heart disease
- Cardiomyopathy (hypertrophic or dilated)
- Long QT syndrome
- Myocarditis
- Drugs
- Apparently normal heart: idiopathic

It is only possible to make a confident diagnosis that an arrhythmia is the cause of palpitations or syncope if an ECG recording of the arrhythmia can be obtained at the time of the patient's symptoms. If the patient is asymptomatic at the time of examination it may be worth arranging for an ECG to be recorded during an attack of palpitations, or to be recorded continuously on a tape recorder (the 'Holter' technique), in the hope that an episode of the arrhythmia will be detected.

THE ECG BETWEEN ATTACKS OF PALPITATIONS OR SYNCOPE

Even when the patient is asymptomatic, the resting ECG can be very helpful, as summarized in Table 2.4.

SYNCOPE DUE TO CARDIAC DISEASE OTHER THAN ARRHYTHMIAS

The ECG may indicate that syncopal attacks have a cardiovascular cause other than an arrhythmia.

ECG evidence of left ventricular hypertrophy or of left bundle branch block may suggest that syncope is due to aortic stenosis. The ECGs in Figures 2.1 and 2.2 were recorded from patients who had syncopal attacks on exercise due to severe aortic stenosis.

ECG evidence of right ventricular hypertrophy suggests thromboembolic pulmonary hypertension. The ECG in Figure 2.3 is that of a middle-aged woman with dizziness on exertion, due to multiple pulmonary emboli.

Fig. 2.1

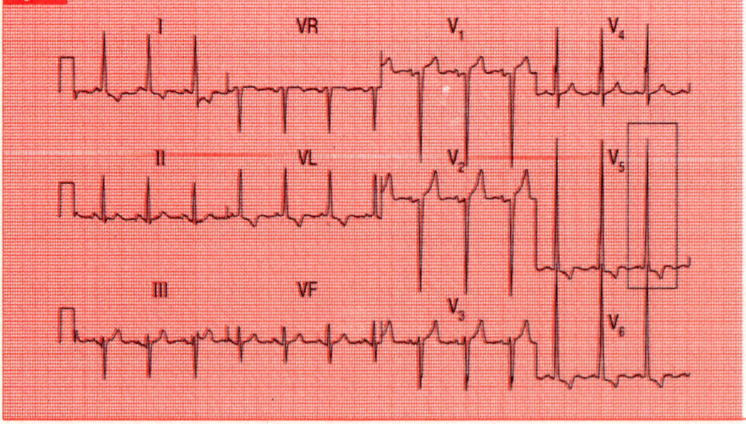

Table 2.4 ECG features between attacks of palpitations or syncope

ECG appearance	Possible cause of symptoms
ECG completely normal	Symptoms may not be due to a primary arrhythmia – consider anxiety, epilepsy, atrial myxoma or carotid sinus hypersensitivity
ECGs that suggest cardiac disease	Left ventricular hypertrophy or left bundle branch block – aortic stenosis Right ventricular hypertrophy – pulmonary hypertension Anterior T wave inversion – hypertrophic cardiomyopathy
ECGs that suggest intermittent tachyarrhythmia	Left atrial hypertrophy – mitral stenosis, so possibly atrial fibrillation Pre-excitation syndromes Long QT syndrome Flat T waves suggest hypokalaemia Digoxin effect – ?digoxin toxicity
ECGs that suggest intermittent bradyarrhythmia	Second degree block First degree block plus bundle branch block Digoxin effect

Left ventricular hypertrophy

Note

- Sinus rhythm
- Bifid P waves suggest left atrial hypertrophy (best seen in lead V_4)
- Normal axis
- Tall R waves and deep S waves
- T waves inverted in leads I, VL, V_5–V_6

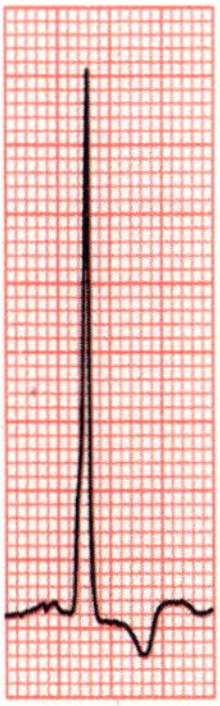

Tall R wave, inverted T wave in lead V_5

Fig. 2.2

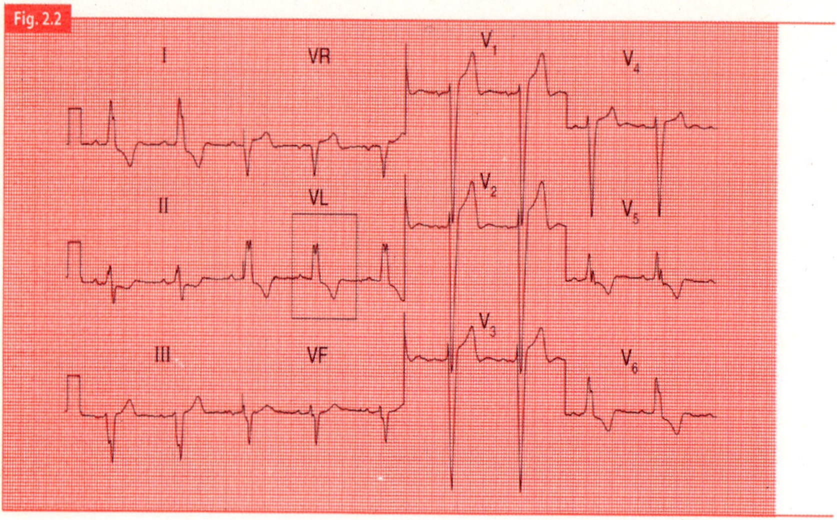

Fig. 2.3

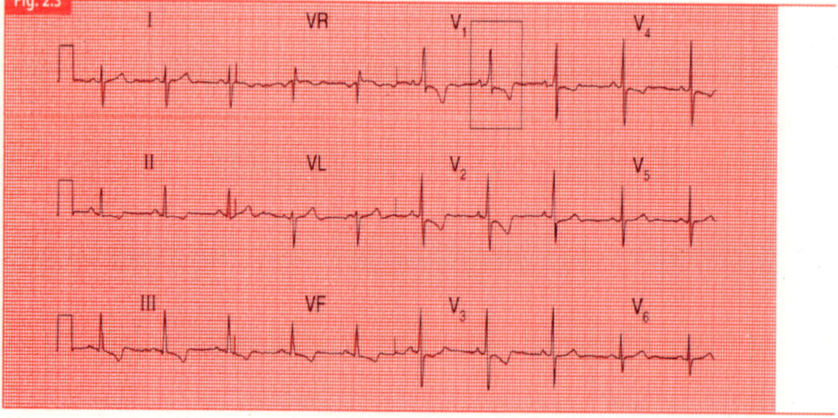

Left bundle branch block

Note

- Sinus rhythm
- Slight PR interval prolongation (212 ms)
- Broad QRS complexes
- 'M' pattern in lateral leads
- T wave inversion in leads I, VL, V_5–V_6

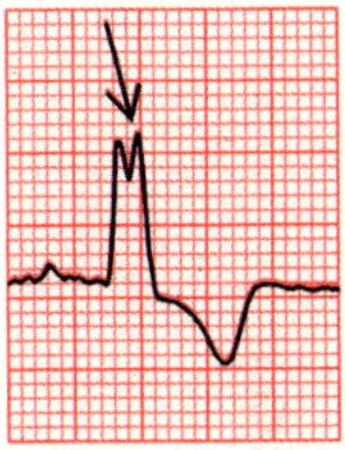

M pattern of left bundle branch block in lead VL

Right ventricular hypertrophy

Note

- Sinus rhythm
- Right axis deviation
- Dominant R waves in lead V_1
- Inverted T waves in leads V_1–V_4

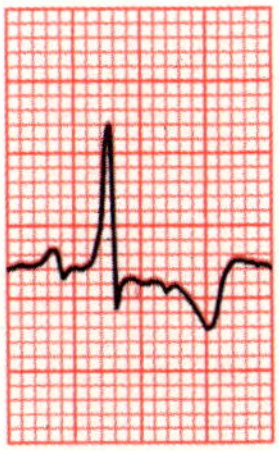

Dominant R wave in lead V_1

Fig. 2.4

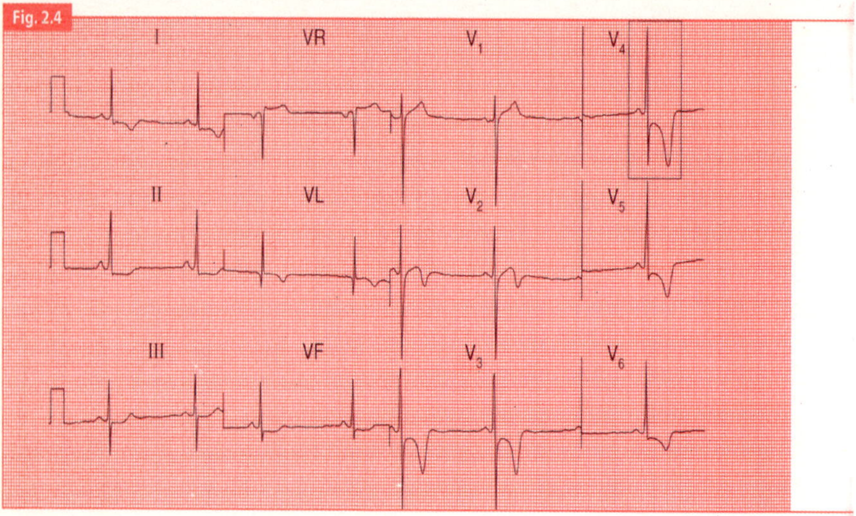

Fig. 2.5

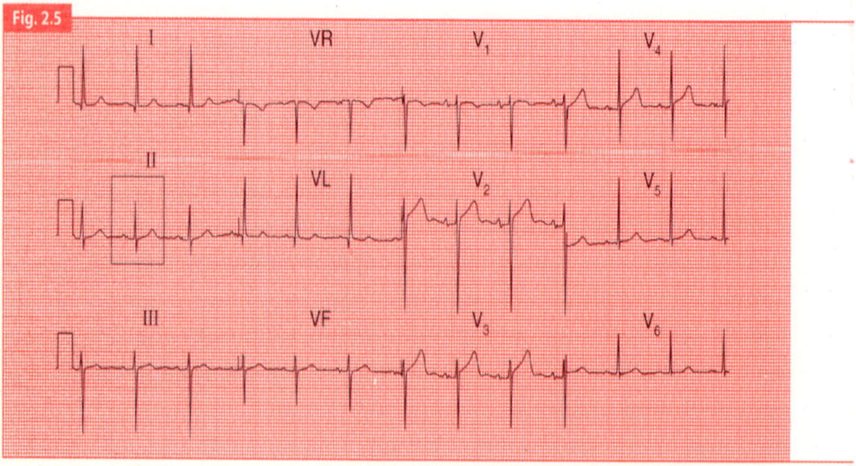

Hypertrophic cardiomyopathy

Note

- Sinus rhythm
- Marked T wave inversion in leads V_3–V_6

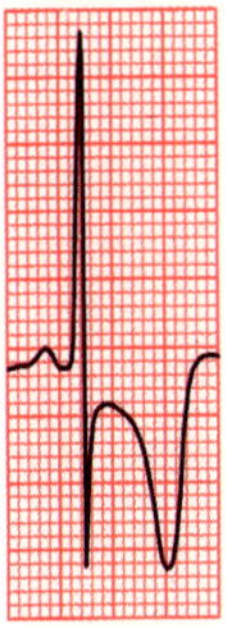

Inverted T wave in lead V_4

Left atrial hypertrophy

Note

- Sinus rhythm
- Bifid P waves most clearly seen in leads I, II, V_3–V_5

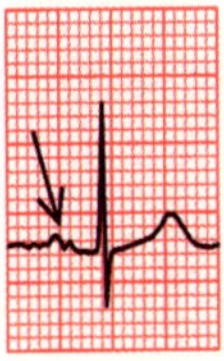

Bifid P wave in lead II

Syncope due to hypertrophic cardiomyopathy may be associated with a characteristic ECG (Fig. 2.4) that resembles that of patients with an anterior non-ST segment elevation myocardial infarction (NSTEMI) (compare with Fig. 3.23). With hypertrophic cardiomyopathy, the T wave inversion is usually more pronounced than with an NSTEMI, but differentiation really depends on the clinical picture, not on the ECG appearance. Hypertrophic cardiomyopathy can cause syncope due to obstruction to outflow from the left ventricle, or can cause symptomatic arrhythmias.

PATIENTS WITH POSSIBLE TACHYCARDIAS

MITRAL STENOSIS

Mitral stenosis leads to atrial fibrillation, but when the heart is still in sinus rhythm the presence of the characteristics of left atrial hypertrophy on the ECG may give a clue that paroxysmal atrial fibrillation is occurring (Fig. 2.5).

PRE-EXCITATION SYNDROMES

In the pre-excitation syndromes, abnormal pathways connect the atria and ventricles, forming an anatomical basis for re-entry tachycardia.

Normal conduction results in the uniform spread of the depolarization wave front in a constant direction. Should the direction of depolarization be reversed in some part of the heart, it becomes possible for a circular or 're-entry' pathway to be set up (Fig. 2.6). Depolarization reverberates round the pathway, causing a tachycardia. The anatomical requirement for this is the branching and rejoining of a conduction pathway. Normally, conduction is anterograde (forward) in both limbs of such a pathway, but an anterograde impulse may pass normally

Fig. 2.6

Re-entry mechanism causing tachycardia

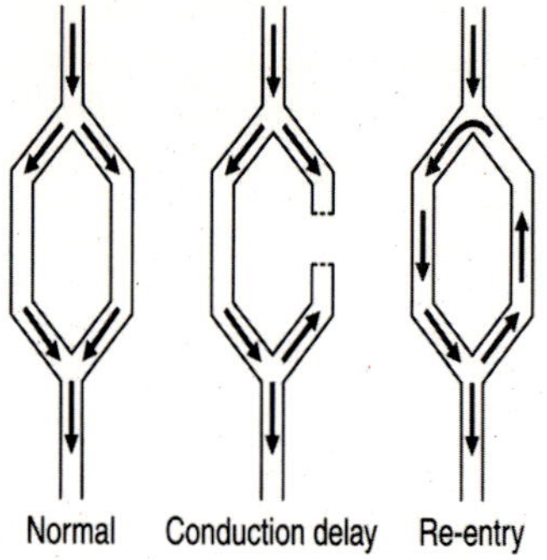

Fig. 2.7

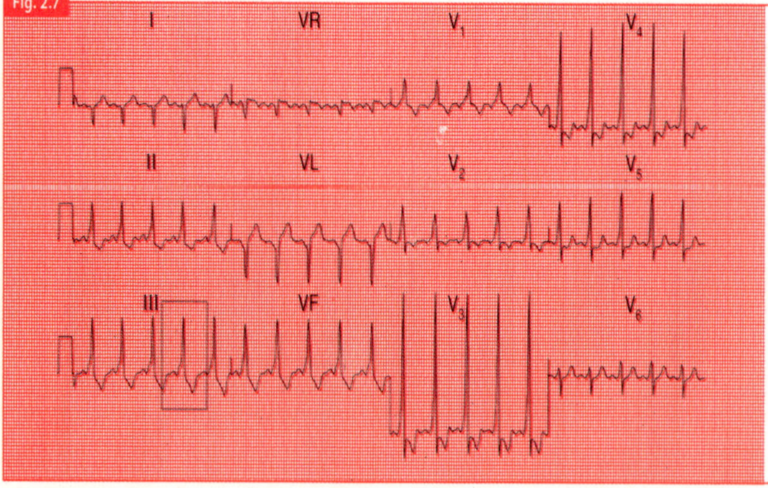

down one branch and be blocked in the other. From the point at which the pathways rejoin, the depolarization wave can spread retrogradely (backwards) up the abnormal branch. If it arrives when that pathway is not refractory to conduction, it can then pass right around the circuit and reactivate it.

Once established, a circular wave of depolarization may continue until some part of the pathway fails to conduct. The conduction of a depolarization wave round a circular pathway may also be interrupted by the arrival of another depolarization wave, set up by an ectopic focus (i.e. an extrasystole).

The Wolff–Parkinson–White syndrome

In the Wolff–Parkinson–White (WPW) syndrome, an accessory pathway connects either the left atrium and left ventricle, or the right atrium and right ventricle. In either case the normal atrioventricular (AV) nodal delay is bypassed, so the PR interval is short. Ventricular activation is initially abnormal, causing a slurred upstroke of the R wave (delta wave), but later activation spreading through the AV node and His bundle is normal.

The re-entry circuit comprises the normal AV node–His bundle connection between the atria and the ventricles, and the accessory pathway. Depolarization can spread down the normal pathway and back (i.e. retrogradely) up through the accessory pathway to reactivate the atria. This is called an 'orthodromic reciprocating tachycardia', and it causes narrow QRS complexes, with P waves sometimes visible just after each QRS complex. Alternatively, depolarization can pass down the accessory pathway and retrogradely up the His bundle to cause an 'antidromic reciprocating tachycardia', in which the QRS complexes are broad and slurred, and P waves may or may not be seen.

With a left-sided accessory pathway, the ECG shows a dominant R wave in lead V_1. This is called the 'type A' pattern (Fig. 2.7). This pattern of WPW conduction can easily be mistaken for right ventricular hypertrophy, the differentiation being made by the presence or absence of a short PR interval.

The ECG in Figure 2.8 is from a young man who complained of symptoms that sounded like paroxysmal tachycardia. His ECG shows the WPW syndrome type A, but it would be quite easy to miss the short PR interval unless the whole of the 12-lead trace were carefully inspected. The short PR interval and delta waves are most obvious in leads V_4 and V_5.

When the accessory pathway is on the right side of the heart, there is no dominant R wave in lead V_1 and this is called the 'type B' pattern (Fig. 2.9).

The Wolff–Parkinson–White syndrome, type A

Note

- Sinus rhythm
- Short PR interval
- Broad QRS complexes
- Dominant R wave in lead V_1
- Slurred upstroke to QRS complexes – the delta wave
- Inverted T waves in leads II, III, VF, V_1–V_4

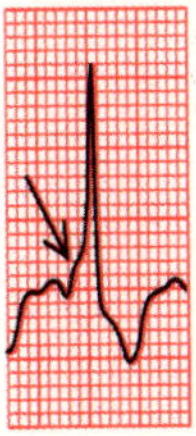

Delta wave in lead III

Fig. 2.8

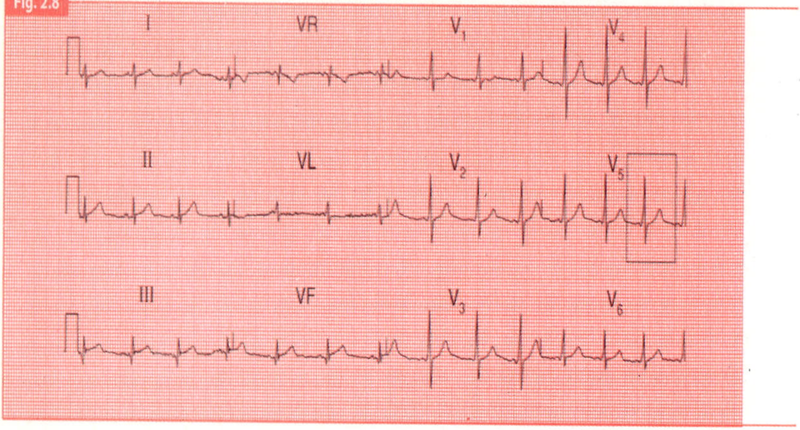

Fig. 2.9

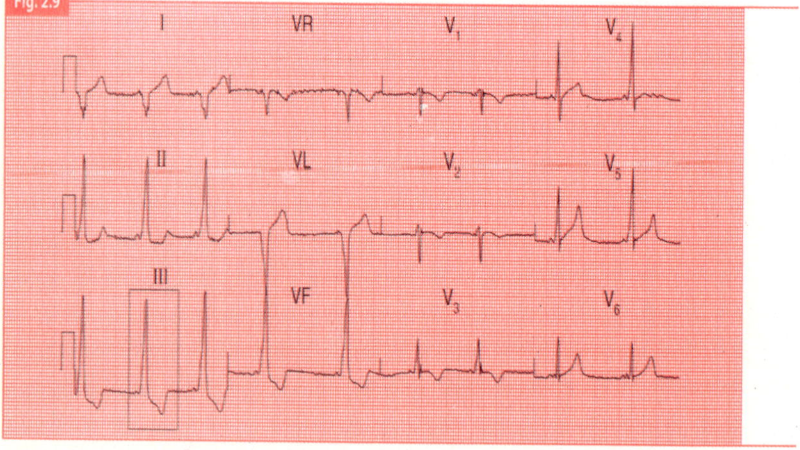

The Wolff–Parkinson–White syndrome, type A

Note

- Sinus rhythm
- Short PR interval, especially obvious in leads V_3–V_5
- Slurred upstroke to QRS complexes, obvious in leads V_3–V_5 but not obvious in the limb leads
- Dominant R wave in lead V_1
- No T wave inversion in the anterior leads (cf. Fig. 2.7)

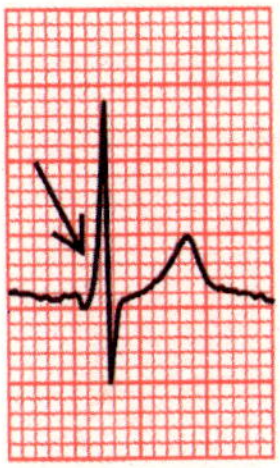

Delta wave in lead V_5

The Wolff–Parkinson–White syndrome, type B

Note

- Sinus rhythm
- Short PR interval
- Broad QRS complexes with delta waves
- No dominant R waves in lead V_1 (cf. Figs 2.7 and 2.8)
- T wave inversion in leads III, VF, V_3

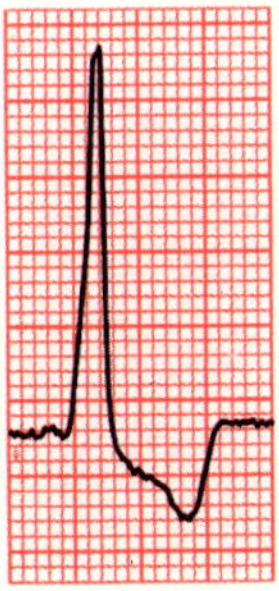

Short PR interval; broad QRS complex in lead III

Fig. 2.10

Tachycardias in the Wolff–Parkinson–White syndrome

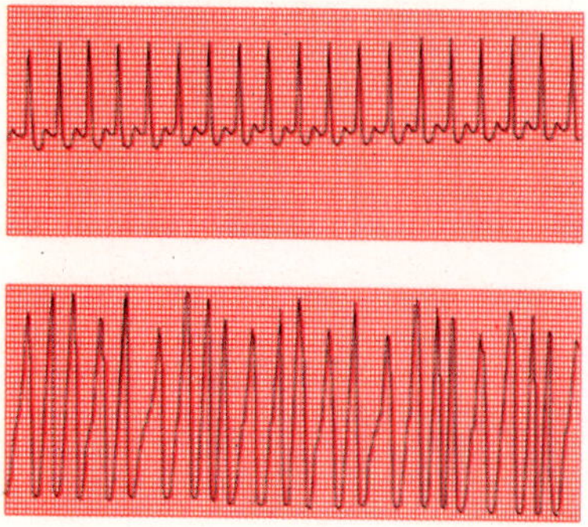

Note

- The upper trace shows a narrow complex (orthodromic) tachycardia
- The lower trace shows a wide complex (antidromic) tachycardia
- In the lower trace the marked irregularity and variation of the complexes suggest that the rhythm is atrial fibrillation
- The underlying diagnosis of the WPW syndrome is not apparent from either trace

Fig. 2.11

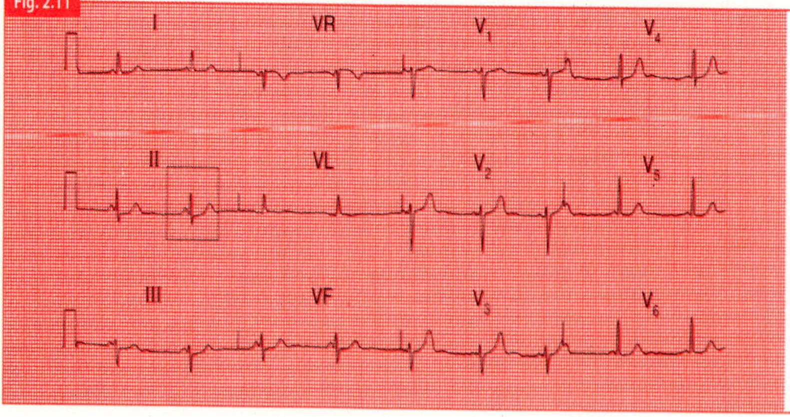

Box 2.4 The Wolff–Parkinson–White syndrome: ECG features

- Short PR interval
- Slight widening of QRS complexes: delta wave with normal terminal segment
- ST segment/T wave changes
- Arrhythmias (narrow or wide complex)
- Arrhythmia with wide, irregular complex suggests the WPW syndrome with atrial fibrillation
- Right-sided pathway: sometimes, anterior T wave inversion
- Left-sided pathway: dominant R waves in leads V_1–V_6

ECGs indicating pre-excitation of the WPW type are found in approximately 1 in every 3000 healthy young people. Only half of these ever have an episode of tachycardia, and many have only very occasional attacks.

When an episode of re-entry tachycardia is associated with a narrow QRS complex, the pattern resembles a junctional (AV nodal re-entry) tachycardia and the presence of a pre-excitation syndrome may not be suspected.

The broad complex (antidromic reciprocating) tachycardias which occur in patients with the WPW syndrome may resemble ventricular tachycardia. In most cases, the underlying rhythm is probably atrial fibrillation with anomalous atrioventricular conduction. This is a serious arrhythmia because ventricular fibrillation may occur (Fig. 2.10).

The ECG features associated with the WPW syndrome are summarized in Box 2.4.

The Lown–Ganong–Levine syndrome

Note

- Sinus rhythm
- Short PR interval
- Normal QRS complexes and P waves

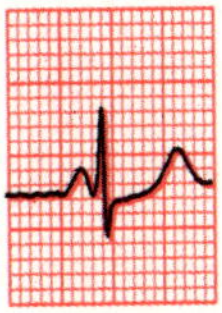

Short PR interval in lead II

The Lown–Ganong–Levine syndrome

Where an accessory pathway connects the atria to the bundle of His rather than to the right or left ventricle, there will be a short PR interval but the QRS complex will be normal. This is called the Lown–Ganong–Levine (LGL) syndrome (Fig. 2.11).

The short and fixed PR interval of pre-excitation must be distinguished from the short and varying PR interval of an 'accelerated idionodal rhythm' ('wandering pacemaker'), shown in Figure 2.12. Here the sinus node rate has slowed, and the heart is controlled by the AV node, which is discharging faster than the SA node. This ECG was recorded from an asymptomatic athlete.

Fig. 2.12

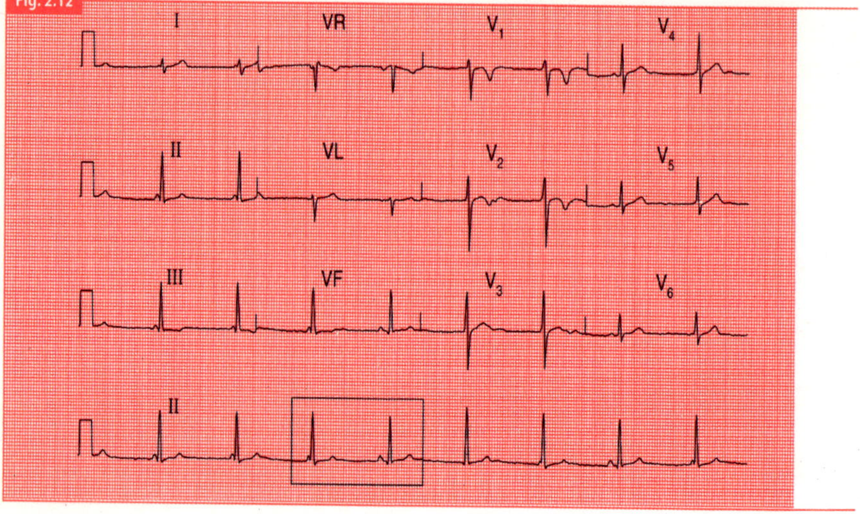

THE LONG QT SYNDROME

Delayed repolarization occurs for a variety of reasons, and causes a long QT interval. A prolonged QT interval is associated with paroxysmal ventricular tachycardia, and therefore can be the cause of episodes of collapse or even sudden death. Some causes of a prolonged QT interval are shown in Box 2.5.

Several genetic abnormalities have been described that lead to familial prolongation of the QT interval. The ECG in Figure 2.13 is from a 10-year-old girl who suffered from 'fainting' attacks. Her sister had died suddenly; three other siblings and both parents had normal ECGs.

The most common cause of QT prolongation is drug therapy. The ECG in Figure 2.14 is from a patient who had a posterior myocardial infarction (see Ch. 3). He was treated with amiodarone because of recurrent ventricular tachycardias, and developed a prolonged QT interval. Figure 2.15 shows his record 4 months later: the prolonged QT interval reverted to normal when the amiodarone treatment was stopped.

When a prolonged QT interval is associated with ventricular tachycardia, this usually involves a continual change from upright to downward QRS complexes. This is called 'torsade de pointes'. The congenital long QT syndrome causes episodes of

Accelerated idionodal rhythm

Note

- SA node stimulates the atria at a constant rate of 50/min
- Ventricular rate is slightly faster than the atrial rate
- Narrow QRS complexes, originating in the AV node
- QRS complexes appear to 'overtake' the P waves, which are not suppressed – causing an apparent variation in the PR interval

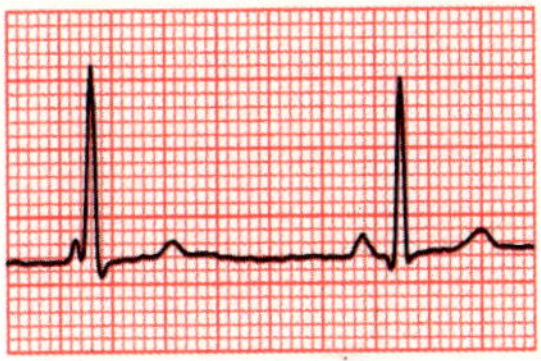

Variation of PR interval

loss of consciousness at times of increased sympathetic nervous system activity. Such episodes occur in about 8% of affected subjects each year, and the annual death rate due to arrhythmias is about 1% of patients with a long QT syndrome. The ECG in Figure 2.16 was recorded from a young girl with congenital long QT syndrome.

The precise relationship between QT_c interval prolongation and the risk of sudden death is unknown; neither is it clear whether prolongation of the QT or QT_c interval is more significant. There is no absolute threshold of risk. However, torsade de pointes ventricular tachycardia seems rare when the QT or QT_c interval is less than 500 ms.

Box 2.5 Possible causes of prolonged QT interval

Congenital
- Jervell–Lange–Nielson syndrome
- Romano–Ward syndrome

Antiarrhythmic drugs
- Quinidine
- Procainamide
- Disopyramide
- Amiodarone
- Sotalol

Other drugs
- Tricyclic antidepressants
- Erythromycin
- Thioridazine

Plasma electrolyte abnormality
- Low potassium
- Low magnesium
- Low calcium

Fig. 2.13

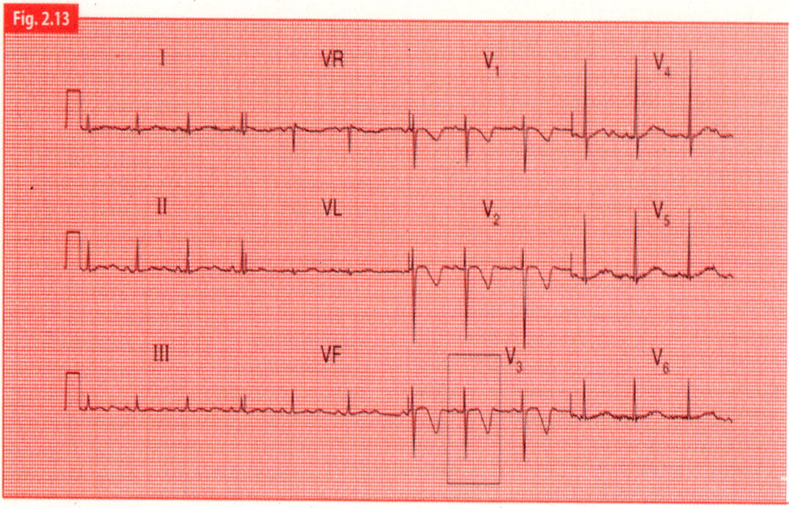

Fig. 2.14

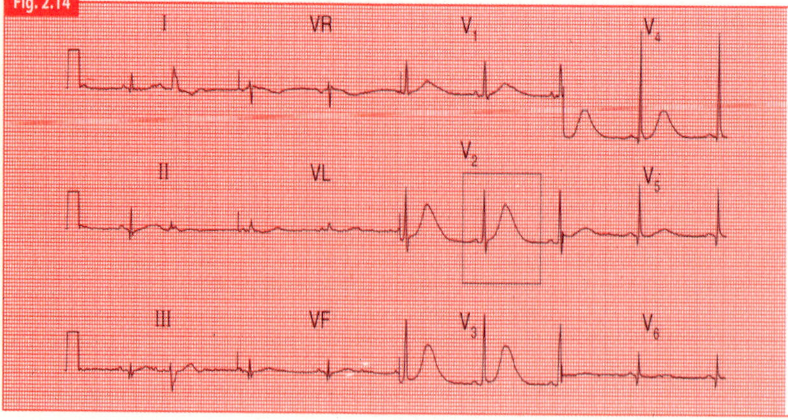

Congenital long QT syndrome

Note

- Sinus rhythm
- Normal axis
- QT interval 520 ms
- Marked T wave inversion in leads V_2–V_4

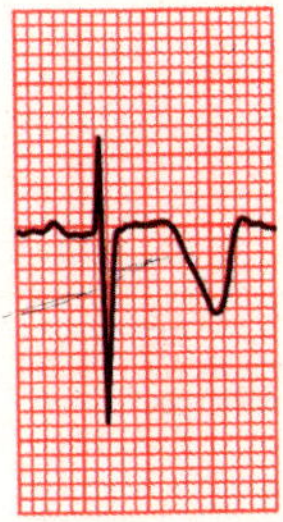

Long QT interval and inverted T wave in lead V_3

Prolonged QT interval due to amiodarone

Note

- Sinus rhythm
- Normal axis
- Dominant R waves in lead V_1 due to posterior infarction
- QT interval 652 ms
- Bizarre T wave shape in anterior leads

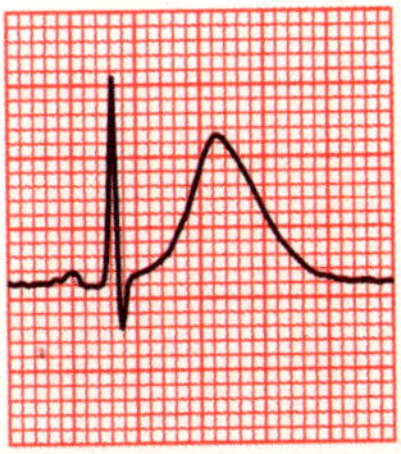

Long QT interval and bizarre T wave in lead V_2

Fig. 2.15

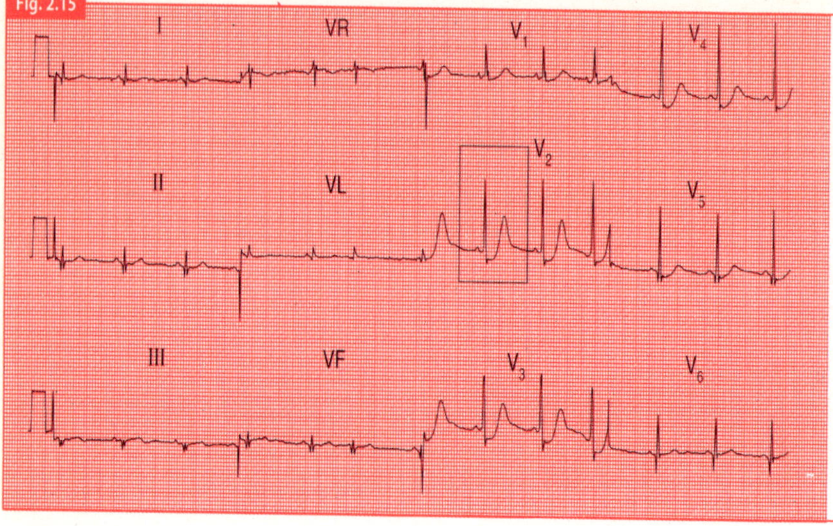

Fig. 2.16

Torsade de pointes ventricular tachycardia

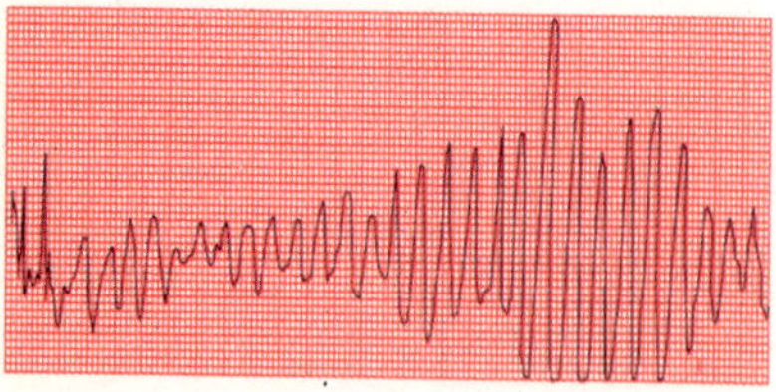

Note

- Broad complex tachycardia at 300/min
- Continually changing shape of QRS complexes

Posterior infarct with normal QT interval

Note

- Same patient as in Figure 2.14
- Sinus rhythm
- Normal axis
- Dominant R waves in lead V_1
- Ischaemic ST segment depression
- Normal QT interval

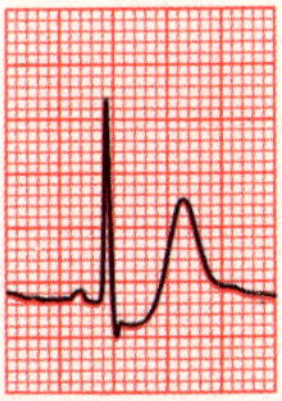

ST segment depression in lead V_2

THE BRUGADA SYNDROME

Sudden collapse due to ventricular tachycardia and fibrillation occurs in a congenital disorder of sodium ion transport called the Brugada syndrome. Between attacks, the ECG superficially resembles that associated with right bundle branch block (RBBB), with an RSR^1 pattern in leads V_1 and V_2 (Fig. 2.17). However, the ST segment in these leads is raised, and there is no wide S wave in lead V_6 as in RBBB. The changes are seen in the right ventricular leads because the abnormal sodium channels are predominantly found in the right ventricle. The ECG abnormality can be transient – the ECG in Figure 2.18 was taken a day later from the same patient.

Fig. 2.17

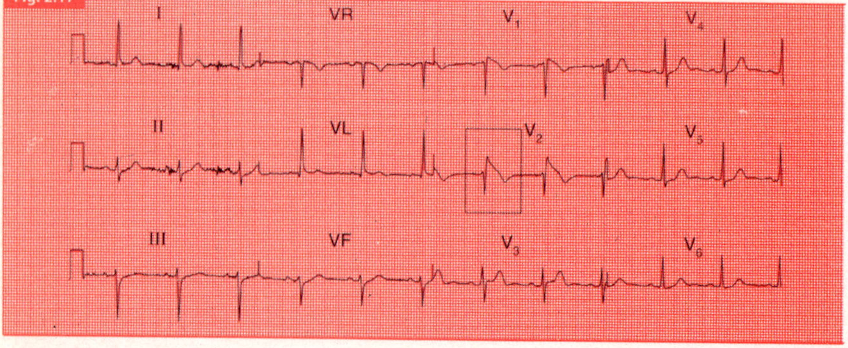

Fig. 2.18

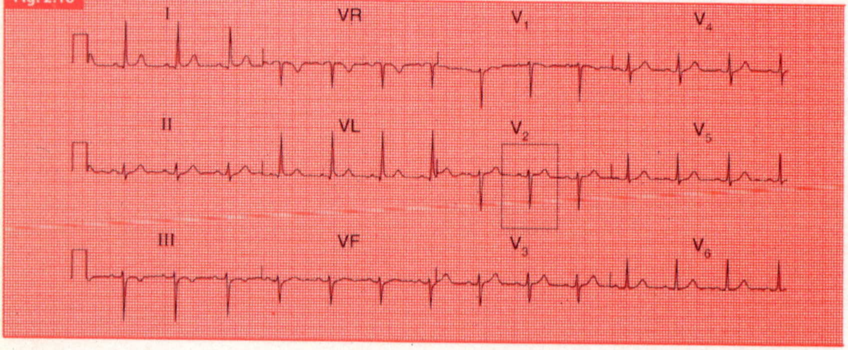

Brugada syndrome

Note

- Sinus rhythm
- Normal axis
- Normal QRS complex duration
- RSR[1] pattern in leads V_1–V_2
- No wide S wave in lead V_6
- Raised, downward-sloping ST segment in leads V_1–V_2

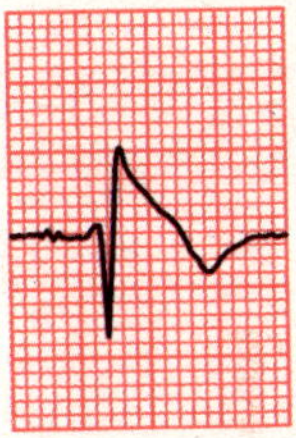

RSR[1] pattern and raised ST segment in lead V_2

Brugada syndrome

Note

- Same patient as in Figure 2.17
- Normal ECG

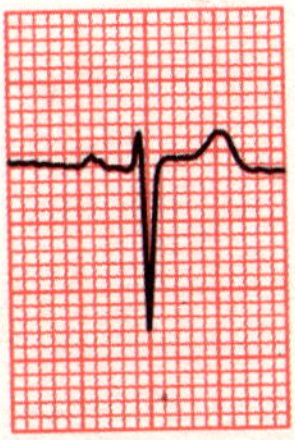

Normal appearance in lead V_2

PATIENTS WITH POSSIBLE BRADYCARDIAS

When a patient is asymptomatic, an intermittent bradycardia can be suspected if the ECG shows any evidence of a conduction defect. However, it must be remembered that conduction defects and escape rhythms are quite common in healthy people and their presence may be coincidental.

ESCAPE RHYTHMS

Myocardial cells are only depolarized when they are stimulated, but the cells of the SA node, those around the AV node (the 'junctional' cells) and those of the conducting pathways all possess the property of spontaneous depolarization or 'automaticity'.

The automaticity of any part of the heart is suppressed by the arrival of a depolarization wave, and so the heart rate is controlled by the region with the highest automatic depolarization frequency. Normally the SA node controls the heart rate because it has the highest frequency of discharge, but if for any reason this fails, the region with the next highest intrinsic depolarization frequency will emerge as the pacemaker and set up an 'escape' rhythm. The atria and the junctional region have automatic depolarization frequencies of about 50/min, compared with the normal SA node frequency of 60–70/min. If both the SA node and the junctional region fail to depolarize, or if conduction to the ventricles fails, a ventricular focus may emerge, with a rate of 30–40/min; this is classically seen in complete heart block.

Escape beats may be single or may form sustained rhythms. They have the same ECG appearance as the corresponding extrasystoles, but appear late rather than early (Fig. 2.19).

In sustained junctional escape rhythms, atrial activation may be seen as a P wave following the QRS complex (Fig. 2.20). This occurs if depolarization spreads in the opposite direction from normal, from the AV node to the atria, and is called 'retrograde' conduction. Figure 2.21 also shows a junctional escape rhythm.

Figure 2.22 shows a ventricular escape beat.

SYNCOPE

In a patient with syncopal attacks, ECG changes that would be ignored in a healthy person take on a greater significance. First degree block, itself of no clinical importance, may point to intermittent complete block, and complete block is much more

Fig. 2.19

Junctional escape beat

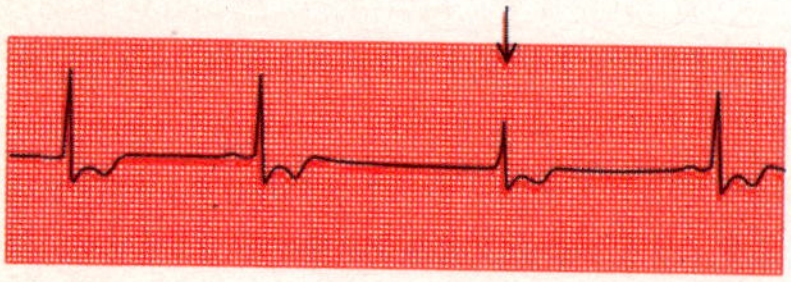

Note

- After two sinus beats there is no P wave
- After an interval there is a narrow QRS complex, with the same configuration as that of the sinus beats but without a preceding P wave
- This is a junctional beat (arrowed)
- Sinus rhythm then reappears

likely when the ECG of a currently asymptomatic patient shows second degree block. The ECGs in Figures 2.23, 2.24 and 2.25 are from patients with syncopal attacks, all of whom eventually needed permanent pacemakers.

Fig. 2.20

Junctional (escape) rhythm

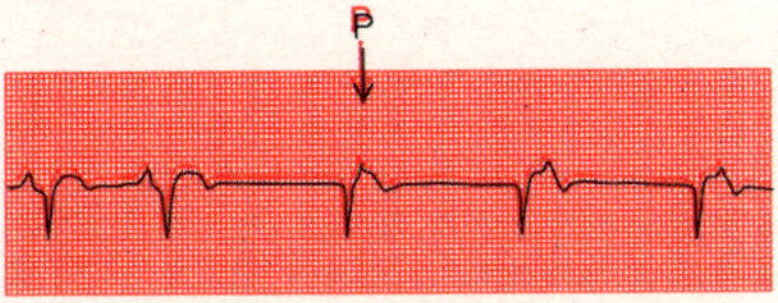

Note

- Two sinus beats are followed by an interval with no P waves
- A junctional rhythm then emerges (with QRS complexes the same as in sinus rhythm)
- A P wave (arrowed) can be seen as a hump on the T wave of the junctional beats: the atria have been depolarized retrogradely

Fig. 2.21

Junctional (escape) rhythm

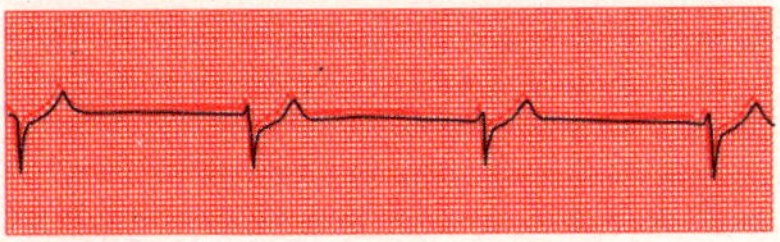

Note

- No P waves
- Narrow QRS complexes and normal T waves

Fig. 2.22

Ventricular escape beat

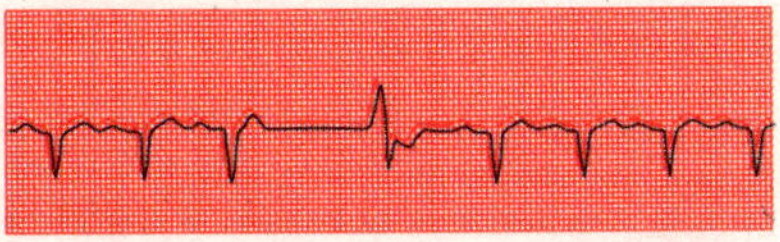

Note

- Three sinus beats are followed by a pause
- There is then a single ventricular beat with a wide QRS complex and an inverted T wave
- Sinus rhythm is then restored

Fig. 2.23

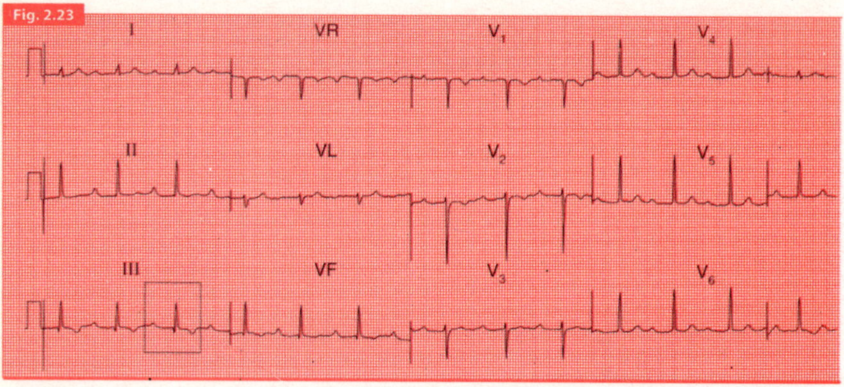

Fig. 2.24

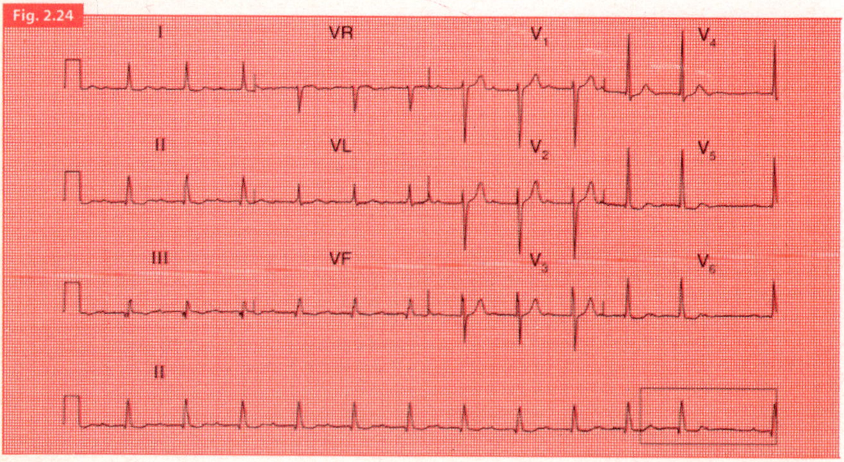

First degree block

Note

- Sinus rhythm
- PR interval 380 ms
- T wave inversion in leads III and VF suggests ischaemia

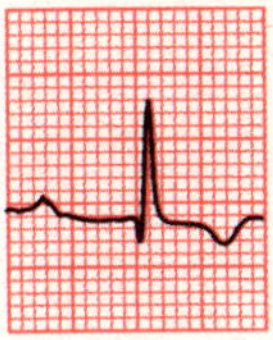

Long PR interval in lead III

Second degree block (Wenckebach)

Note

- Sinus rhythm
- PR interval lengthens progressively from 360 ms to 440 ms and then a P wave is not conducted
- Small Q wave and inverted T wave in leads III and VF suggest an old inferior infarct

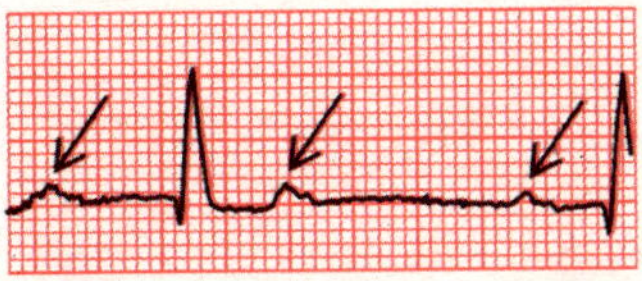

P waves

Fig. 2.25

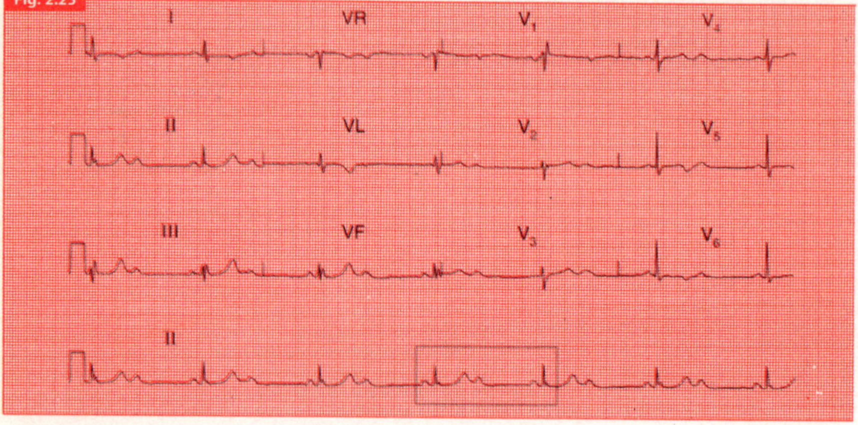

Fig. 2.26

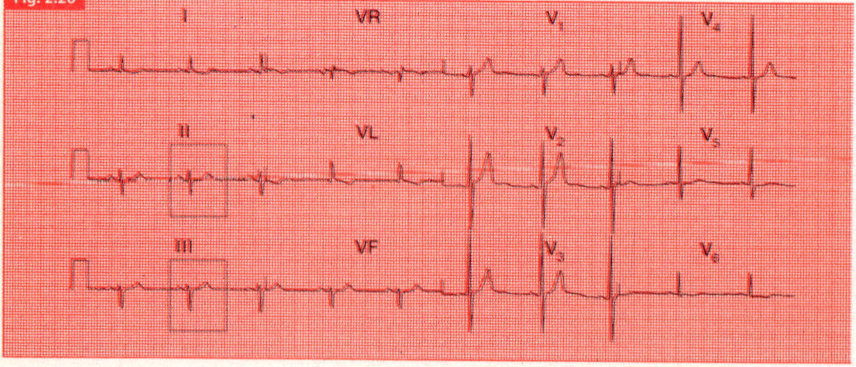

Second degree block (2:1)

Note

- Sinus rhythm
- Alternate beats conducted and not conducted
- Lateral T wave inversion in leads I, VL, V_6 suggests ischaemia

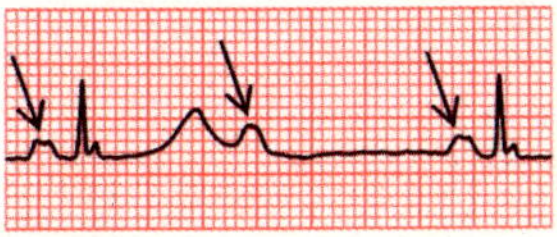

P waves

Left axis deviation

Note

- Sinus rhythm
- Dominant S waves in leads II and III: left axis deviation
- Normal QRS complex duration
- Lateral T wave inversion

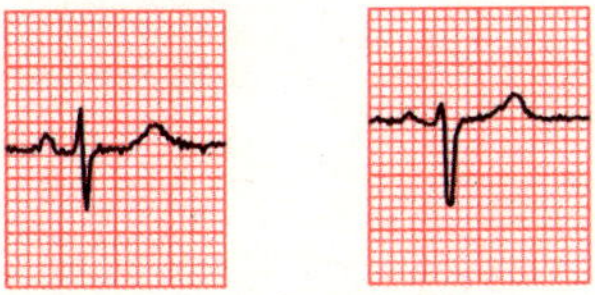

Dominant S waves in leads II and III

COMBINATIONS OF CONDUCTION ABNORMALITIES

Left axis deviation usually indicates left anterior hemiblock, but when the QRS complex is narrow it can be accepted as a normal variant (Fig. 2.26).

A widened QRS complex with marked left axis deviation represents the full pattern of left anterior hemiblock (Fig. 2.27).

When left anterior hemiblock is associated with first degree block and left bundle branch block (Fig. 2.28), both fascicles of the left bundle are failing to conduct and conduction is also delayed in either the AV node, the His bundle or the right bundle branch.

Alternatively, the combination of first degree block and right bundle branch block (RBBB) (Fig. 2.29) shows that conduction has failed in the right bundle branch and is also beginning to fail elsewhere.

A combination of left anterior hemiblock and RBBB means that conduction into the ventricles is only passing through the posterior fascicle of the left bundle branch (Fig. 2.30). This is called 'bifascicular block'.

A combination of left anterior hemiblock, RBBB and first degree block suggests that there is disease in the remaining conducting pathway – either in the main His bundle or in the posterior fascicle of the left bundle branch. This is sometimes called 'trifascicular block' (Fig. 2.31). Complete conduction block in the right bundle and in both fascicles of the left bundle would, of course, cause complete (third degree) heart block.

Right axis deviation is not necessarily a feature of left posterior hemiblock, but when combined with other evidence of conducting tissue disease such as first degree block (Fig. 2.32), it usually is.

A combination of second degree (2:1) block with left anterior hemiblock (Fig. 2.33) or with both left anterior hemiblock and RBBB (Fig. 2.34) suggests widespread conduction tissue disease.

Fig. 2.27

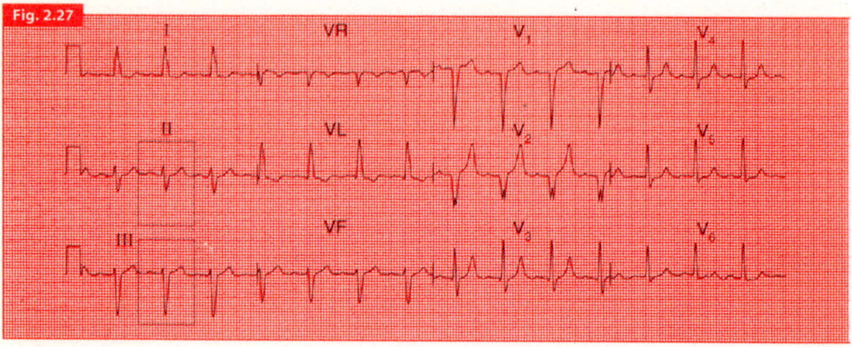

Fig. 2.28

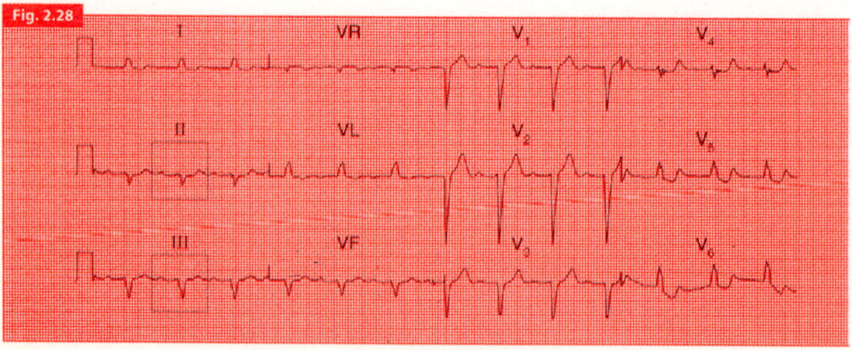

Left anterior hemiblock

Note

- Sinus rhythm
- Left axis deviation
- Broad QRS complexes (122 ms)
- Inverted T waves in lead VL

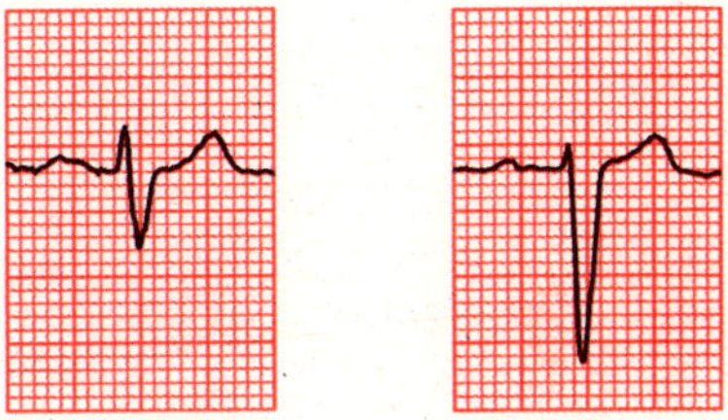

Dominant S waves and broad QRS complexes in leads II and III

First degree block and left anterior hemiblock

Note

- Sinus rhythm
- PR interval 300 ms
- Left anterior hemiblock
- Broad QRS complexes

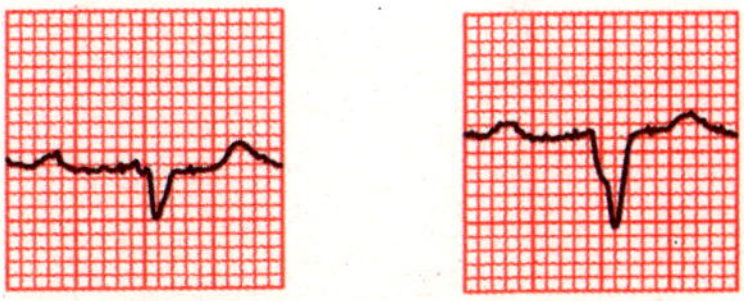

Long PR interval in leads II and III

Fig. 2.29

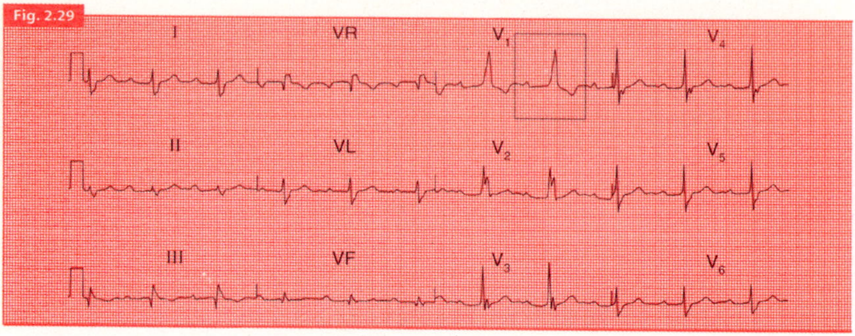

Fig. 2.30

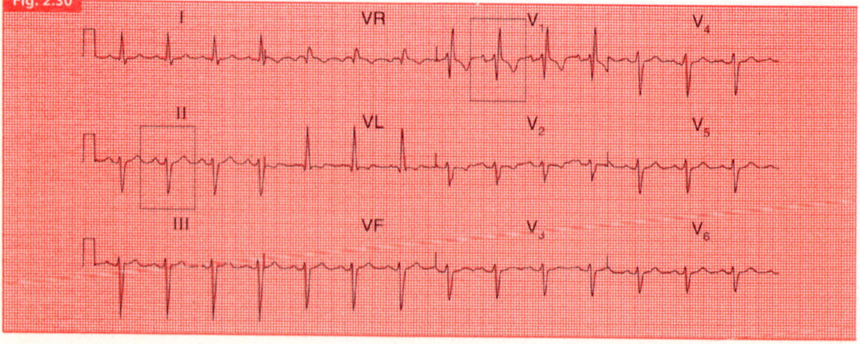

First degree block and right bundle branch block (RBBB)

Note

- Sinus rhythm
- PR interval 328 ms
- Right axis deviation
- Broad QRS complexes
- RBBB pattern

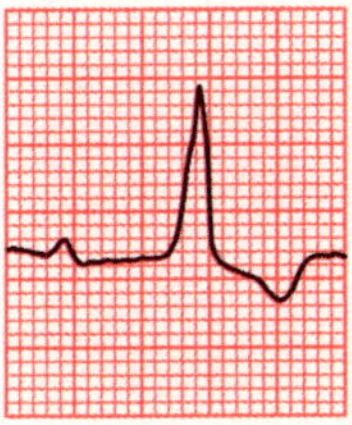

Long PR interval and RBBB pattern in lead V_1

Bifascicular block

Note

- Sinus rhythm
- PR interval normal (176 ms)
- Left anterior hemiblock
- Right bundle branch block (RBBB)

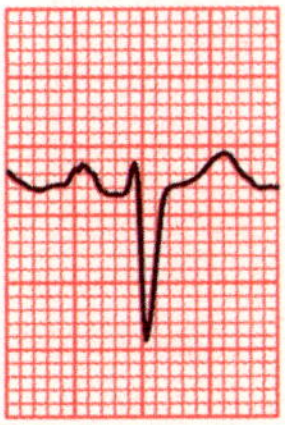

Left axis deviation and broad QRS complex in lead II

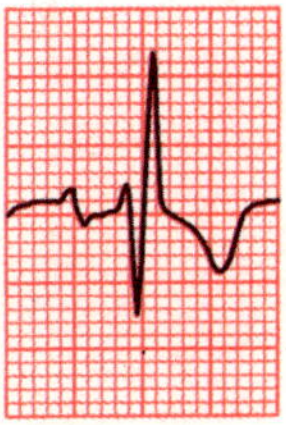

RBBB in lead V_1

Fig. 2.31

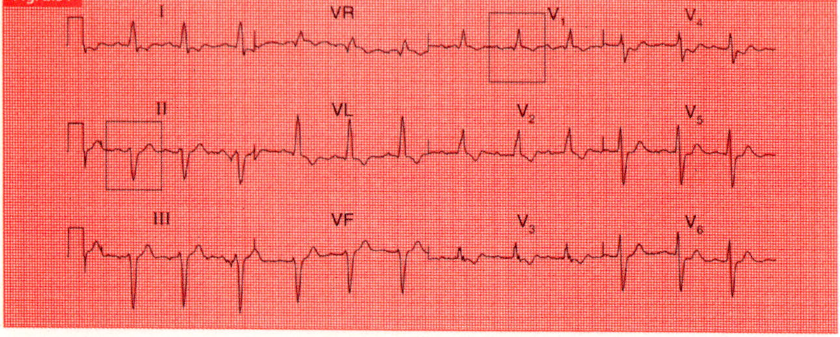

Fig. 2.32

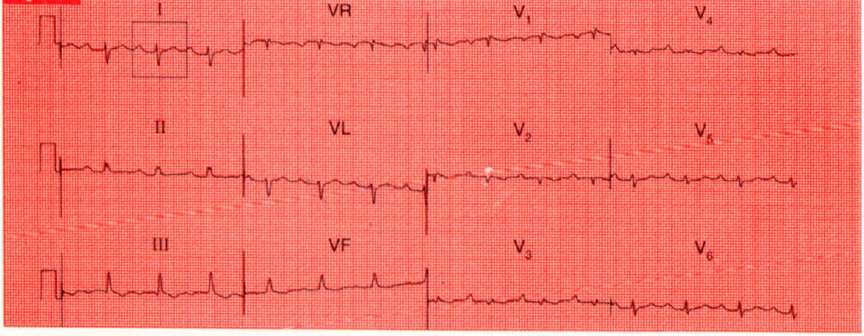

Trifascicular block

Note

- Sinus rhythm
- PR interval 224 ms
- Left anterior hemiblock
- Right bundle branch block (RBBB)

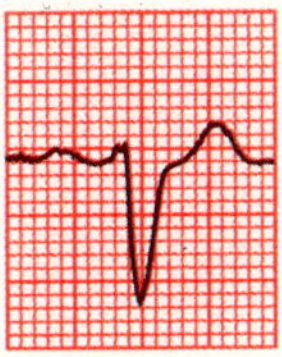

Left axis deviation in lead II

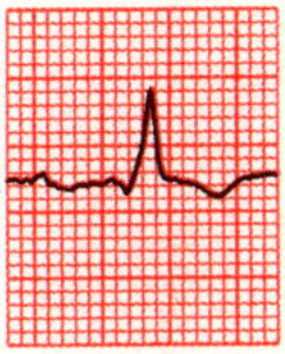

RBBB in lead V_1

Left posterior hemiblock

Note

- Sinus rhythm
- First degree block (PR interval 320 ms)
- Right axis deviation
- This could represent right ventricular hypertrophy, but there is no dominant R wave in lead V_1

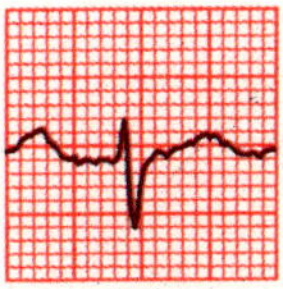

Long PR interval and deep S wave in lead I

Fig. 2.33

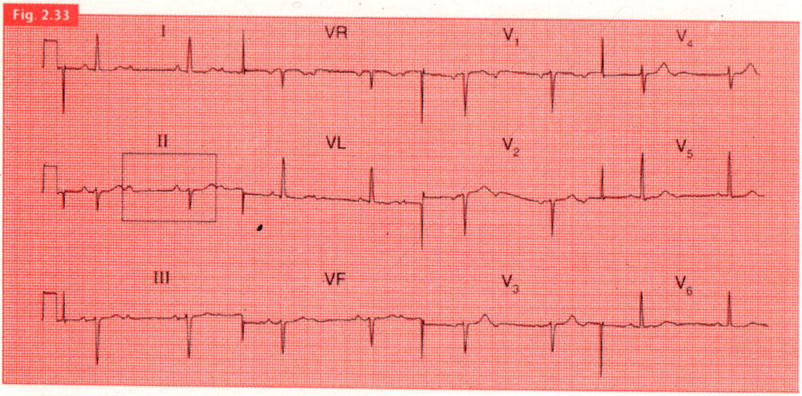

Fig. 2.34

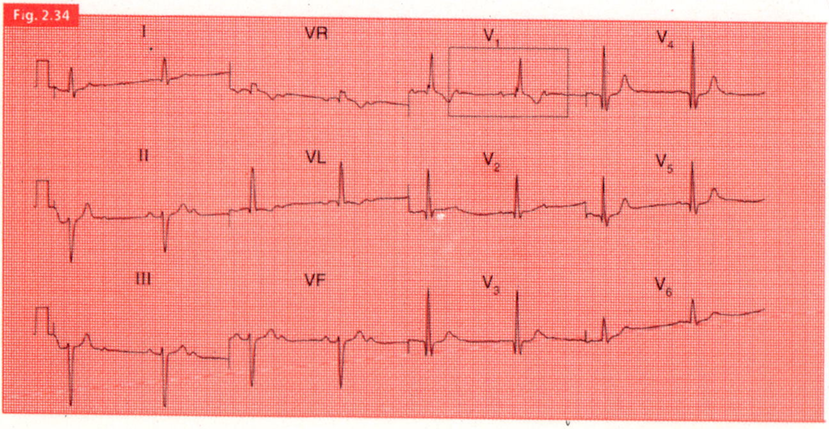

Second degree block and left anterior hemiblock

Note

- Sinus rhythm
- Second degree block (2:1 type)
- Left anterior hemiblock
- Poor R wave progression suggests possible old anterior infarct

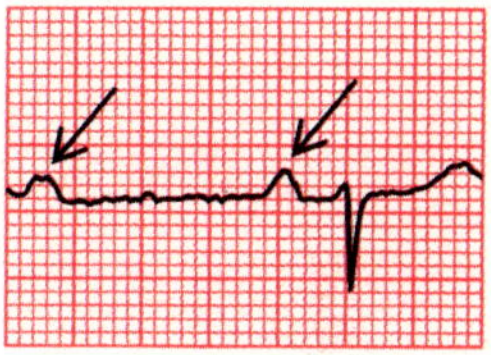

P waves in lead II

Second degree block, left anterior hemiblock and right bundle branch block (RBBB)

Note

- Sinus rhythm
- Second degree block (2:1 type)
- Left anterior hemiblock
- RBBB

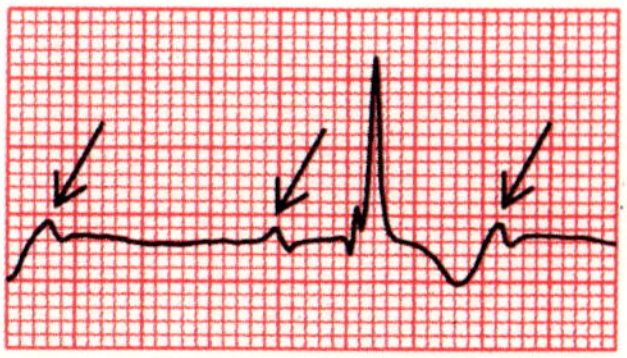

P waves and RBBB in lead V_1

Fig. 2.35

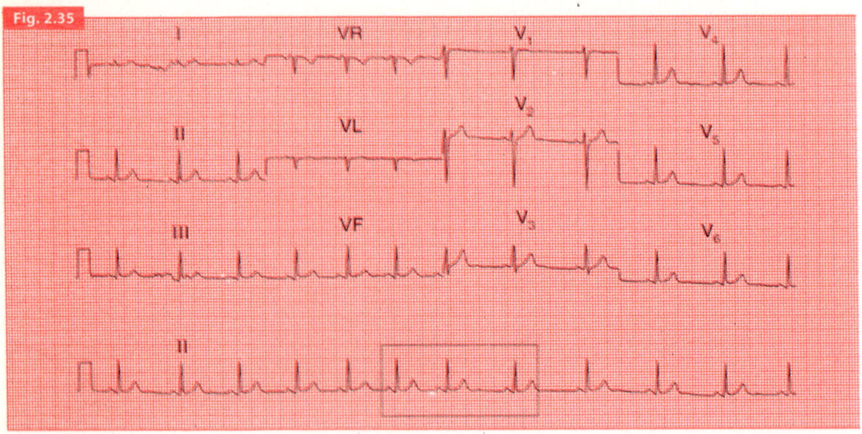

Fig. 2.36

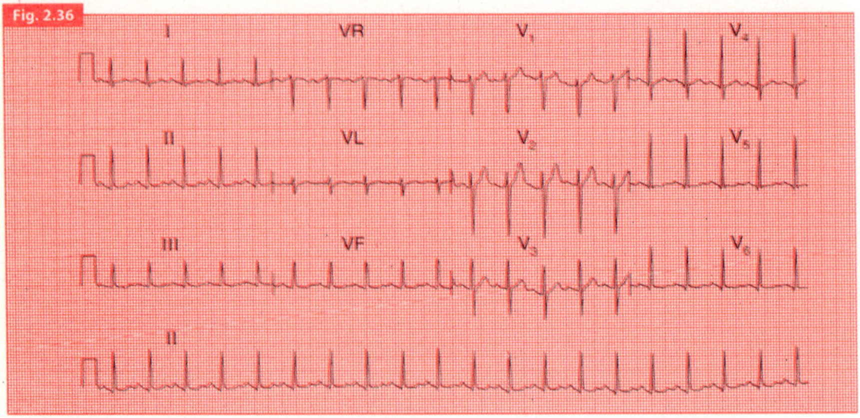

Sinus arrhythmia

Note

- Sinus rhythm
- All P waves identical
- Progressive shortening then lengthening of the R–R interval

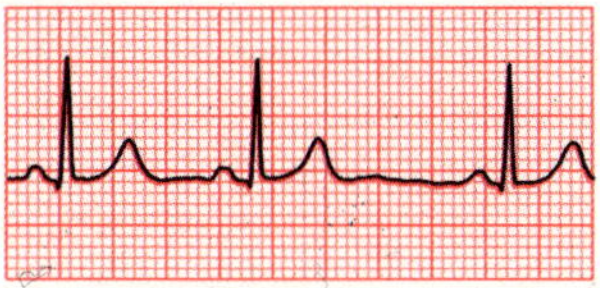

Identical P waves and irregular R–R interval

Sinus tachycardia

Note

- Sinus rhythm at the rate of 120/min
- Nonspecific ST segment changes in leads III, VF, V_6

THE ECG WHEN THE PATIENT HAS SYMPTOMS

If an ECG can be recorded at the time when the patient has symptoms, then there can be little doubt about the relationship between the symptoms and the cardiac rhythm.

SINUS RHYTHM IN PATIENTS WITH SYMPTOMS

Sinus rhythm can be irregular (sinus arrhythmia) but the patient is never aware of this. The ECG of a patient with sinus arrhythmia (Fig. 2.35) may suggest atrial extrasystoles – but in sinus rhythm, P wave morphology is constant while with atrial extrasystoles it varies.

Patients often complain of palpitations that are due to sinus tachycardia: the main causes are exercise, anxiety, thyrotoxicosis and the treatment of asthma with beta-adrenergic agonists, and other causes are summarized in Box 1.1 (p. 3). The ECG in Figure 2.36 shows sinus tachycardia from an unusual cause – the habitual drinking of large quantities of Coca-Cola.

When sinus tachycardia results from anxiety, heart rates of up to 150/min are possible and the rhythm may be mistaken for an atrial tachycardia. Pressure on the carotid sinus will cause transient slowing of the heart rate and the P waves will become more obvious.

Marked sinus bradycardia is characteristic of athletic training, but is also part of the cause of symptoms in fainting (the 'vasovagal' attack). It may also contribute to hypotension and heart failure in patients with an inferior myocardial infarction. Possible causes of sinus bradycardia are listed in Box 1.2 (p. 5).

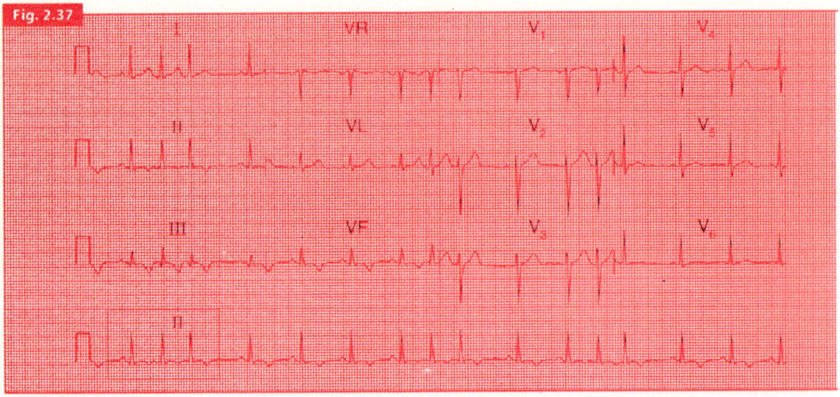

Fig. 2.37

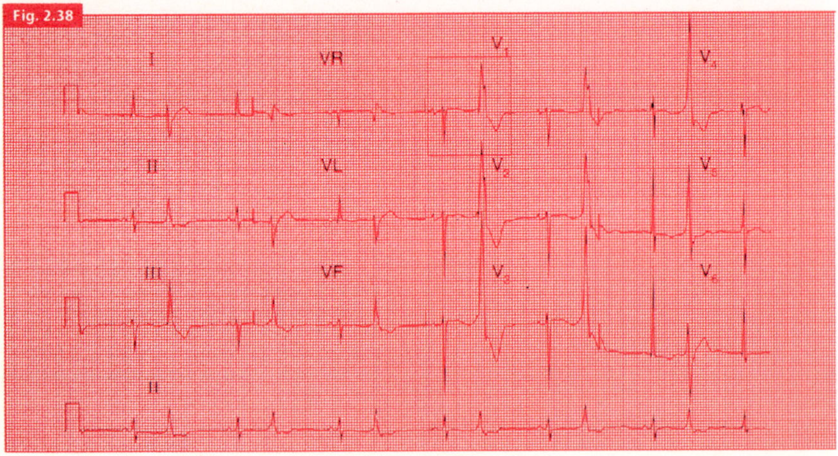

Fig. 2.38

Supraventricular extrasystoles

Note

- Sinus rhythm with atrial and junctional extrasystoles
- Normal axis
- Normal QRS complexes
- Inverted T waves in leads III, VF

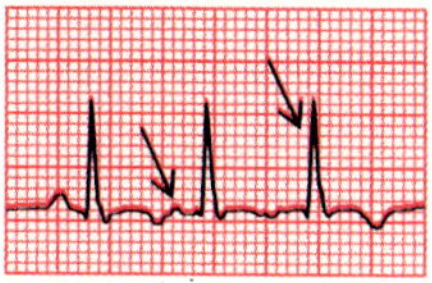

First beat: normal; second beat: atrial extrasystole, with abnormal P wave; third beat: AV nodal (junctional) extrasystole, with no P wave

Ventricular extrasystoles

Note

- Sinus rhythm with coupled ventricular extrasystoles
- Sinus beats show tall R waves and inverted T waves in leads V_5–V_6 (indicating left ventricular hypertrophy)
- Extrasystoles are of right bundle branch block (RBBB) configuration, and their T wave inversion has no other significance

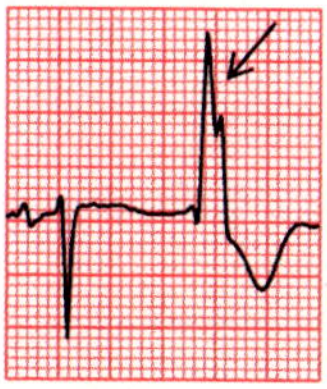

Extrasystole with RBBB configuration in lead V_1

EXTRASYSTOLES IN PATIENTS WITH SYMPTOMS

An ECG is necessary to differentiate between supraventricular and ventricular extrasystoles.

When extrasystoles have a supraventricular origin (Fig. 2.37), the QRS complex is narrow and both it and the T wave have the same configuration as in the sinus beat. Atrial extrasystoles have abnormal P waves. Junctional extrasystoles either have a P wave very close to the QRS complex (in front of it or behind it) or have no visible P waves.

Ventricular extrasystoles produce wide QRS complexes of abnormal shape, and the T wave is also usually abnormal. No P waves are present (Fig. 2.38).

When a ventricular extrasystole appears on the upstroke of the preceding beat, the 'R on T' phenomenon is said to be present (Fig. 2.39). This can initiate ventricular fibrillation, but usually it does not do so.

Fig. 2.39

R on T phenomenon

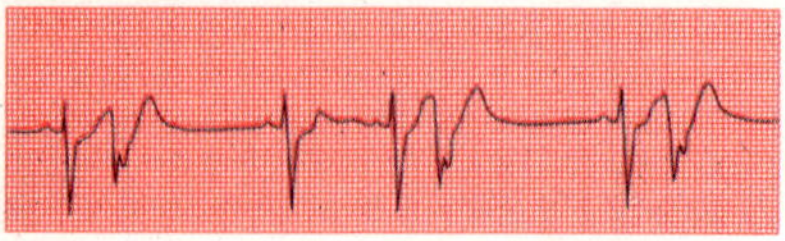

Note

- Ventricular extrasystoles occurring near the peak of the preceding T wave

Fig. 2.40

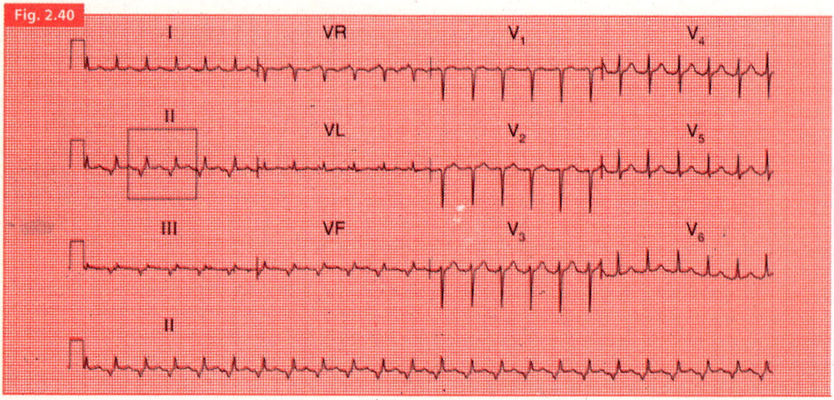

Box 2.6 Narrow complex tachycardias

A regular narrow complex tachycardia may be:
- Sinus rhythm
- Atrial tachycardia
- Atrial flutter
- AV nodal re-entry tachycardia (ANVRT) – the commonest type of supraventricular tachycardia
- AV re-entry tachycardia (AVRT), caused by the WPW syndrome

An irregular narrow complex tachycardia is usually:
- Atrial fibrillation

NARROW COMPLEX TACHYCARDIAS IN PATIENTS WITH SYMPTOMS

A tachycardia can be described as 'narrow complex' if the QRS complex is of normal duration, i.e. < 120 ms. Properly speaking, sinus, atrial and junctional arrhythmias are all supraventricular, but the term 'supraventricular tachycardia' is often inappropriately used interchangeably with 'junctional tachycardia'. All these supraventricular rhythms have QRS complexes of normal shape and width, and the T waves have the same shape as in the sinus beat.

Types of narrow complex tachycardias are listed in Box 2.6.

ATRIAL TACHYCARDIA

In atrial tachycardia (Fig. 2.40), P waves are present but they have an abnormal shape. They are sometimes hidden in the T wave of the preceding beat.

In atrial tachycardia the P wave rate is in the range 130–250/min. When the atrial rate exceeds about 180/min, physiological block will occur in the AV node, so that the ventricular rate becomes half that of the atria. Atrial tachycardia with 2:1 block is characteristic of (but not commonly seen with) digoxin toxicity.

Atrial tachycardia

Note
- Narrow complex tachycardia, heart rate 140/min
- Abnormally shaped P waves, one per QRS complex
- Short PR interval
- ECG otherwise normal

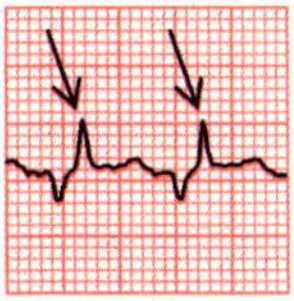

Abnormal P waves in lead II

Fig. 2.41

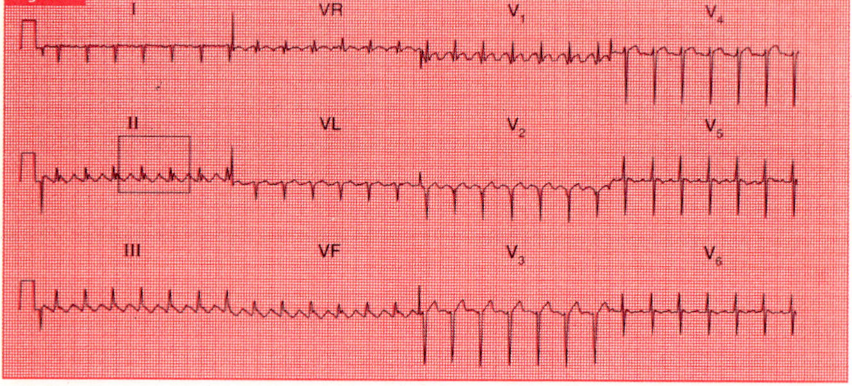

Fig. 2.42

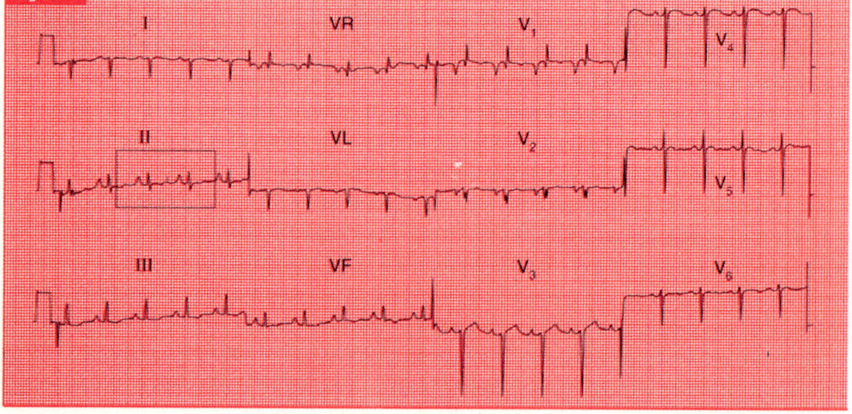

Atrial flutter with 2:1 block

Note

- Regular narrow complex tachycardia
- 'Sawtooth' of atrial flutter most easily seen in lead II

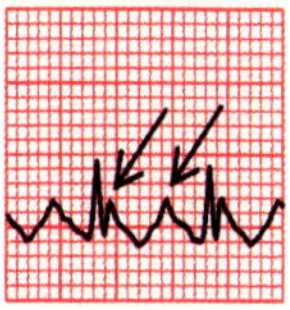

'Flutter' waves in lead II

Sinus rhythm, post-cardioversion

Note

- Same patient as in Figure 2.41
- Sinus rhythm
- Right axis deviation
- Dominant R waves in lead V_1
- Deep S waves in lead V_6, suggesting right ventricular hypertrophy
- The cardiac axis and QRS complexes have not been changed by cardioversion

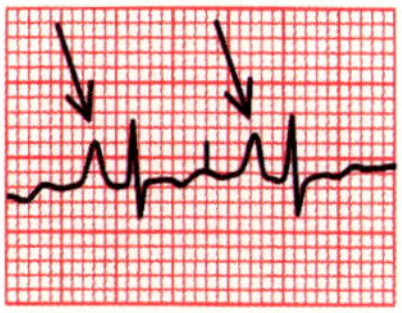

P waves in lead II

ATRIAL FLUTTER

In atrial flutter, the atrial rate is 300/min and the P waves form a continuous 'sawtooth' line. As the AV node usually fails to conduct all the P waves, the relationship between P waves and QRS complexes is usually 2:1, 3:1, or 4:1. Figure 2.41 shows atrial flutter with 2:1 block, giving a ventricular rate of 150/min. The ECG in Figure 2.42 is from the same patient after reversion to sinus rhythm.

The ECG in Figure 2.43 shows atrial flutter with 4:1 block.

The ECG in Figure 2.44 shows a narrow complex (therefore supraventricular) rhythm with a rate of 300/min. This is almost certainly atrial flutter with 1:1 conduction.

If the ventricular rate is rapid and P waves cannot be seen, carotid sinus pressure will usually increase the block in the AV node and make the 'sawtooth' more obvious (see Fig. 2.97 on p. 157).

Fig. 2.43

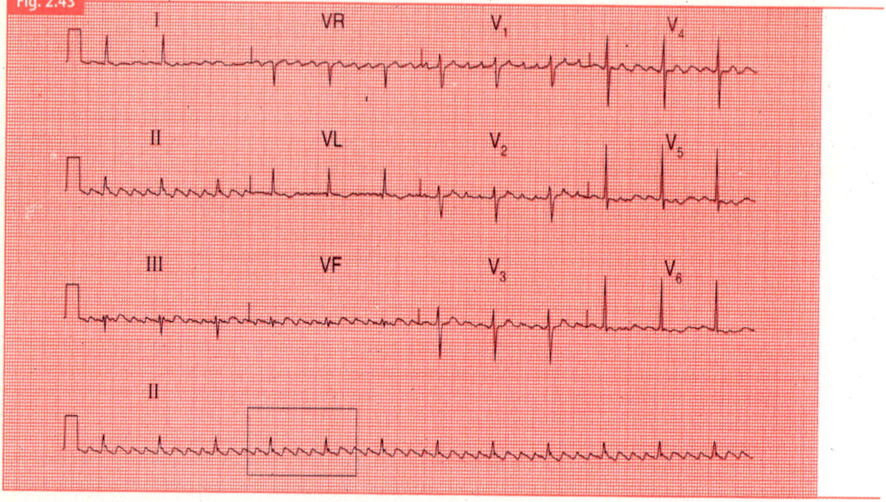

Fig. 2.44

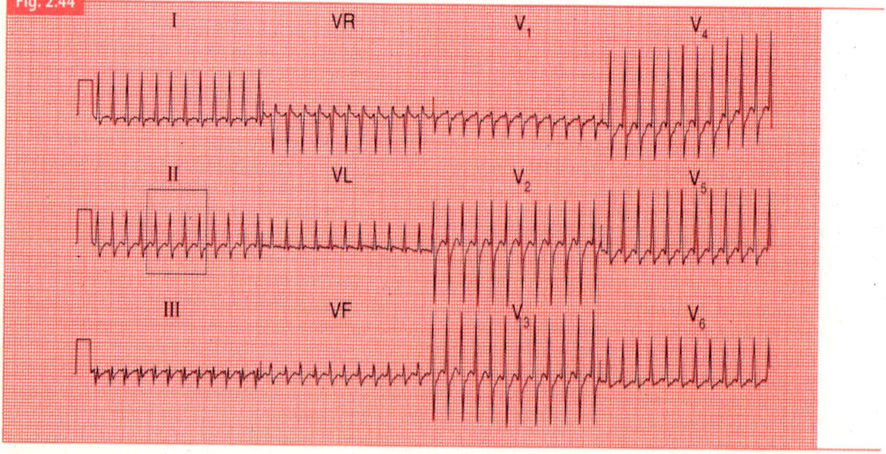

Atrial flutter with 4:1 block

Note

- With 4:1 block and a ventricular rate of 72/min, flutter waves can be seen in all leads

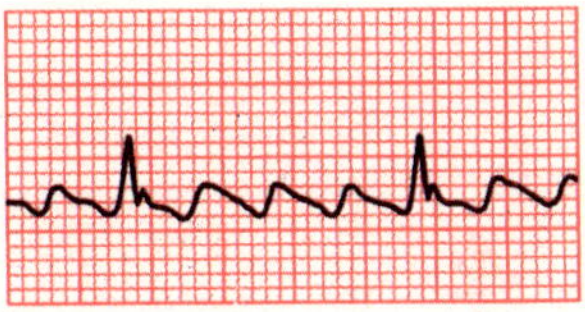

Flutter waves

Atrial flutter with 1:1 conduction

Note

- Narrow complex tachycardia at nearly 300/min
- No P waves visible
- Ventricular rate suggests that the underlying rhythm is atrial flutter

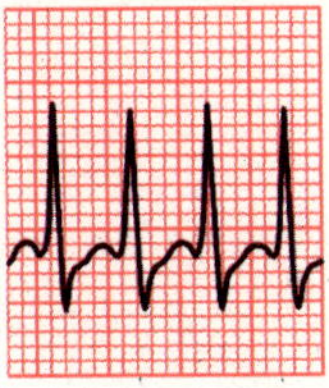

Narrow complex tachycardia at 300/min in lead II

Fig. 2.45

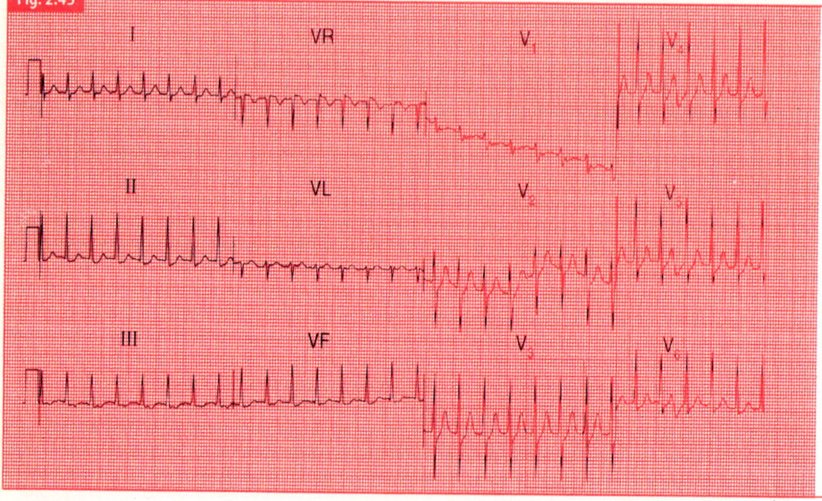

Fig. 2.46

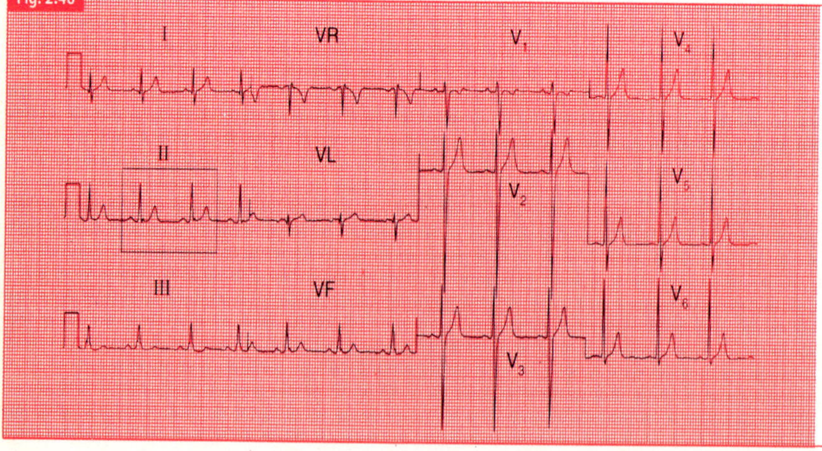

Atrioventricular nodal re-entry tachycardia

Note

- Regular narrow complex tachycardia, rate 150/min
- No P waves visible
- ST segment depression in leads II–III, VF suggests ischaemia

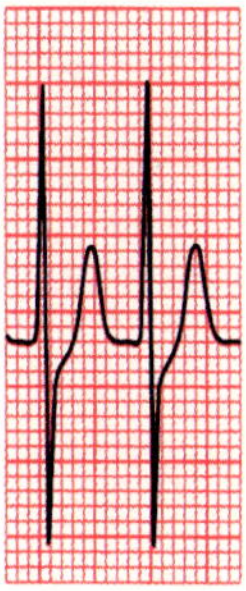

Narrow complexes at 150/min in lead V_3

Sinus rhythm following cardioversion

Note

- Sinus rhythm
- QRS complexes and T waves are the same shape as in AVNRE tachycardia (Fig. 2.45)
- Now no suggestion of ischaemia

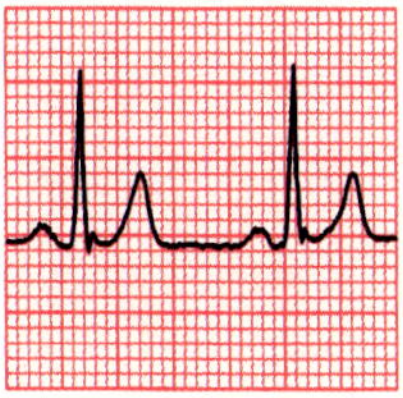

Sinus rhythm in lead II

ATRIOVENTRICULAR NODAL RE-ENTRY OR JUNCTIONAL TACHYCARDIA

Atrioventricular nodal re-entry tachycardia (AVNRE) is caused by re-entry of the electrical impulse via a double conducting channel within, or very close to, the AV node. An older term is junctional tachycardia. In this rhythm no P waves can be seen. Carotid sinus pressure either reverts the heart to sinus rhythm or has no effect.

The ECG in Figure 2.45 shows a narrow complex tachycardia at 150/min, without any obvious P waves. After reversion to sinus rhythm (Fig. 2.46), the shape of the QRS complexes does not change.

The ECG in Figure 2.47 shows what appears to be a straightforward AVNRE tachycardia, but on return to sinus rhythm (Fig. 2.48) it shows a Wolff–Parkinson–White pattern. The tachycardia was therefore orthodromic, with the re-entry circuit involving anterograde (normal) conduction down the AV node and His bundle.

Fig. 2.47

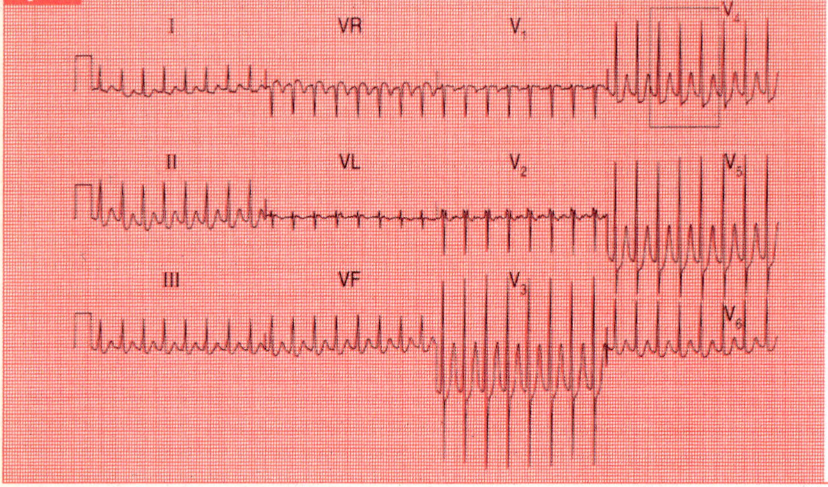

Fig. 2.48

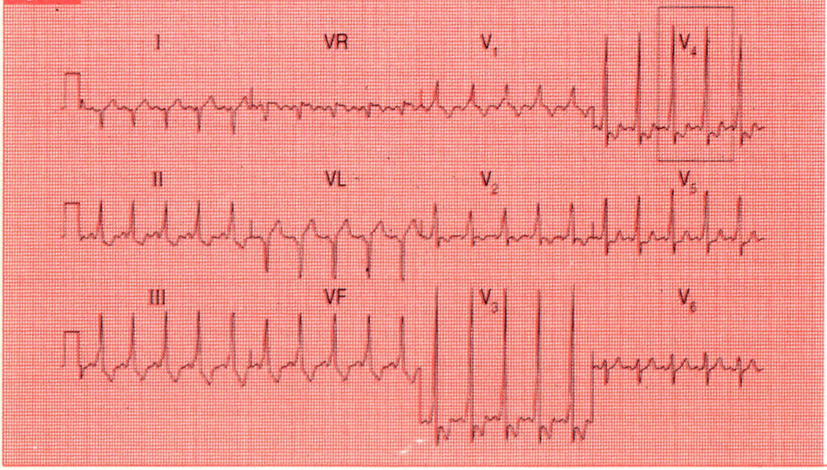

Supraventricular tachycardia

Note

- Narrow complex tachycardia
- No P waves visible
- Some ST segment depression, suggesting ischaemia

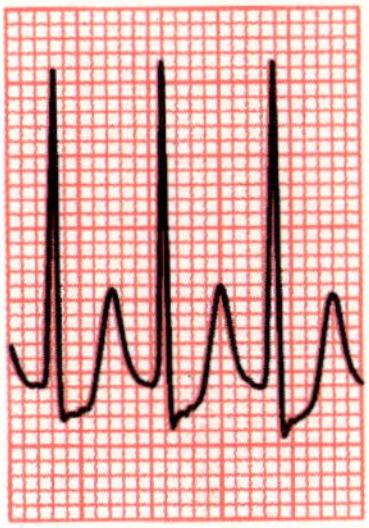

Narrow complexes with ST segment depression in lead V_4

Sinus rhythm, the Wolff–Parkinson–White syndrome

Note

- Same patient as in Figure 2.47
- Sinus rhythm
- Short PR interval
- Broad QRS complexes with delta wave
- Dominant R wave in lead V_1 shows the WPW syndrome type A

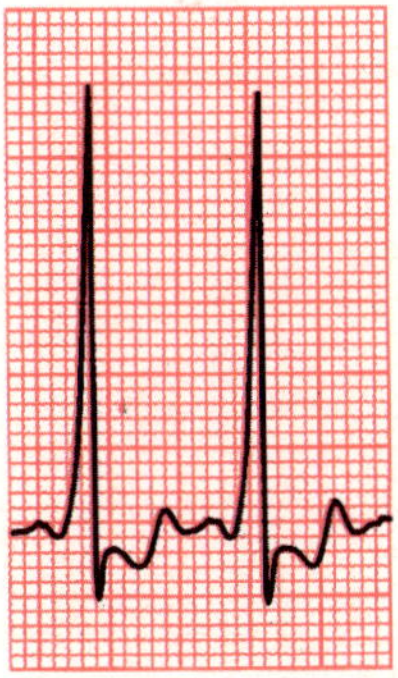

Short PR interval and delta wave in lead V_4

Fig. 2.49

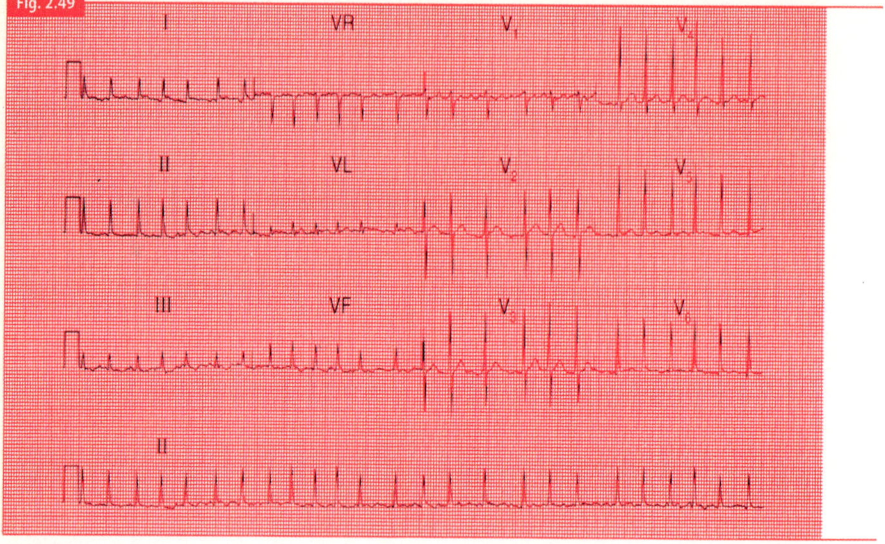

Fig. 2.50

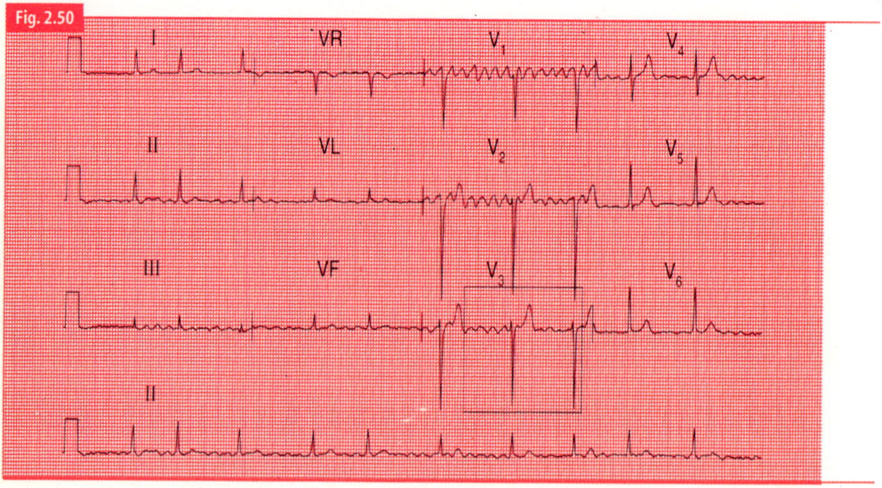

Atrial fibrillation

Note

- Irregular narrow complex tachycardia at 150/min
- During long R–R intervals, irregular baseline can be seen
- Suggestion of flutter waves in lead V_1

ATRIAL FIBRILLATION

In atrial fibrillation, disorganized atrial activity causes the P waves to disappear and the ECG baseline becomes totally irregular (Fig. 2.49). At times atrial activity may become sufficiently synchronized for a 'flutter-like' pattern to appear, but this rapidly breaks up (Fig. 2.50). In atrial fibrillation, as opposed to atrial flutter, the QRS complexes are totally irregular.

Some causes of atrial fibrillation are summarized in Box 2.7.

Atrial fibrillation

Note

- Irregular narrow complex rhythm
- Apparent flutter waves in lead V_1, but these are not constant and from leads II and V_3 it is clear that this is atrial fibrillation

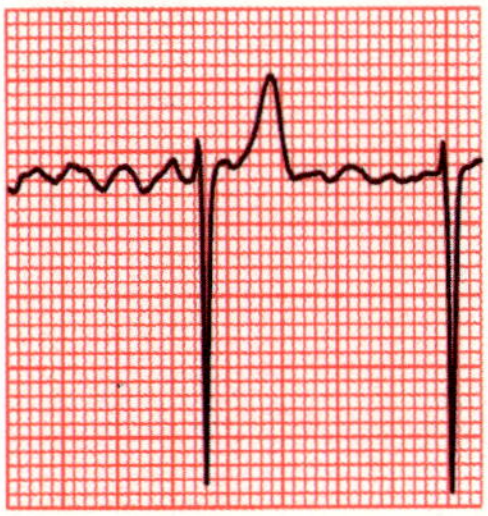

Atrial fibrillation in lead V_3

Box 2.7 Causes of atrial fibrillation (paroxysmal or persistent)

- Rheumatic heart disease
- Thyrotoxicosis
- Alcoholism
- Cardiomyopathy
- Acute myocardial infarction
- Chronic ischaemic heart disease
- Hypertension
- Myocarditis
- Pericarditis
- Pulmonary embolism
- Pneumonia
- Cardiac surgery
- The Wolff–Parkinson–White syndrome
- 'Lone' (i.e. no cause found)

BROAD COMPLEX TACHYCARDIAS IN PATIENTS WITH SYMPTOMS

'Broad complex' tachycardias are those in which the QRS complex duration exceeds 120 ms and which are not due to sinus rhythm with bundle branch block. Broad complex tachycardias can be either supraventricular, with bundle branch block or the Wolff–Parkinson–White syndrome, or ventricular. The types of broad complex tachycardia are listed in Box 2.8.

A supraventricular origin for a broad complex tachycardia can only be diagnosed with certainty when there is intermittent sinus rhythm with the same QRS complex configuration as is seen in the tachycardia (Fig. 2.51).

Here we are concerned with broad complex rhythms without obvious P waves. These could be atrial fibrillation or junctional rhythms with bundle branch block, or could be ventricular rhythms. The differentiation of broad complex tachycardias can be difficult (see Box 2.10 on p. 129). You cannot distinguish between supraventricular and ventricular rhythms by the clinical state of the patient. Either type of rhythm can be well tolerated, and either can lead to cardiovascular collapse. However, broad complex tachycardias occurring in the course of an acute myocardial infarction (which is when they are most often seen) are almost always ventricular in

Fig. 2.51

Junctional tachycardia with bundle branch block

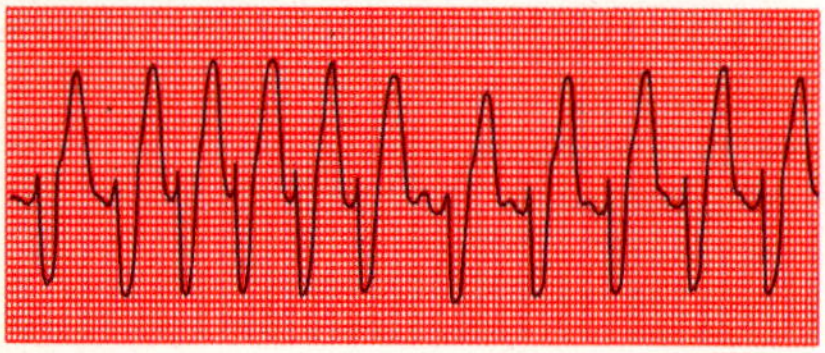

Note

- A single sinus beat with a broad QRS complex is followed by five beats without P waves, but with the same broad QRS pattern
- Sinus rhythm is then restored and the QRS complex remains unchanged
- The tachycardia must be supraventricular with bundle branch block

origin. Other causes of ventricular tachycardia are listed in Box 2.9.

With these things in mind, the ECG should be analysed logically. Look in turn for the following features:

1. The presence of P waves. If there is one P wave per QRS complex, it must be sinus rhythm with bundle branch block. If P waves can be seen at a slower rate than the QRS complexes, it must be ventricular tachycardia (VT).
2. The QRS complex duration. If longer than 160 ms, it is probably VT.
3. QRS complex regularity. VT is usually regular. An irregular broad complex tachycardia usually means atrial fibrillation with abnormal conduction.
4. The cardiac axis. VT is usually associated with left axis deviation.
5. QRS complex configuration. If the QRS complexes in the V leads all point either upwards or downwards ('concordance') it is probably VT.
6. When the QRS complex shows a right bundle branch block pattern, a supraventricular tachycardia with abnormal conduction is more likely if the second R peak is higher than the first. VT is likely if the first R peak is higher.
7. The presence of fusion and capture beats indicates that the broad complexes are due to VT (see p. 126).

Box 2.8 Broad complex tachycardias

- Any supraventricular rhythm with bundle branch block
- Accelerated idioventricular rhythm (rate < 120/min)
- Ventricular tachycardia
- Torsade de pointes ventricular tachycardia
- The Wolff–Parkinson–White (WPW) syndrome

An irregular broad complex tachycardia is likely to be:

- Atrial fibrillation with bundle branch block
- Atrial fibrillation with the WPW syndrome

Box 2.9 Causes of ventricular tachycardia

- Acute myocardial infarction
- Chronic ischaemia
- Cardiomyopathy:
  - — hypertrophic
  - — dilated
- Mitral valve prolapse
- Myocarditis
- Electrolyte imbalance
- Congenital long QT syndrome
- Drugs:
  - — antiarrhythmic
  - — digoxin
- Idiopathic

Fig. 2.52

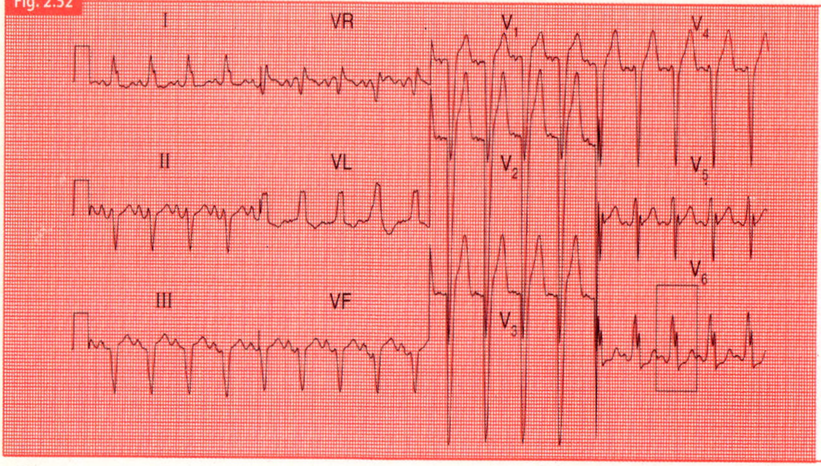

Fig. 2.53

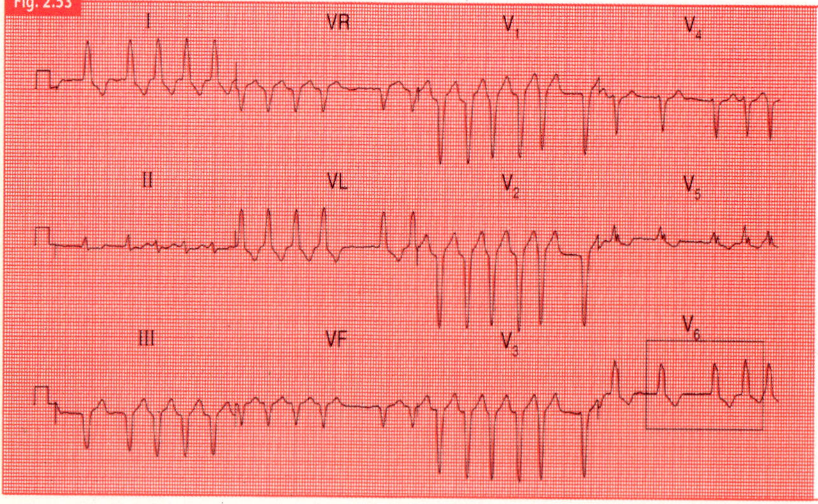

Sinus rhythm with left bundle branch block (LBBB)

Note

- Sinus rhythm
- Left axis deviation
- Wide QRS complexes of LBBB configuration

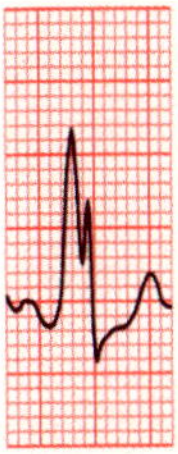

M wave of LBBB in lead V_6

P WAVES

The ECG in Figure 2.52 is from a patient with an acute infarction, and shows a broad complex rhythm at about 110/min. One P wave per QRS complex can clearly be seen, and this is obviously sinus rhythm with left bundle branch block (LBBB).

The ECG in Figure 2.53 shows a very irregular broad complex rhythm with no obvious P waves. There is an obvious LBBB pattern in leads V_5 and V_6. Whether the R–R interval is short or long, the appearance of the QRS complex is the same. The irregularity is the key to the diagnosis of atrial fibrillation with LBBB.

The ECG in Figure 2.54 is also an example of atrial fibrillation and LBBB, but this is not quite as obvious as in Figure 2.53. The QRS complexes at

Atrial fibrillation with left bundle branch block (LBBB)

Note

- Recorded at half sensitivity (0.5 cm = 1 mV)
- Irregular broad complex tachycardia
- No obvious P waves, but irregular baseline in lead VR
- LBBB configuration of QRS complexes

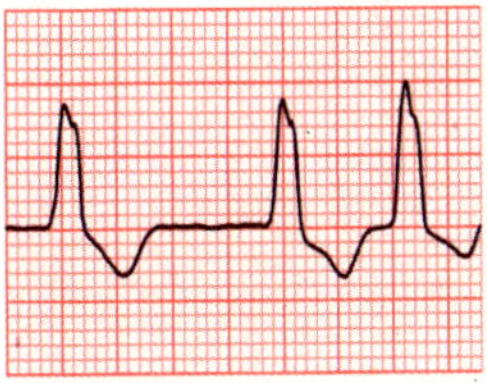

M wave of LBBB in lead V_6

Fig. 2.54

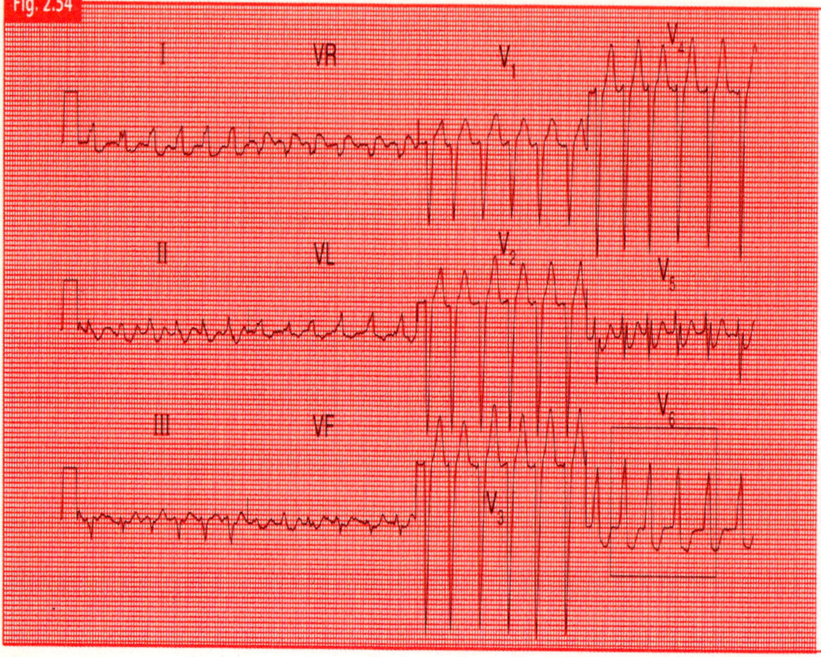

first sight may appear regular, but on close inspection they are not. The LBBB is also not so obvious, but can be seen in lead I.

Occasionally it may be possible to identify P waves with a slower rate than the QRS complexes, indicating that the QRS complexes must be ventricular in origin. A 12-lead ECG during the tachycardia is important for this, because P waves may be visible in some leads but not in others (Fig. 2.55).

Atrial fibrillation with left bundle branch block (LBBB)

Note

- Broad complex rhythm at 140/min
- Slightly irregular rhythm, best seen in lead V_6
- LBBB pattern, most obvious in lead I

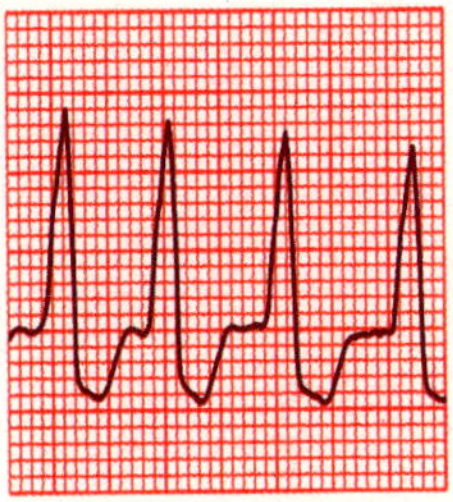

Irregular rhythm in lead V_6

Fig. 2.55

Ventricular tachycardia

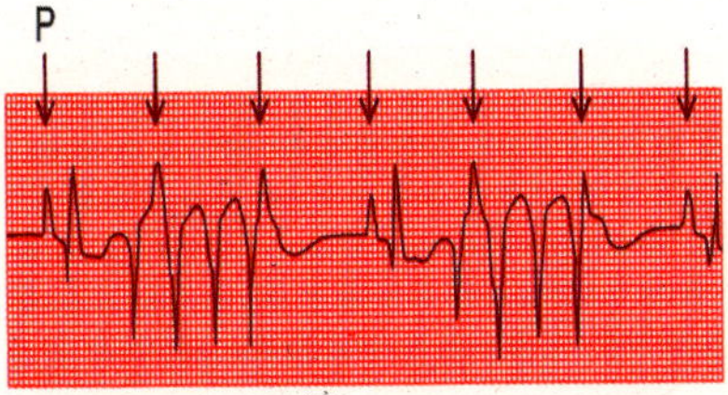

Note

- A single sinus beat is followed by a broad complex tachycardia
- During the tachycardia, P waves can still be seen at a normal rate (arrowed)
- So the broad complex tachycardia must have a ventricular origin

Fig. 2.56

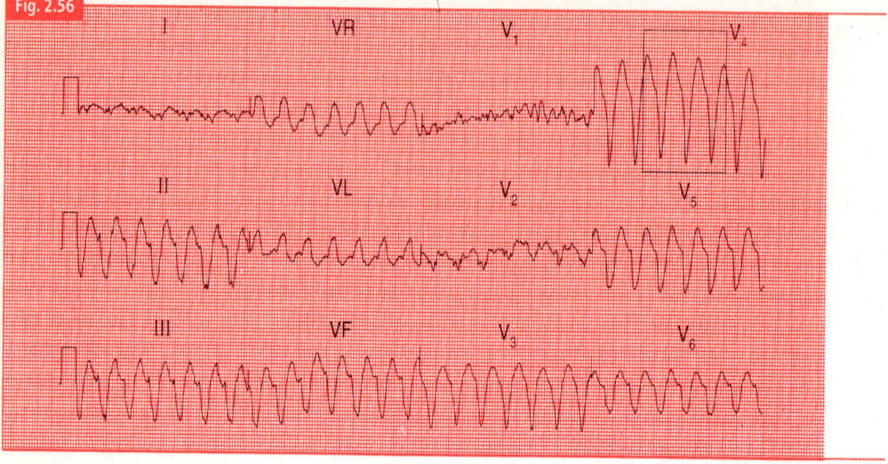

Fig. 2.57

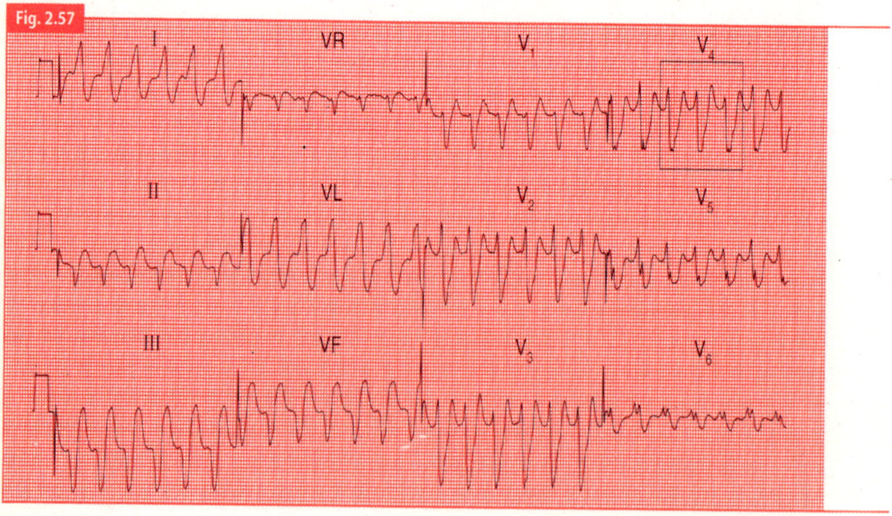

Ventricular tachycardia

Note

- Regular broad complex tachycardia at 160/min
- Appearance of lead V_1 is clearly an artefact
- Left axis deviation
- All complexes point downwards (concordance)
- There are no R waves in the chest leads, so the complexes are sometimes known as 'QS' complexes

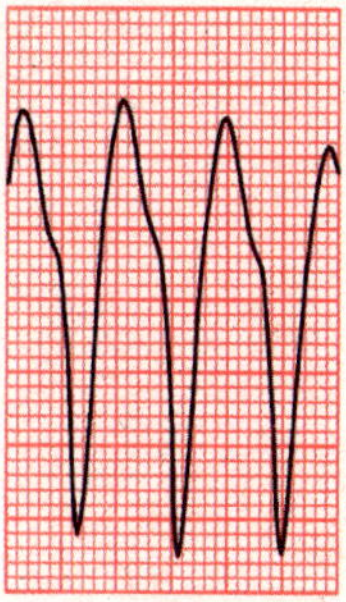

Broad complexes in lead V_4

Ventricular tachycardia

Note

- Regular broad complex tachycardia at 150/min
- No P waves visible
- Left axis deviation
- Concordance of QRS complexes in chest leads

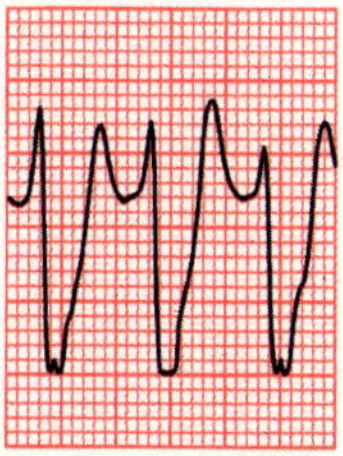

Broad complexes in lead V_4

THE QRS COMPLEX

The ECG in Figure 2.56 shows a broad complex tachycardia recorded from a patient with an acute infarction, and there is no question that this represents ventricular tachycardia (VT). The important features are:

- regular rhythm at 160/min (a fairly typical rate)
- very broad complexes of 360 ms duration (when the QRS complex duration is > 160 ms, VT is likely)
- left axis deviation
- in the V leads the QRS complexes all point in the same direction (in this case downwards). This is called 'concordance'.

The ECG in Figure 2.57 shows an ECG from another patient with an acute infarction. The shape

Fig. 2.58

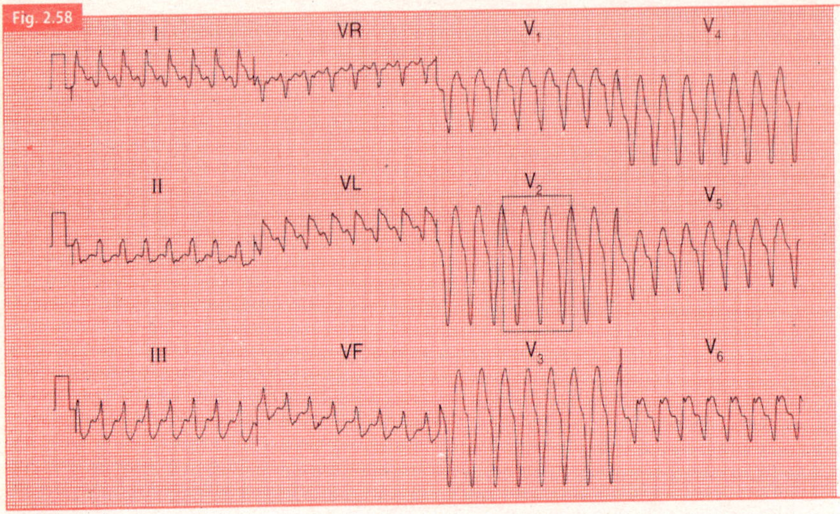

Fig. 2.59

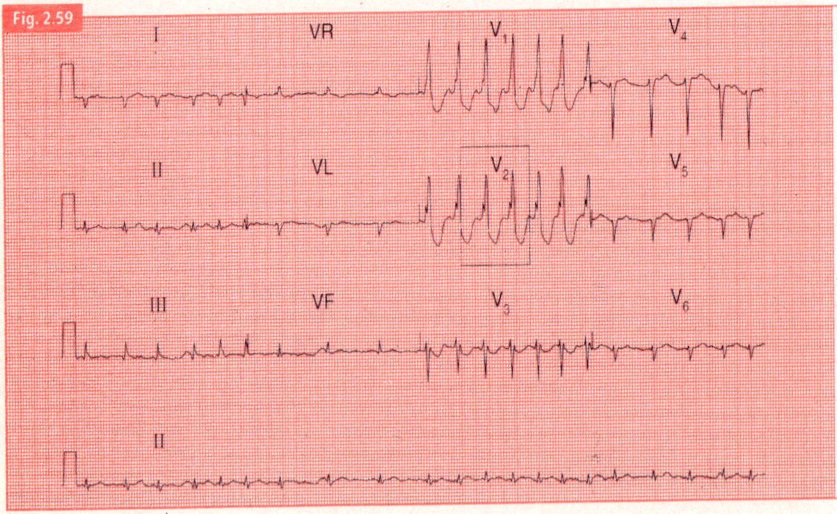

Ventricular tachycardia

Note

- Regular broad complex tachycardia
- No P waves
- Normal axis
- Concordance (downward) of QRS complexes

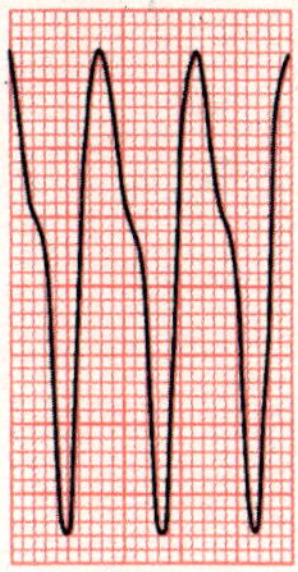

Broad complexes in lead V_2

Atrial fibrillation with right bundle branch block (RBBB)

Note

- Irregular broad complex tachycardia
- Right axis deviation
- QRS complexes show RBBB pattern, with second R peak higher than the first

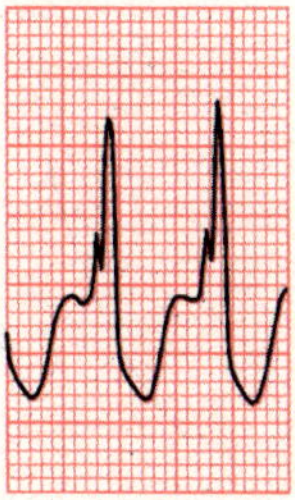

R^1 taller than R peak in lead V_2

of the QRS complexes is different from that in Figure 2.56, but the principles are the same:

- The rhythm is regular.
- The complexes are very broad.
- There is left axis deviation.
- The complexes show concordance.

The ECG in Figure 2.58 shows another example of VT, but this time the axis is normal. Unfortunately the ‘rules’ for diagnosing VT are not absolute and one or more of the features above may not be present.

The ECG in Figure 2.59 shows atrial fibrillation with an abnormal QRS complex, the duration of which (116 ms) is just within the normal range. The RSR^1 pattern, most obviously seen in lead V_2, and the slurred S wave in lead V_6, show that this is ‘partial right bundle branch block (RBBB)’. Note that the second R peak of the QRS complex (R^1) is higher than first peak. This is characteristic of RBBB. These features show that this is a supraventricular rhythm.

The ECG in Figure 2.60 shows a regular tachycardia with no P waves and a QRS complex showing an RBBB pattern. The duration of the QRS complex is at the upper limit of normal, at 120 ms. This might be a supraventricular (probably junctional) tachycardia with RBBB conduction, or it may be a fascicular tachycardia. A fascicular tachycardia usually arises in the posterior fascicle of the left bundle branch. Typically there is left axis deviation (not present here). This is an unusual rhythm with a benign prognosis, and it typically responds to verapamil.

The ECG in Figure 2.61 shows how difficult differentiation between supraventricular and ventricular rhythms can be. Some features suggest a supraventricular, and some a ventricular, origin of the rhythm.

Fig. 2.60

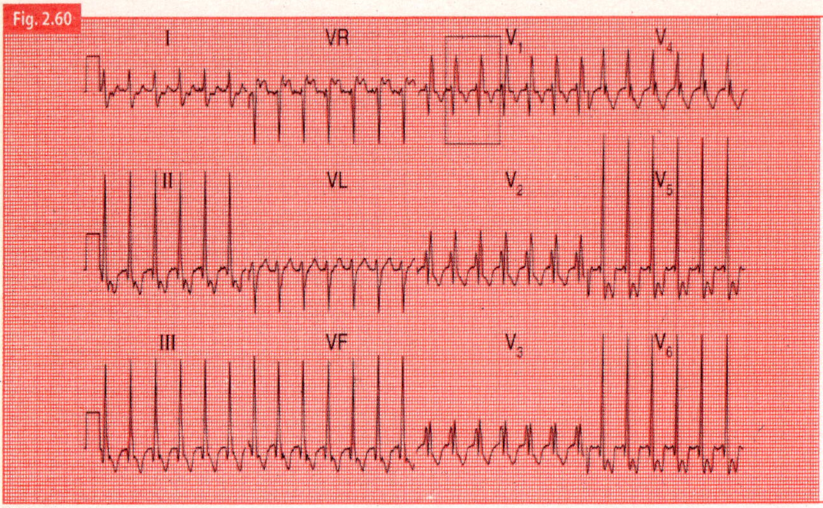

Fig. 2.61

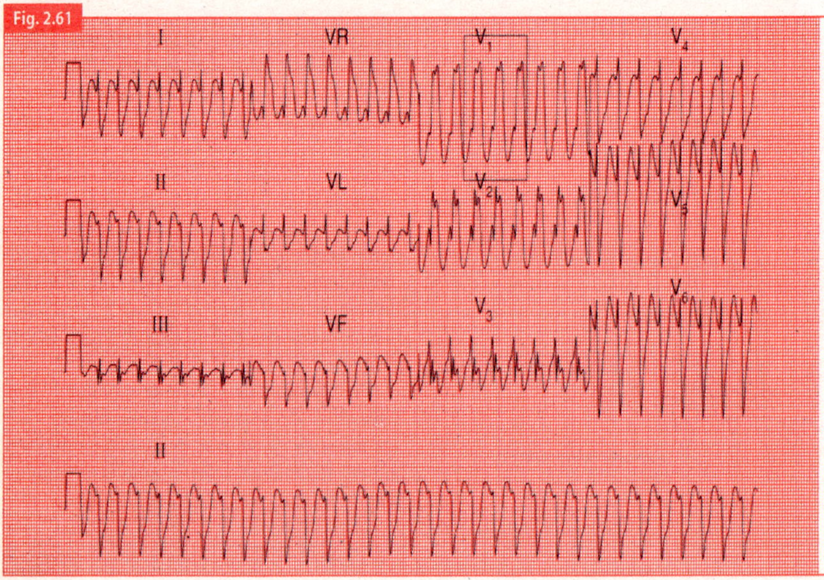

?Junctional tachycardia with right bundle branch block or ?fascicular tachycardia

Note

- Regular rhythm at 150/min
- Normal axis (R and S waves equal in lead I)
- QRS complex duration 120 ms (upper limit of normal)
- The second R peak (R') is taller than the R peak

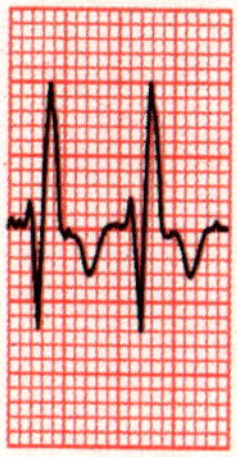

R' taller than R peak in lead V_1

Often only a comparison of the patient's ECGs taken when the tachycardia is present and when the patient is in sinus rhythm will establish the nature of the tachycardia. In the case of any patient with a tachycardia it is essential to look through the old notes, to see if any ECGs have been recorded previously. The ECG in Figure 2.62 shows a broad complex tachycardia rather similar to that shown in Figure 2.61. This patient was in pain and was hypotensive, so he was cardioverted, and Figure 2.63 shows the post-cardioversion record. The QRS complexes are narrow, so the arrhythmia must have been VT.

Broad complex tachycardia of uncertain origin

Note

- Regular rhythm at 195/min
- Right axis deviation (suggests a supraventricular tachycardia with bundle branch block)
- Very broad complexes, with QRS duration 200 ms (the primary evidence for ventricular tachycardia)
- QRS complexes in lead V_1 point upwards, while complexes in V_6 point downwards: no concordance (suggests a supraventricular tachycardia)
- The second R peak (R') is greater than the R peak in lead V_1 (suggests a supraventricular tachycardia)

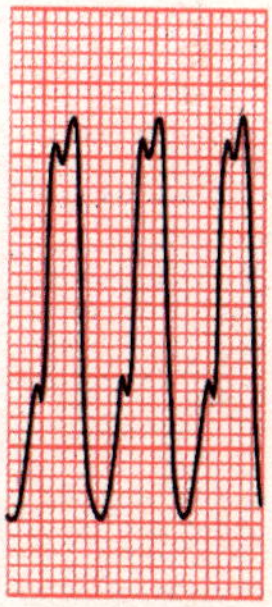

Broad complexes in lead I

Fig. 2.62

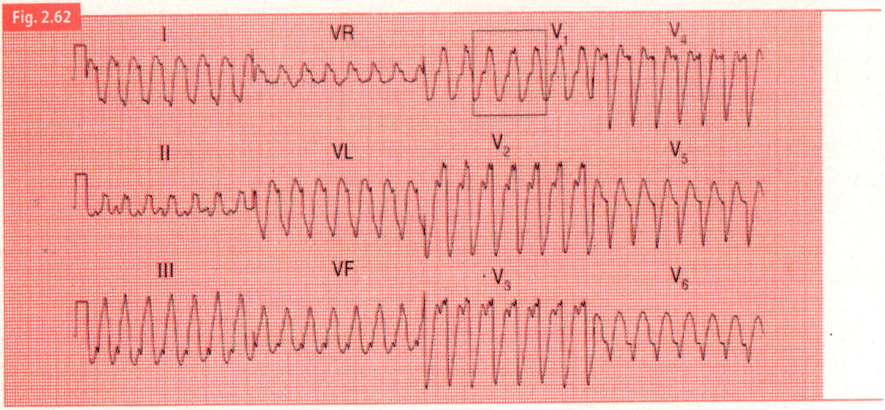

Fig. 2.63

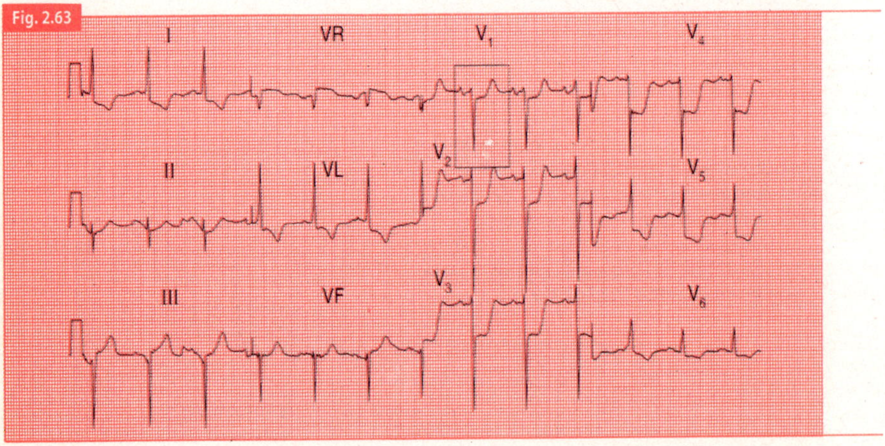

Broad complex tachycardia: ?ventricular; ?supraventricular

Note

- Regular rhythm at 180/min
- Right axis deviation
- Very broad complexes with QRS complex duration 200 ms
- R and R[1] peaks are variable
- No concordance

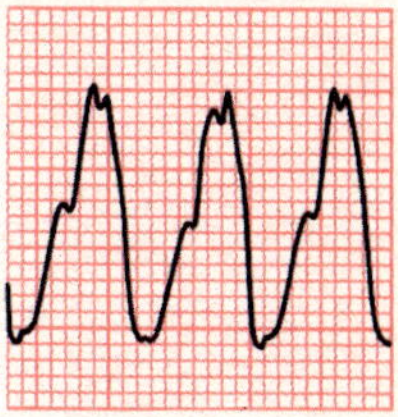

Variable R and R[1] peaks in lead V_1

Post-cardioversion: sinus rhythm with normal conduction

Note

- Same patient as in Figure 2.62
- Sinus rhythm
- Axis now shows left deviation
- Narrow QRS complexes
- Widespread ST segment depression, indicating ischaemia
- The narrow QRS complexes, with a change of axis, show that the original rhythm (shown in Fig. 2.62) must have been ventricular

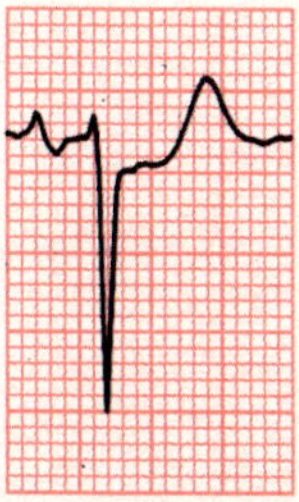

Narrow QRS complexes in lead V_1

Fig. 2.64

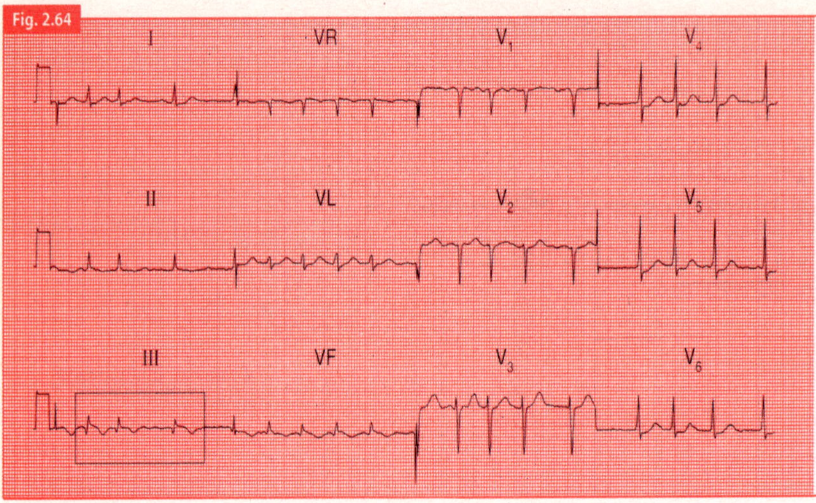

Fig. 2.65

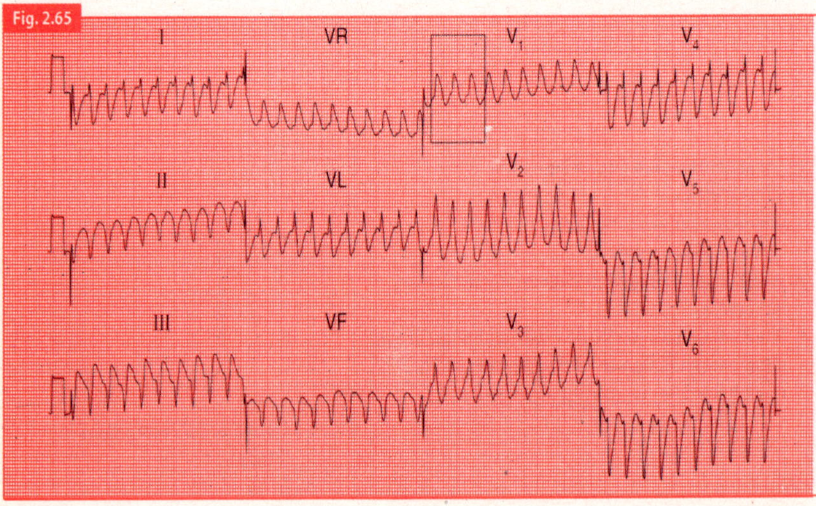

Atrial fibrillation and inferior infarction

Note

- Irregular, narrow complex rhythm
- Irregular baseline indicates atrial fibrillation
- Normal axis
- Small Q waves in leads III and VF with inverted T waves, suggesting inferior infarction
- Slight ST segment depression in leads V_4–V_5 suggests ischaemia

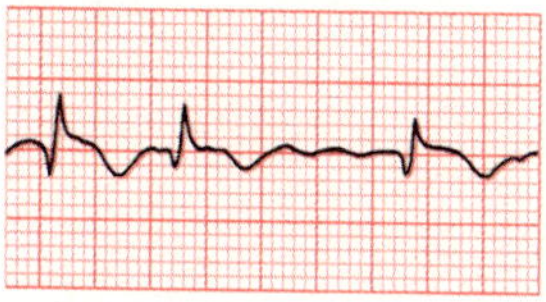

Small Q waves and inverted T waves in lead III

Figure 2.64 shows the ECG from a patient admitted to hospital with an inferior myocardial infarction, initially with atrial fibrillation.

The patient then developed a broad complex tachycardia (Fig. 2.65). In the context of an acute infarction this would almost certainly be VT. A comparison of Figure 2.65 with the ECG in atrial fibrillation (Fig. 2.64) shows the combination of a different, indeterminate, axis and RBBB. The change of axis is a strong pointer to a ventricular origin of the rhythm.

Ventricular tachycardia (VT) and inferior infarction

Note

- Same patient as in Figure 2.64
- Broad complex tachycardia
- Indeterminate axis
- Right bundle branch block (RBBB) pattern, but in lead V_1, R peak greater than R^1 peak (not very clearly defined)
- No concordance
- With acute myocardial infarction, this will be VT

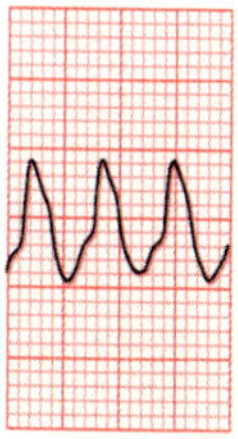

RBBB pattern in lead V_1

Fig. 2.66

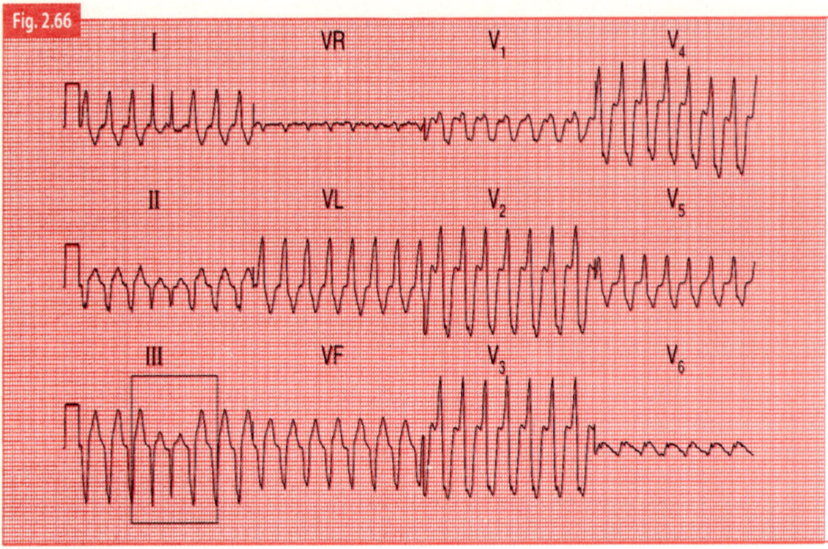

FUSION BEATS AND CAPTURE BEATS

If an early beat can be found with a narrow QRS complex, it can be assumed that a wide complex tachycardia is ventricular in origin. The narrow early beat demonstrates that the bundle branches will conduct supraventricular beats normally, even at high heart rates.

A 'fusion beat' is said to occur when the ventricles are activated simultaneously by a supraventricular and a ventricular impulse, so that a QRS complex with an intermediate pattern is seen (Fig. 2.66).

A 'capture beat' occurs when the ventricles are activated by an impulse of supraventricular origin during a run of VT (Fig. 2.66). Figure 2.67 shows another example of a capture beat, indicating that the broad complex tachycardia is VT.

Ventricular tachycardia

Note

- Broad complex tachycardia at 180/min
- Left axis deviation
- Probable right bundle branch block (RBBB) pattern, with R peak greater than R^1 in lead V_1
- Two narrow complexes in leads I–III – the first is probably a 'fusion' beat and the second a 'capture' beat

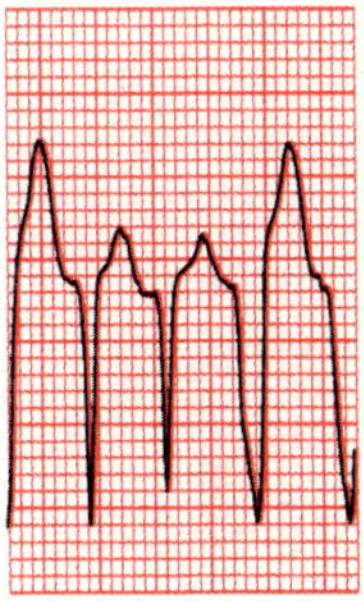

Fusion and capture beats in lead III

Fig. 2.67

Ventricular tachycardia

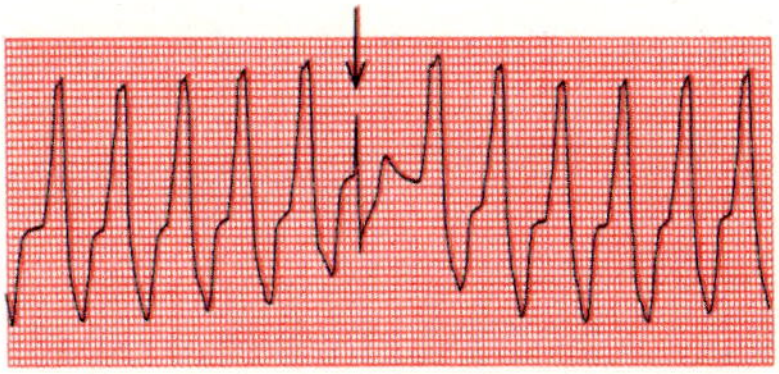

Note

- A single early beat with a narrow QRS complex (arrowed) interrupts a broad complex tachycardia
- A single 'capture' beat must have a supraventricular origin, and by inference the broad complexes must have a ventricular origin

DIFFERENTIATION OF BROAD COMPLEX TACHYCARDIAS

Box 2.10 summarizes some distinguishing features of broad complex tachycardias.

SPECIAL FORMS OF VENTRICULAR TACHYCARDIA IN PATIENTS WITH SYMPTOMS

RIGHT VENTRICULAR OUTFLOW TRACT TACHYCARDIA

This is usually an exercise-induced tachycardia, which originates in the right ventricular outflow tract. It can be treated by ablation (see Ch. 6). It is recognizable because the broad complex tachycardia shows a combination of right axis deviation and left bundle branch block (Fig. 2.68).

TORSADE DE POINTES

Ventricular tachycardia (VT) is called 'monomorphic' when all the QRS complexes have the same appearance, and 'polymorphic' when they vary. A 'twisting' polymorphic VT is called 'torsade de pointes'. This is often seen in patients whose ECG in sinus rhythm shows a long QT interval (see p. 72). Figures 2.69 and 2.70 show the ECGs from a patient with a long QT interval when in sinus rhythm, who

Fig. 2.68

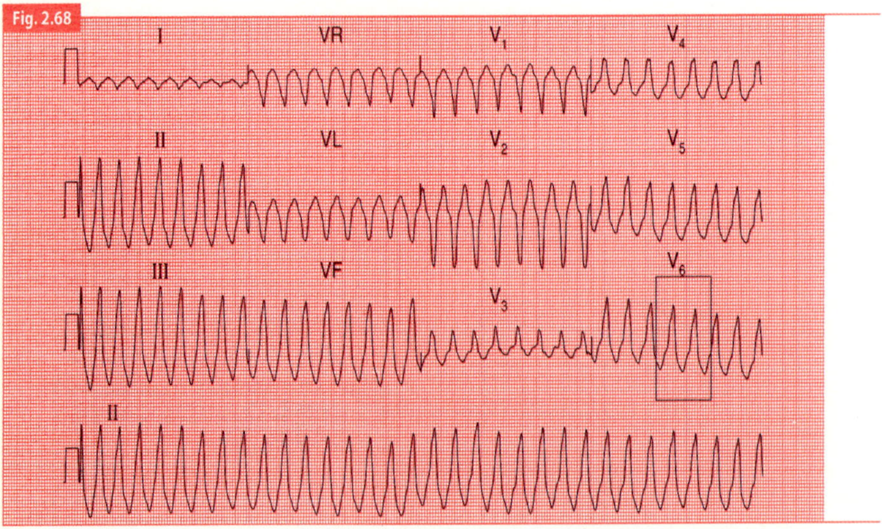

Box 2.10 Differentiation of broad complex tachycardias

- Broad complex tachycardias in patients with acute myocardial infarction are likely to be ventricular
- Compare with record taken in sinus rhythm – change of axis suggests a ventricular rhythm
- Left axis deviation, especially with right bundle branch block, is usually ventricular
- Identify P waves (independent P waves in ventricular tachycardia)
- QRS complex width: if > 160 ms, usually ventricular
- QRS complex regularity: if very irregular, probably atrial fibrillation with conduction defect
- Concordance: ventricular tachycardia is likely if the QRS complexes are predominantly upward, or predominantly downward, in all the chest leads
- With right bundle branch block pattern, ventricular origin is likely if:
  — there is left axis deviation
  — there is a tall R wave in lead V_1
  — the secondary R wave is taller than primary R wave (R^1) in lead V_1
- With left bundle branch block pattern, ventricular origin is likely if there is a QS wave (i.e. no R wave) in lead V_6
- Capture beats: narrow complex following short R–R interval (i.e. an early narrow beat interrupting a broad complex tachycardia) suggests that the basic rhythm is ventricular
- Fusion beats: an intermediate QRS complex pattern arises when the ventricles are activated simultaneously by a supraventricular and a ventricular impulse

Right ventricular outflow tract tachycardia

Note

- Broad complex tachycardia
- Right axis deviation
- Left bundle branch block (LBBB) pattern

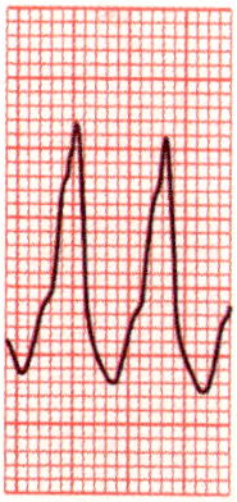

Broad QRS complexes and LBBB pattern in lead V_6

Fig. 2.69

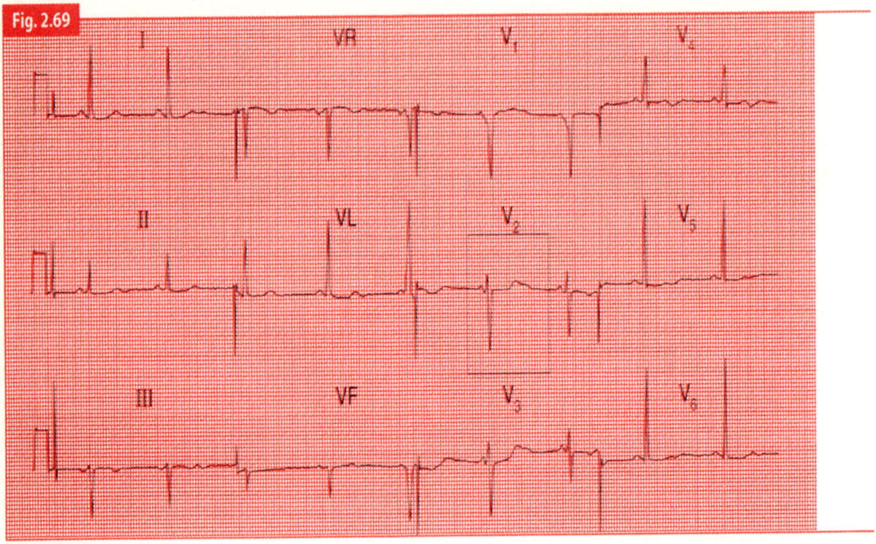

Fig. 2.70

Torsade de pointes ventricular tachycardia

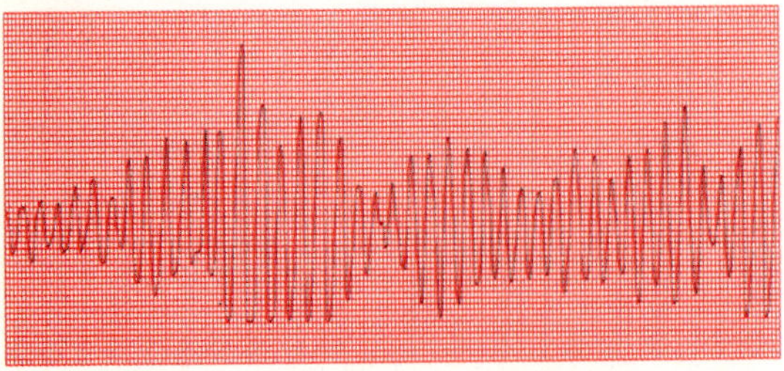

Note

- Broad complex, polymorphic tachycardia with continual change of shape

Long QT syndrome: drug toxicity

Note

- Sinus rhythm
- Third complex in lead VL is probably a 'fusion' beat
- QT interval difficult to measure because of U waves, but probably about 540 ms

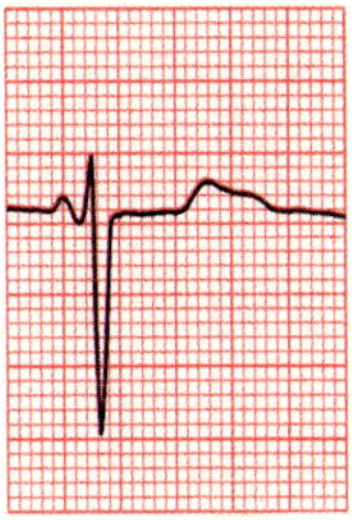

Long QT interval in lead V_2

Fig. 2.71

Ventricular tachycardia (torsade de pointes)

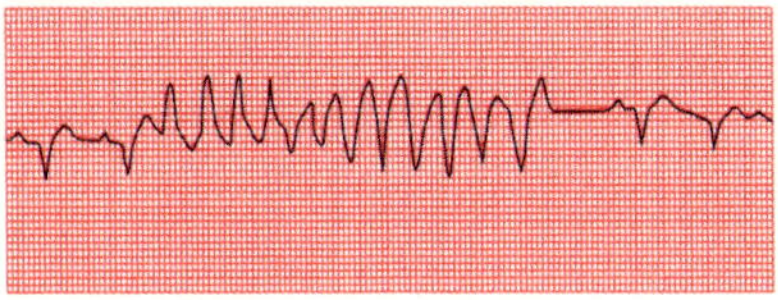

Note

- Two sinus beats are followed by ventricular tachycardia
- The complexes initially point upwards, but then become inverted; the QRS complex rate is variable

developed torsade de pointes VT. This pattern immediately raises the possibility of drug toxicity, and in this case the cause was thioridazine (see p. 73).

Figure 2.71 shows another example of torsade de pointes VT, in this case due to a Class I antiarrhythmic drug.

Possible causes of torsade de pointes VT due to drugs are listed in Box 2.11.

Box 2.11 Drugs causing torsade de pointes ventricular tachycardia

- Class I antiarrhythmic drugs
- Amiodarone
- Sotalol
- Tricyclic antidepressants
- Many other drugs

Fig. 2.72

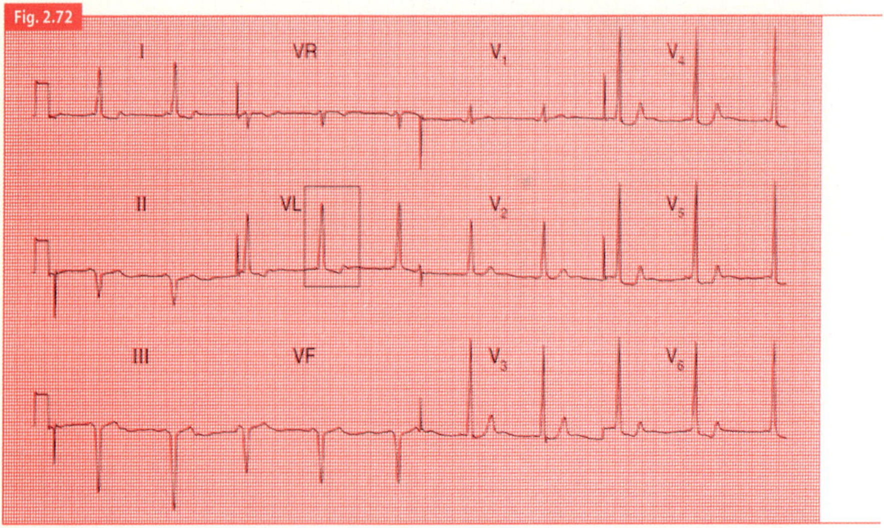

Fig. 2.73

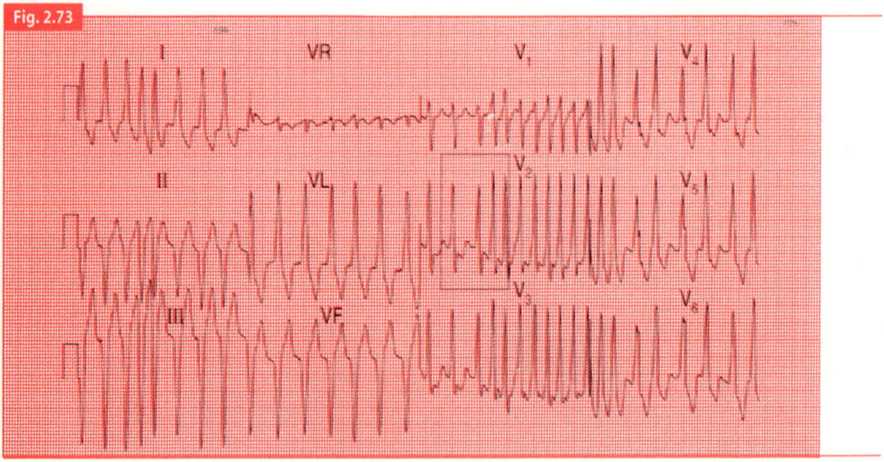

The Wolff–Parkinson–White syndrome

Note

- Sinus rhythm
- Short PR interval
- Left axis deviation
- Prominent delta wave
- Dominant R waves in lead V_1

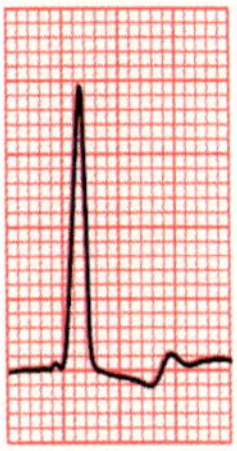

Short PR interval and delta wave in lead VL

BROAD COMPLEX TACHYCARDIAS ASSOCIATED WITH THE WOLFF–PARKINSON–WHITE SYNDROME

Remember that the Wolff–Parkinson–White (WPW) syndrome causes a wide QRS complex because of the delta wave. When a re-entry tachycardia occurs with depolarization down the accessory pathway, the ECG will show a wide QRS complex which can look remarkably like VT. However, if depolarization spreads down the His bundle and then back up the accessory pathway, the QRS complexes will be narrow and resemble a supraventricular tachycardia.

When the broad complex tachycardia is polymorphic (variable-shape QRS complexes) and very irregular, the rhythm is likely to be atrial fibrillation with the WPW syndrome. This is extremely dangerous, as it can degenerate into ventricular fibrillation (Figs 2.72 and 2.73).

The Wolff–Parkinson–White syndrome with atrial fibrillation

Note

- Same patient as in Figure 2.72
- Irregular broad complex tachycardia
- Rate up to 300/min
- Delta waves still apparent
- Marked irregularity suggests atrial fibrillation

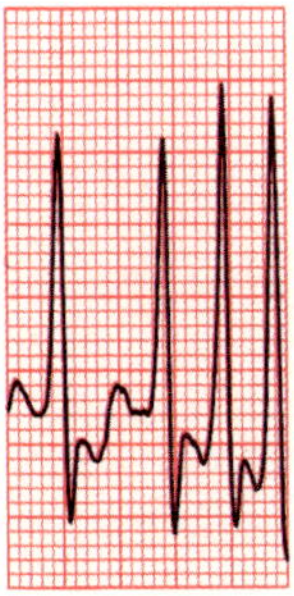

Delta waves in lead V_2

Fig. 2.74

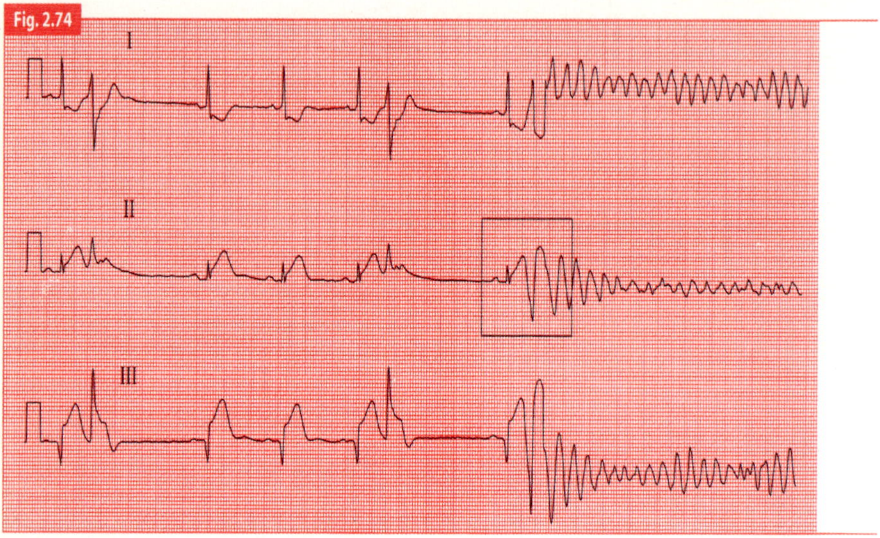

VENTRICULAR FIBRILLATION

The ECG in Figure 2.74 was being recorded from a patient with an acute inferior myocardial infarction when he collapsed due to VF.

BRADYCARDIAS IN PATIENTS WITH SYMPTOMS

ESCAPE RHYTHMS

Escape rhythms are usually asymptomatic, but symptoms occur when the automaticity that generates the escape rhythm is inadequate to maintain a cardiac output.

SINOATRIAL DISEASE – THE 'SICK SINUS SYNDROME'

Abnormal function of the SA node may be associated with failure of the conduction system. Many patients with sinoatrial disease are asymptomatic, but all the symptoms associated with bradycardias – dizziness, syncope and the symptoms of heart failure – can occur.

The abnormal rhythms seen in the sick sinus syndrome are listed below in Box 2.12.

Disordered SA node function can be familial or congenital and can occur in ischaemic, rheumatic, hypertensive or infiltrative cardiac disease. It is, however, frequently idiopathic. Because atrial and

Ventricular fibrillation

Note

- Leads I, II and III, continuous records
- Initially sinus rhythm, with occasional ventricular extrasystoles
- 'R on T' ventricular extrasystole followed by ventricular fibrillation

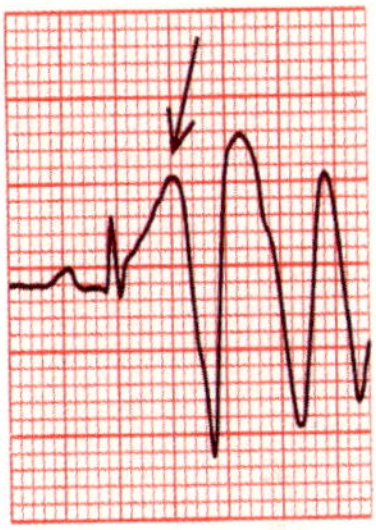

R on T phenomenon in lead II

junctional tachycardias often occur together, the patient may present with palpitations. The combination of sick sinus syndrome and tachycardias is sometimes called the 'bradycardia–tachycardia syndrome'. The ECGs in Figures 2.75 and 2.76 are from a young man who had a normal ECG with a slow sinus rate when asymptomatic, but who intermittently became extremely dizzy when he developed a profound sinus bradycardia.

The ECG in Figure 2.77 shows an ambulatory record from a young woman who complained of short-lived attacks of dizziness. When she had these, the ECG showed sinus pauses.

Box 2.12 Cardiac rhythms in sick sinus syndrome

- Unexplained or inappropriate sinus bradycardia
- Sudden changes in sinus rate
- Sinus pauses (sinoatrial arrest or exit block)
- Atrial standstill ('silent atrium')
- Atrioventricular junctional escape rhythms
- Atrial tachycardia alternating with junctional escape (bradycardia–tachycardia syndrome)
- Junctional tachycardia alternating with junctional escape
- Atrial fibrillation with a slow ventricular response
- Prolonged pauses after premature atrial beats

Fig. 2.75

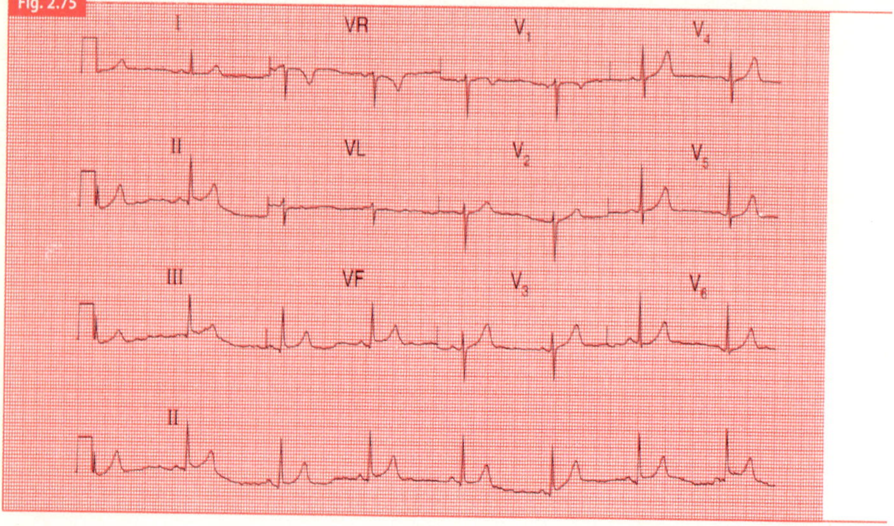

Fig. 2.76

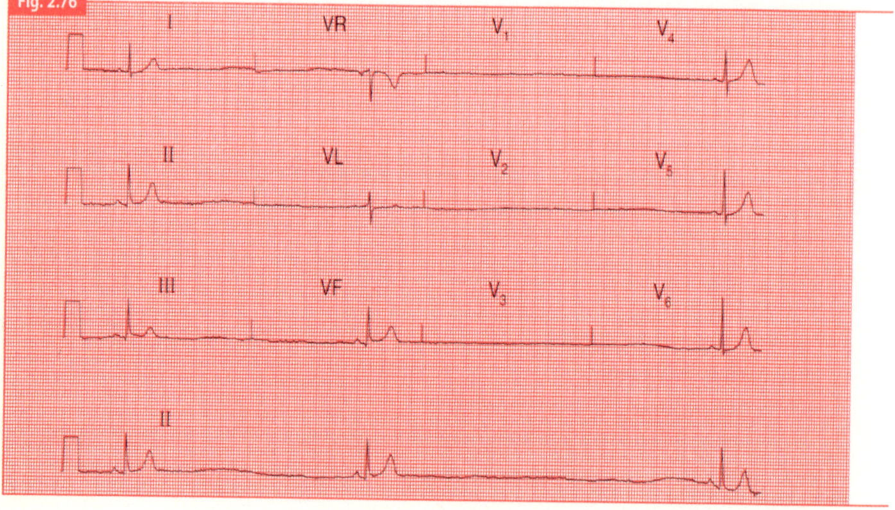

Sinus bradycardia

Note

- Sinus rhythm
- Rate 45/min, ECG otherwise normal

Sick sinus syndrome: sinus bradycardia

Note

- Same patient as in Figure 2.75
- Sinus rhythm
- Rate down to 12/min at times
- No complexes recorded in leads V_1–V_3

Fig. 2.77

Sinus pauses

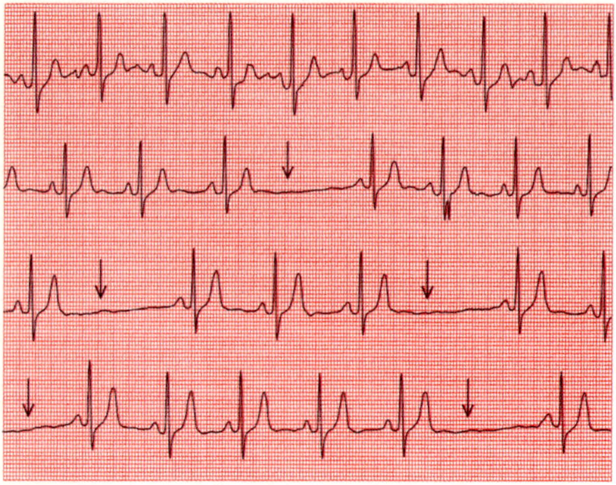

Note

- Ambulatory record
- Sinus rhythm throughout, but marked pauses (arrowed) at time of symptoms
- In the pause, the P–P interval is exactly twice the P–P interval of the preceding beat. There has therefore been 'exit block' from the SA node

Fig. 2.78

Sinus arrest

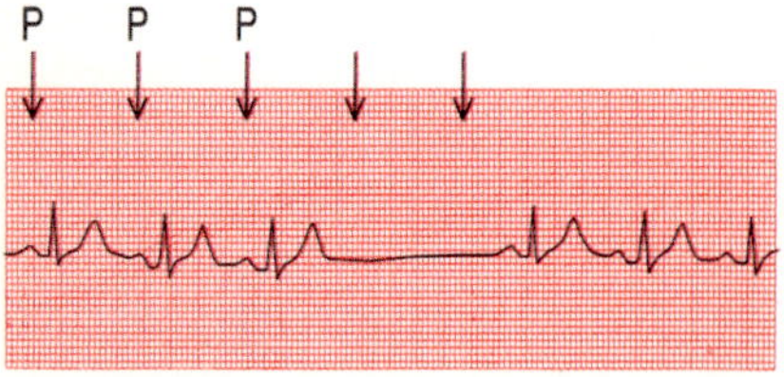

Note

- Sinus rhythm
- After three beats there is a 'sinus pause' with no P wave
- Arrows mark where the next two P waves should have been
- Sinus rhythm is then restored, but the cycle has been reset

Figure 2.78 shows the other variety of sinus pause – sinus arrest.

The ECG in Figure 2.79 shows an example of a 'silent atrium', when the heart rhythm depends on the irregular depolarization of a focus in the AV node.

Figure 2.80 shows the rhythm of a patient with the 'bradycardia–tachycardia' syndrome. This patient

Fig. 2.79

Sick sinus syndrome: silent atrium

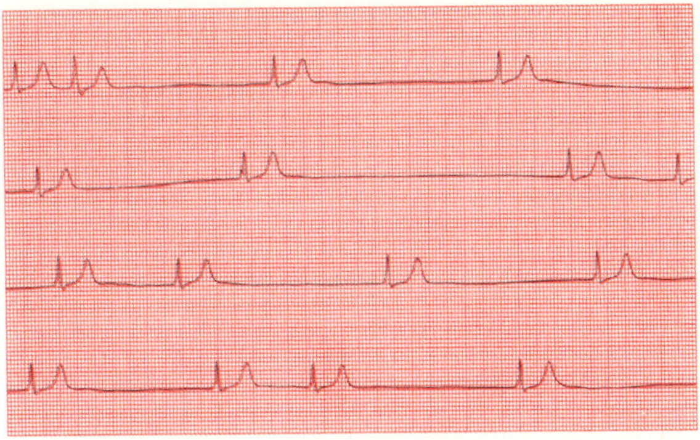

Note
- Ambulatory recording from lead II
- Irregular, narrow complex rhythm
- No P waves visible
- Nodal escape, with rate down to 16/min at times

Fig. 2.80

Sick sinus syndrome: bradycardia–tachycardia syndrome

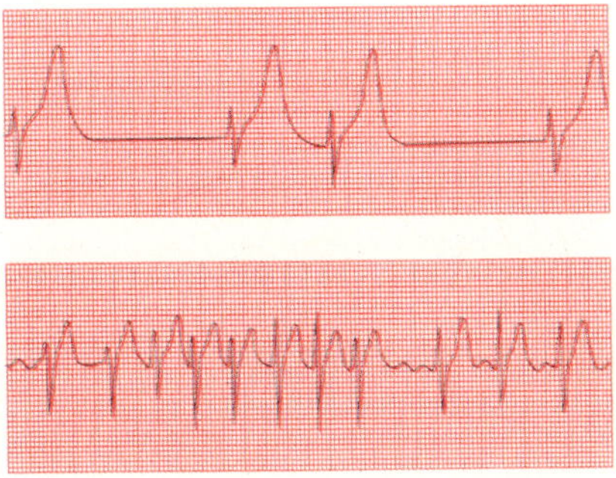

Note
- Upper trace: a silent atrium with irregular junctional escape beats
- Lower trace: junctional tachycardia is followed by a period of sinus rhythm

Fig. 2.81

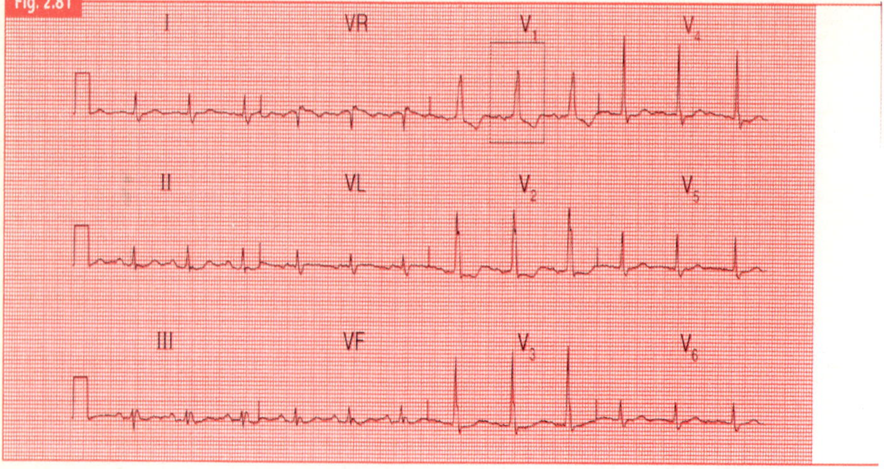

Fig. 2.82

Sinus arrest and atrioventricular nodal escape

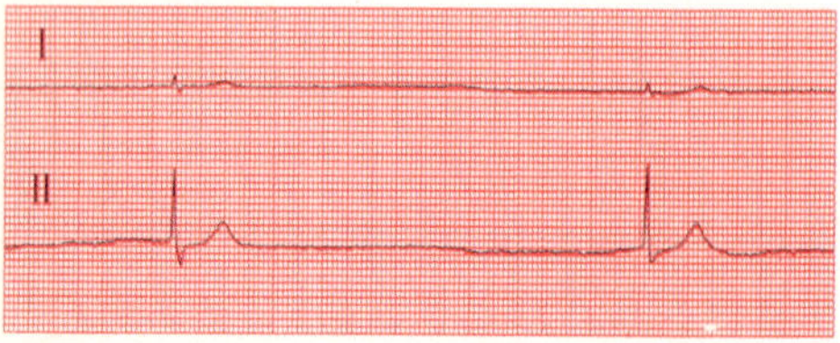

Note

- Same patient as in Figure 2.81
- Ambulatory record
- No P waves
- Narrow complex rhythm
- Rate 15/min, due to AV nodal (junctional) escape

First degree block and right bundle branch block

Note

- Sinus rhythm
- PR interval 220 ms (first degree block)
- Right bundle branch block (RBBB)

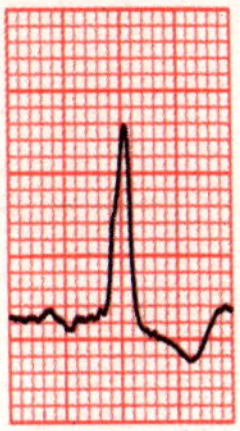

Long PR interval and RBBB pattern in lead V_1

was asymptomatic at times when his ECG shows a 'silent atrium' with a slow and irregular junctional (AV nodal) escape rhythm, but complained of palpitations when he had an AV nodal tachycardia.

Figure 2.81 shows the ECG from a patient who, when asymptomatic, showed first degree block and right bundle branch block. He complained of fainting attacks, and an ambulatory recording (Fig. 2.82) showed that this was due to sinus arrest with a very slow AV nodal escape rhythm, giving a ventricular rate of 15/min. This is an example of the combination of conduction system disease and sick sinus syndrome.

Possible causes of sick sinus syndrome are listed in Box 2.13.

Box 2.13 Sick sinus syndrome

Familial

- Isolated
- With atrioventricular conduction disturbance
- With QT interval prolongation
- Congenital

Acquired

- Idiopathic
- Coronary disease
- Rheumatic disease
- Cardiomyopathy
- Neuromuscular disease:
  - Friedreich's ataxia
  - peroneal muscular atrophy
  - Charcot–Marie–Tooth disease
- Infiltration:
  - amyloidosis
  - haemochromatosis
- Collagen diseases:
  - rheumatoid
  - scleroderma
  - SLE
- Myocarditis:
  - viral
  - diphtheria
- Drugs:
  - lithium
  - aerosol propellants

Fig. 2.83

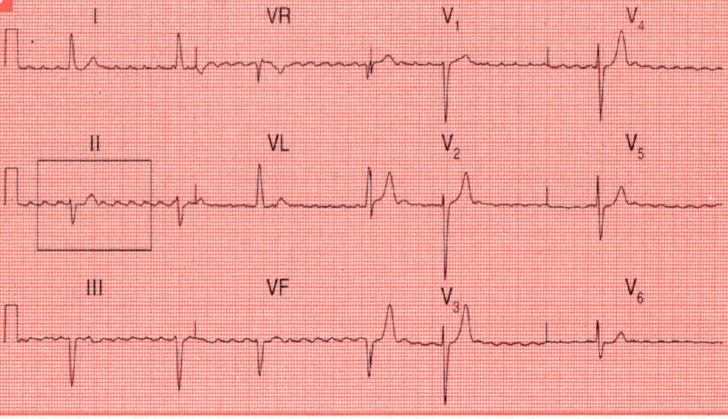

Fig. 2.84

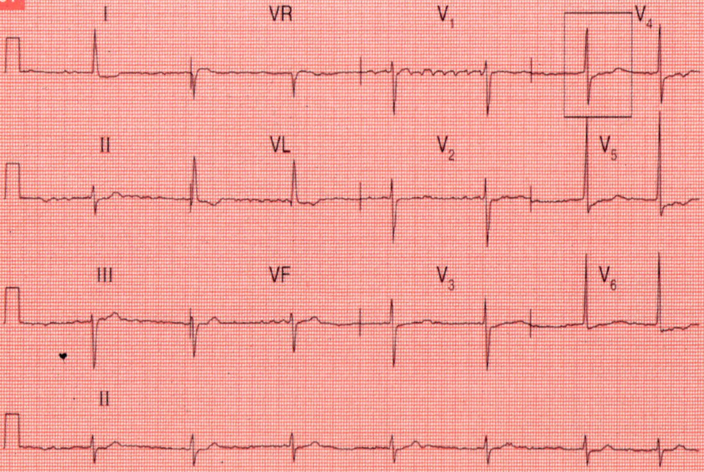

Atrial flutter with variable block

Note

- Irregular bradycardia
- Flutter waves at 300/min obvious in all leads
- Ventricular rate varies, range 30–55/min
- QRS complex duration slightly prolonged (128 ms), indicating partial right bundle branch block
- There is not complete block, as shown by the irregular QRS complexes

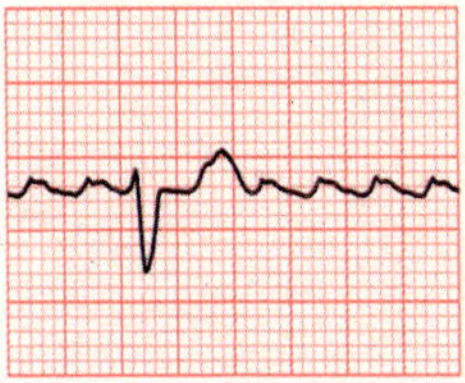

Flutter waves in lead II

Atrial fibrillation

Note

- Irregular rhythm, rate 43/min
- Flutter-like waves in lead V_1 but these are not constant
- Left axis deviation
- QRS complexes otherwise normal
- Prolonged QT intervals of 530 ms: ?hypokalaemia

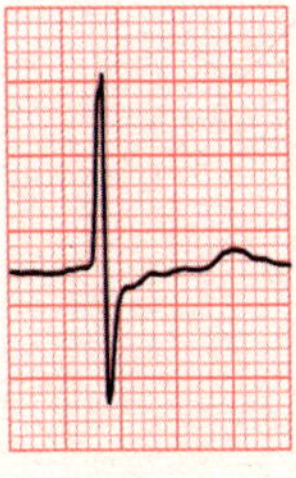

Prolonged QT interval in lead V_4

ATRIAL FIBRILLATION AND FLUTTER

A slow ventricular rate can accompany atrial flutter or atrial fibrillation because of slow conduction through the AV node and His bundle systems (Figs 2.83 and 2.84). This may be the result of treatment with drugs that delay AV nodal conduction, such as digoxin, beta-blockers or verapamil, but can occur because of conducting tissue disease.

Complete block associated with atrial fibrillation is recognized from the regular and wide QRS complexes which originate in the ventricular muscle (Fig. 2.85).

Fig. 2.85

Atrial fibrillation and complete block

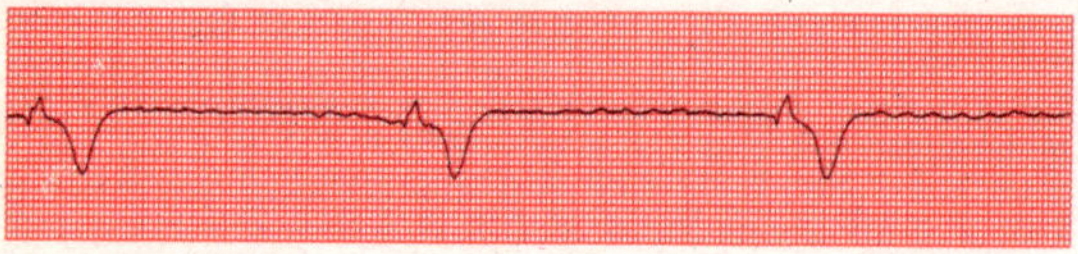

Note

- Irregular baseline suggests atrial fibrillation
- Regular broad complexes, rate about 15/min
- Inverted T waves

Fig. 2.86

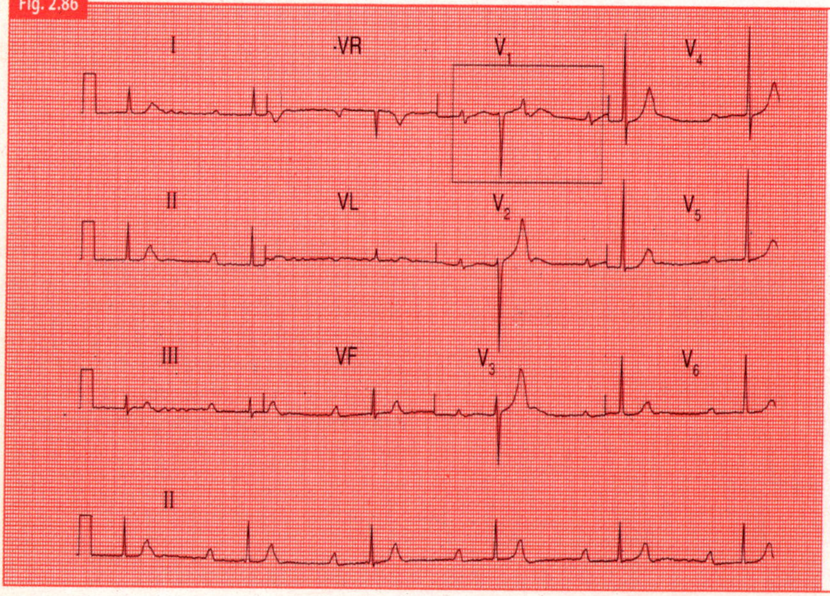

ATRIOVENTRICULAR BLOCK

Symptoms are not caused by first degree block, second degree block of the Wenckebach or Mobitz type 2 varieties, left anterior hemiblock or the bundle branch blocks.

Second degree block will cause dizziness and breathlessness if the ventricular rate is slow enough (Fig. 2.86). Young people tolerate slow hearts better than old people do.

Complete (third degree) block characteristically involves a slow rate, but this may be fast enough to cause only tiredness or the symptoms of heart failure. Figure 2.87 shows the ECG of a 60-year-old man who, despite a heart rate of 40/min, had few complaints.

If the ventricular rate is very slow the patient may lose consciousness in a 'Stokes–Adams' attack, which can cause a seizure and sometimes death. The ECG in Figure 2.88 is from a patient who was asymptomatic while his ECG showed sinus rhythm with first degree block and right bundle branch block, but who then had a Stokes–Adams attack with the onset of complete block (Fig. 2.89).

The possible causes of heart block are summarized in Box 2.14.

Second degree block (2:1)

Note

- Sinus rhythm
- Second degree block, 2:1 type
- Ventricular rate 33/min
- Normal QRS complexes and T waves

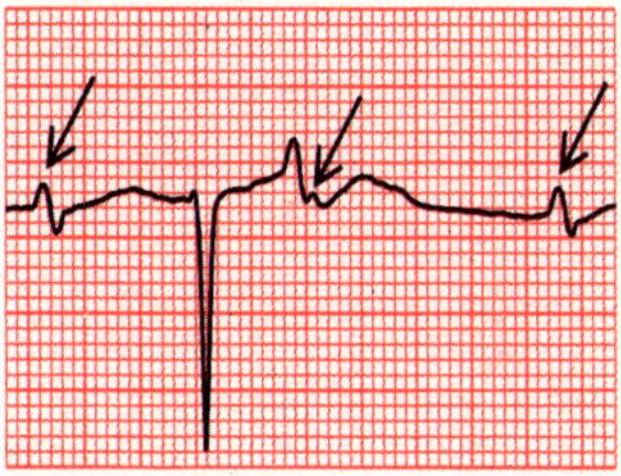

P waves in lead V_1

Fig. 2.87

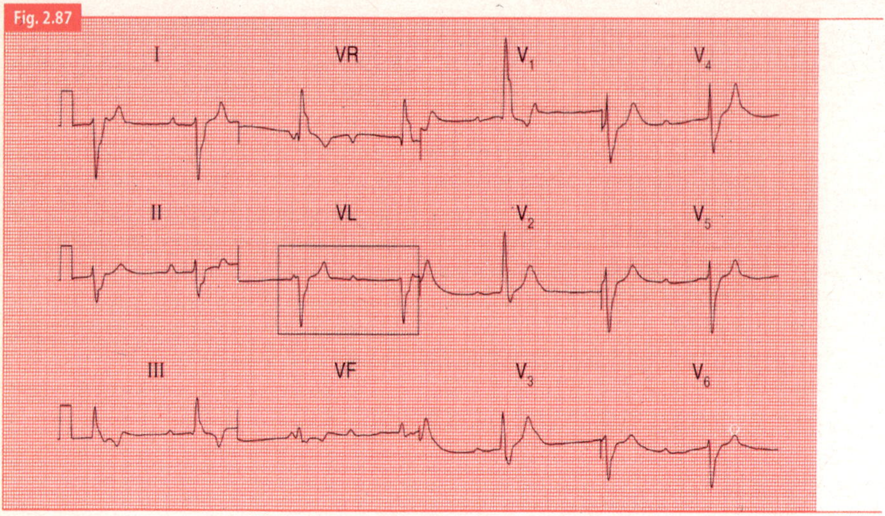

Fig. 2.88

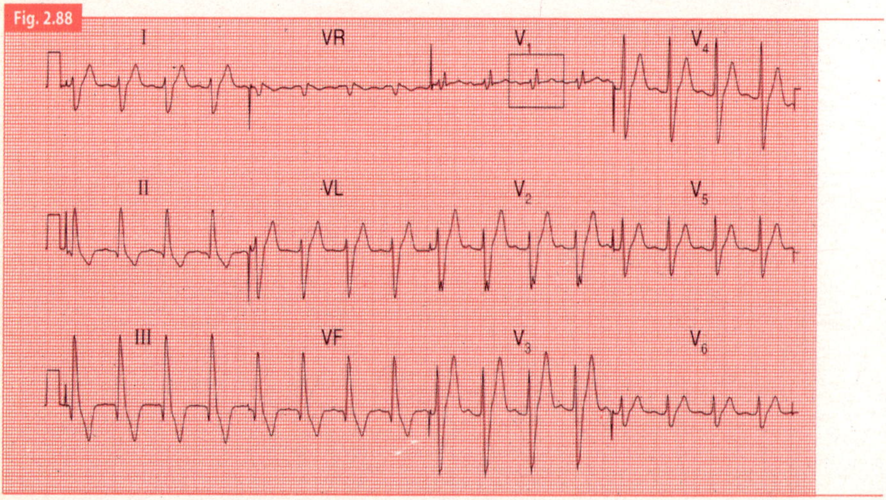

Complete heart block

Note

- Sinus rate 70/min
- Regular ventricular rate, 40/min
- No relationship between P waves and QRS complexes
- Wide QRS complexes
- Right bundle branch block

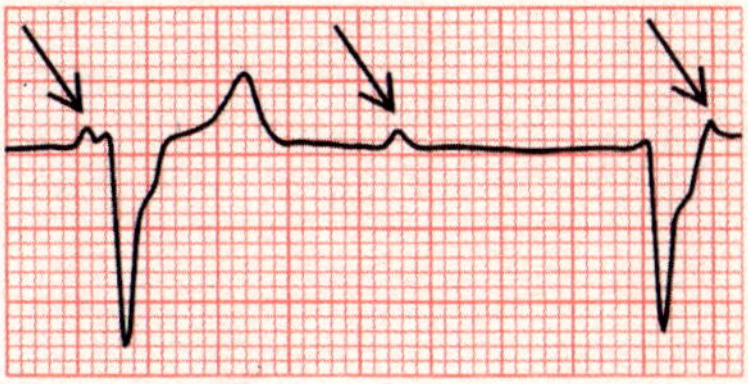

P waves in lead VL

First degree block and right bundle branch block

Note

- Sinus rhythm
- PR interval 240 ms
- Right axis deviation
- Right bundle branch block (RBBB)

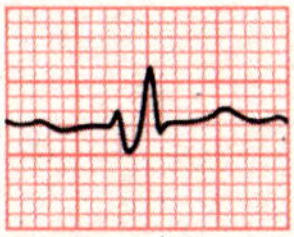

Long PR interval and RBBB pattern in lead V_1

Fig 2.89

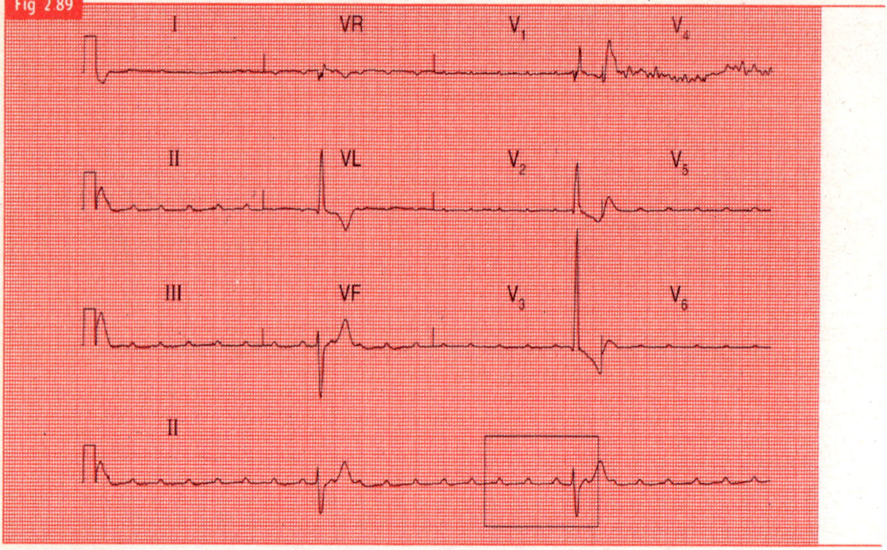

Box 2.14 Causes of heart block

First and second degree block

- Normal variant
- Increased vagal tone
- Athletes
- Sick sinus syndrome
- Acute carditis
- Ischaemic disease
- Hypokalaemia
- Lyme disease (*Borrelia burgdorferi*)
- Digoxin
- Beta-blockers
- Calcium-channel blockers

Complete block

- Idiopathic (conduction tissue fibrosis)
- Congenital
- Ischaemic disease
- Associated with aortic valve calcification
- Cardiac surgery and trauma
- Digoxin intoxication
- Bundle interruption by tumours, parasites, abscesses, granulomas, injury

Complete block and Stokes–Adams attack

Note

- Same patient as in Figure 2.88
- Sinus rate 140/min
- Ventricular rate 15/min
- No relationship between P waves and QRS complexes
- Because of the slow ventricular rate, no QRS complexes were recorded in leads I–III or V_1–V_3, although the rhythm strip shows a complex in lead II

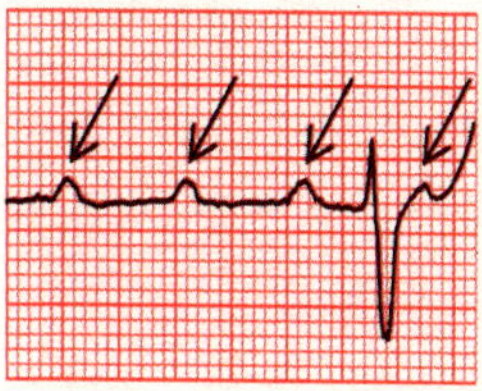

P waves

AMBULATORY ECG RECORDING

The only way to be certain that a patient's symptoms are due to an arrhythmia is to show that an arrhythmia is present at the time. If symptoms occur frequently – say two or three times a week – a 24-hour tape recording (called a 'Holter' record after its inventor) may show the abnormality. When symptoms are infrequent, patient-activated 'event recorders' are more useful.

Figures 2.90, 2.91 and 2.92 show examples of ambulatory records obtained from patients who complained of syncopal attacks, but whose hearts were in sinus rhythm at the time they were seen.

When an ambulatory record shows arrhythmias which are not accompanied by symptoms, it is difficult to be certain of their significance. Table 2.5 (p. 152) shows the arrhythmias that were recorded during two 24-hour periods from a group of 86

Fig. 2.90

Ventricular tachycardia

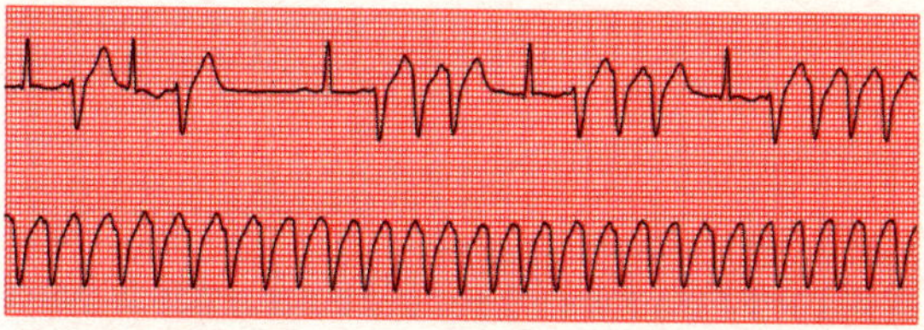

Note

- Ambulatory recording
- Initially sinus rhythm with ventricular extrasystoles
- Then salvos (three beats) of extrasystoles, leading to a broad complex tachycardia
- The change in QRS complex configuration suggests that the tachycardia is ventricular but a 12-lead ECG would be necessary to be certain

Fig. 2.91

Ventricular standstill

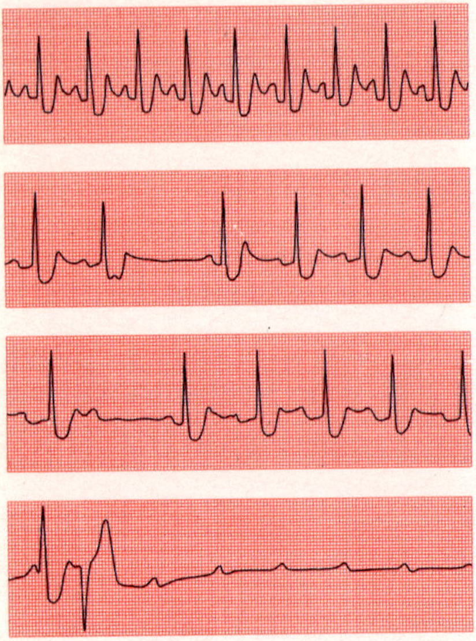

Note

- Ambulatory recording
- Top strip shows sinus rhythm with normal AV conduction
- Second strip shows SA block, which was asymptomatic
- Third strip shows second degree block, which was also asymptomatic
- Bottom strip shows a ventricular extrasystole followed by ventricular standstill. The patient lost consciousness due to this Stokes–Adams attack

volunteers who were apparently completely free of heart disease. This study shows that supposedly dangerous arrhythmias, such as ventricular tachycardia, can occur and pass unnoticed in apparently healthy people.

Ventricular extrasystoles are so common that they can clearly be ignored, although epidemiological evidence suggests that in large groups of patients they can be crude 'markers' of heart disease.

Fig. 2.92

Sudden death due to ventricular fibrillation

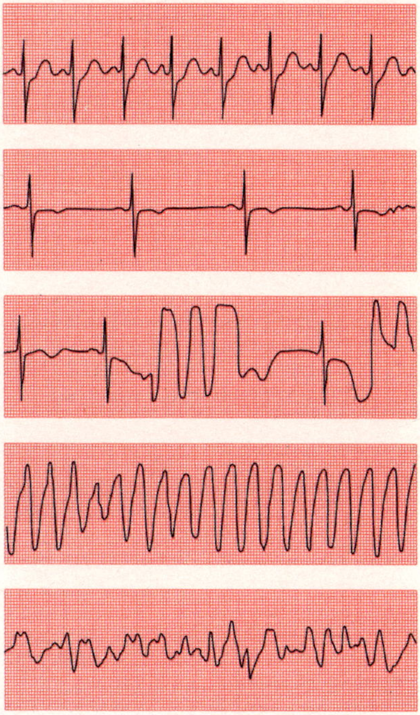

Note

- Ambulatory recording
- First strip shows sinus rhythm
- Sinus bradycardia then develops, with inversion of the T wave suggesting ischaemia
- Short runs of ventricular tachycardia (VT) lead to polymorphic VT
- Ventricular fibrillation then develops

Table 2.5 **Arrhythmias observed during 48 hours of ambulatory recording in 86 healthy subjects aged 16–65 (from Clarke et al 1976 Lancet 2:508–510)**

Type of arrhythmia	No. of individuals with arrhythmia		
Ventricular extrasystoles	63	(Including: • multifocal • bigeminy • R on T	 13 13 3)
Ventricular tachycardia	2		
Supraventricular tachycardia	4		
Junctional escape	8		
Second degree block	2		

WHAT TO DO

WHAT TO DO WHEN AN ARRHYTHMIA IS SUSPECTED

1. Consider possible underlying diagnoses.
2. Simple investigations:
   — Haemoglobin (sinus tachycardia).
   — Thyroid function (sinus tachycardia or bradycardia).
   — Chest X-ray (for heart size and to exclude the possibility of mild heart failure).
3. Ambulatory ECG: 24-hour recording if symptoms are frequent, or event recording when symptoms are infrequent.
4. Echocardiography, to aid diagnosis when any sort of structural heart disease seems possible (e.g. valve disease with atrial fibrillation, or cardiomyopathy with syncope).
5. Tilt testing, when neurocardiogenic syncope or orthostatic hypotension is suspected.

PRECIPITATION OF ARRHYTHMIAS

Arrhythmias are sometimes precipitated by exercise (Fig. 2.93) and if the patient's history suggests that this is so, then treadmill testing may be helpful. Attempts to provoke an arrhythmia by exercise should, however, only be made when full resuscitation facilities are available.

If the patient complains of syncopal attacks, particularly on movement of the head, it is worth pressing the carotid sinus in the neck to see if the patient has carotid sinus hypersensitivity. Complete SA node inhibition may be induced, sometimes with unpleasant effects (Fig. 2.94).

Fig. 2.93

Exercise-induced ventricular tachycardia

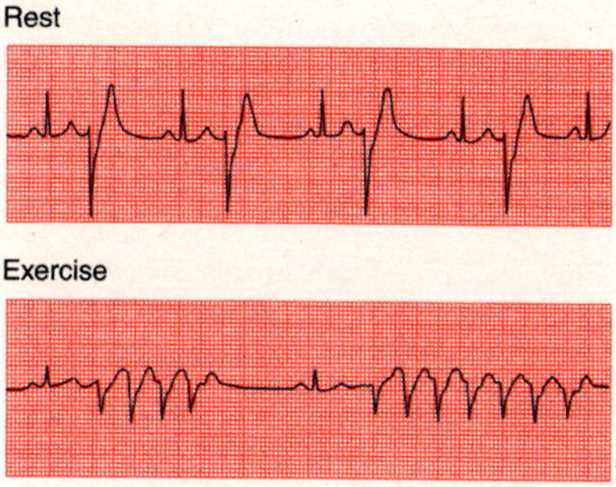

Note

- At rest (upper trace) the ECG shows frequent ventricular extrasystoles
- During exercise (lower trace), ventricular tachycardia occurs

Fig. 2.94

Carotid sinus hypersensitivity

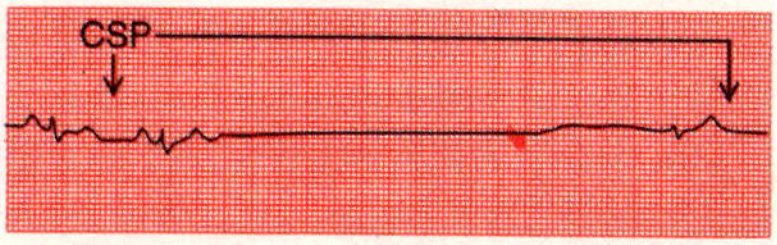

Note

- Carotid sinus pressure causes cessation of all cardiac activity, due to excessive vagal influence

WHAT TO DO WHEN AN ARRHYTHMIA IS RECORDED

1. Does the arrhythmia need treating as an emergency?
   — If there are unpleasant symptoms, or evidence of haemodynamic disturbance – yes.
   — If the patient is asymptomatic – probably not, unless haemodynamic problems seem likely.
2. Does the arrhythmia have an obvious cause? Possible causes are:
   — Myocardial infarction, sometimes following thrombolysis (not usually important).
   — Drugs (especially antiarrhythmic drugs).
   — Alcohol.
   — Thyrotoxicosis.
   — Rheumatic heart disease.
   — Cardiomyopathy.

PRINCIPLES OF ARRHYTHMIA MANAGEMENT

- Any arrhythmia causing significant symptoms or a haemodynamic disturbance must be treated immediately.
- All antiarrhythmic drugs should be considered cardiac depressants, and they are potentially pro-arrhythmic. The use of multiple agents should be avoided.
- Electrical treatment (cardioversion for tachycardias, pacing for bradycardias) should be used in preference to drug therapy when there is marked haemodynamic impairment.

MANAGEMENT OF CARDIAC ARREST

The treatment of an individual patient will depend on the particular arrhythmia involved. Remember, confirm cardiac arrest by checking:

- Airway
- Breathing
- Circulation.

The immediate actions are:

- Begin cardiopulmonary resuscitation (CPR). Ventilation and chest compression should be given in a ratio of 2 breaths to every 30 compressions.
- Defibrillate in cases of ventricular fibrillation and pulseless ventricular tachycardia as soon as possible.
- Intubate as soon as possible.
- Gain or verify IV access.

SHOCKABLE RHYTHMS – VENTRICULAR FIBRILLATION (VF) OR PULSELESS VENTRICULAR TACHYCARDIA (VT)

Actions:

1. Precordial thump (especially useful in VT).
2. Defibrillate at 200 J.
3. 2 min of CPR.
4. If unsuccessful, defibrillate at 360 J.
5. If unsuccessful, give adrenaline (epinephrine) 1 mg i.v.
6. Defibrillate at 360 J.
7. 2 min of CPR.
8. If VF/pulseless VT persists, give amiodarone 300 mg i.v.

Fig. 2.95

DC conversion of ventricular fibrillation

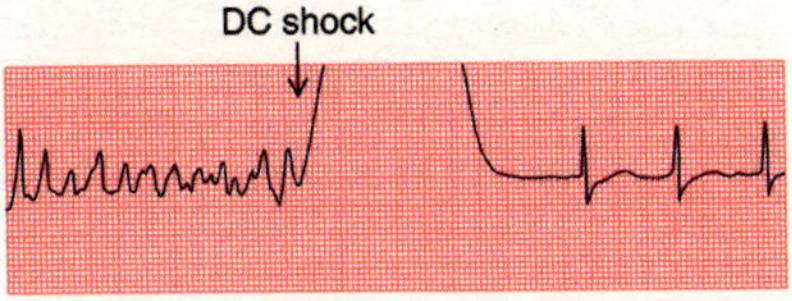

Note

- Ventricular fibrillation is abolished by DC shock
- A supraventricular rhythm (probably sinus in origin) immediately takes control of the heart

9. Give further shocks after 2-min periods of CPR.
10. Give adrenaline (epinephrine) 1 mg i.v. immediately before alternate shocks.
11. For refractory VF, give magnesium sulfate 2 g i.v. bolus (8 mmol).

The ECG in Figure 2.95 shows a successful defibrillation.

Box 2.15 Causes of pulseless electrical activity (PEA)

- Tamponade
- Drug overdose
- Electrolyte imbalance
- Hypothermia
- Pulmonary embolism
- Tension pneumothorax

NON-SHOCKABLE RHYTHMS – ASYSTOLE AND PULSELESS ELECTRICAL ACTIVITY (PEA)

The term PEA has replaced 'electromechanical dissociation' (EMD) because some pulseless patients have some weak myocardial contractions, although insufficient to generate a cardiac output. In cases of PEA, think about the underlying causes (see Box 2.15).

Actions:

- Precordial thump.
- CPR 30:2 (30 chest compressions followed by 2 ventilations).
- If it is unclear whether the rhythm is 'fine ventricular fibrillation' or asystole, treat as VF until three defibrillations have not changed the apparent rhythm.
- Adrenaline (epinephrine) 1 mg i.v.
- CPR 30:2 for 2 min.
- Atropine 3 mg i.v.
- If unsuccessful, continue adrenaline (epinephrine) 1 mg after alternate 2-min cycles of CPR.

- Consider the possibility of a treatable cause (all of which begin with H or T):
  - Hypoxia
  - Hypovolaemia
  - Hyperkalaemia, hypocalcaemia, acidaemia
  - Hypothermia
  - Tension pneumothorax
  - Tamponade
  - Toxic substances, or therapeutic substances in overdose
  - Thromboembolic or mechanical obstruction (*e.g. pulmonary embolus*).

Following resuscitation, check:

- Arterial blood gases – if the pH is < 7.1 or if arrest is associated with tricyclic overdose, give bicarbonate 50 mmol.
- Electrolytes.
- ECG.
- Chest X-ray – principally to exclude a pneumothorax caused by the resuscitation.

MANAGEMENT OF OTHER ARRHYTHMIAS

EXTRASYSTOLES

- Supraventricular: no treatment. If the patient has symptoms, explanation and reassurance. Advise to discontinue smoking and avoid coffee and alcohol.
- Ventricular: usually no treatment, though treatment may be considered:
  - when ventricular extrasystoles are so frequent that cardiac output is impaired
  - when there is a frequent R on T phenomenon
  - when the patient complains of an irregular heartbeat but reassurance and an explanation prove ineffective.
- Three ventricular extrasystoles together (a 'salvo') should be treated as a ventricular tachycardia.

CAROTID SINUS PRESSURE IN THE MANAGEMENT OF TACHYCARDIAS

The first step in the management of any tachycardia is to try carotid sinus pressure (CSP).

In sinus rhythm, CSP will cause transient slowing of the heart rate. This may be useful in identifying the true origin of the rhythm when there is doubt (Fig. 2.96).

In atrial flutter, AV conduction is blocked so the ventricular rate falls. The atrial activity becomes obvious, which helps to identify the rhythm (Fig. 2.97). CSP seldom converts atrial flutter to sinus rhythm.

In atrial tachycardia and junctional tachycardia, CSP may restore sinus rhythm (Fig. 2.98).

In atrial fibrillation and ventricular tachycardia, CSP has no effect.

Fig. 2.96

CSP and sinus rhythm

Without CSP

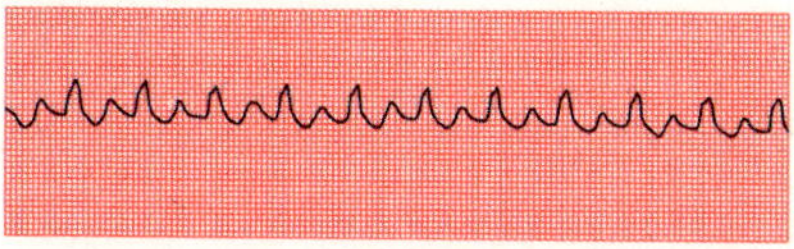

With CSP

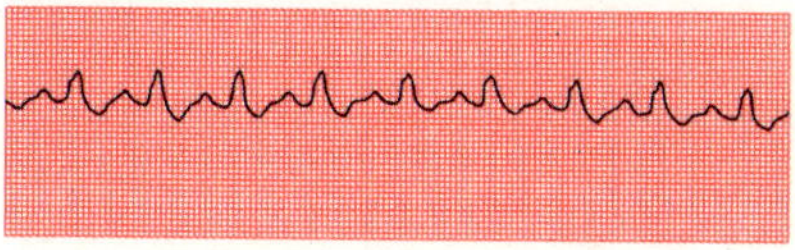

Note

- Upper trace shows a broad complex tachycardia
- It is not obvious whether the deflection before the QRS complex represents a T wave, or a T wave followed by a P wave
- Lower trace shows that with CSP the rate falls, and P waves become obvious

Fig. 2.97

CSP in atrial flutter

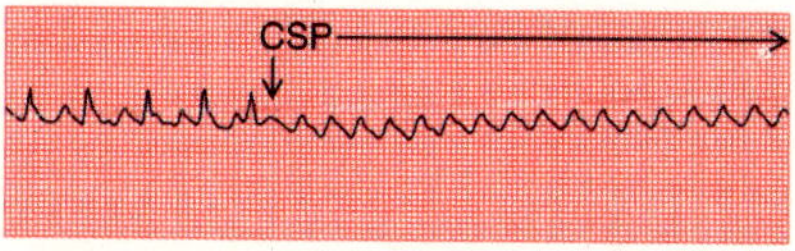

Note

- CSP increases the block at the AV node
- Ventricular activity is completely suppressed
- 'Flutter' waves are obvious

Fig. 2.98

CSP in junctional tachycardia

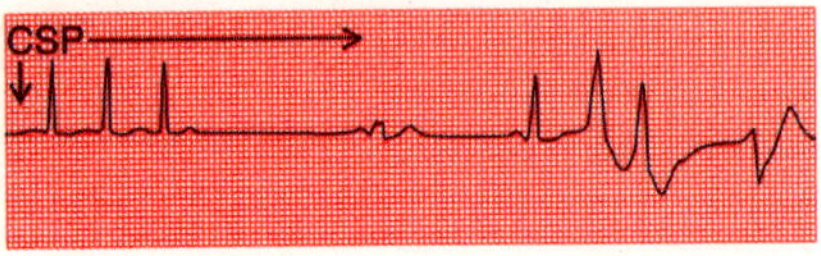

Note

- CSP reverts junctional tachycardia to sinus rhythm, but in this case multifocal ventricular extrasystoles occurred

SINUS TACHYCARDIA

Remember that sinus tachycardia always has a cause (see Box 2.3 on p. 59), and it is the cause that should be treated.

ATRIOVENTRICULAR RE-ENTRY (JUNCTIONAL) TACHYCARDIA

Try in order:

1. Carotid sinus massage.
2. Adenosine 3 mg i.v. bolus, followed if necessary after 2 min by a further 6 mg adenosine and, if necessary after a further 2 min, by a further 12 mg adenosine. Unwanted but transient effects include asthma, flushing, chest tightness and dizziness.
3. Verapamil 2.5–5 mg i.v. or atenolol 2.5 mg i.v., repeated at 5 min intervals to a total of 10 mg. Note: These drugs should not be administered together, and verapamil should not be given to patients receiving a beta-blocker.
4. DC shock.

ATRIAL TACHYCARDIA

Remember that this may be due to digoxin toxicity. Treat as for junctional tachycardia.

ATRIAL FIBRILLATION AND FLUTTER

A choice has to be made between rate control and conversion of atrial fibrillation to sinus rhythm. It should be remembered that long-term success following conversion is very unlikely in patients who:

- have had atrial fibrillation for more than a year
- have cardiac enlargement
- have evidence of left ventricular impairment
- have any form of structural abnormality in the heart.

If a patient has a ventricular rate of > 150/min and chest pain or other evidence of poor perfusion, immediate cardioversion should be attempted. In an emergency, immediate heparin treatment provides adequate prophylaxis against embolism. Cardioversion can be attempted with amiodarone i.v. or flecainide i.v., but electrical cardioversion (100 J– 200 J–360 J) is more reliable.

Patients who are not haemodynamically impaired, and who have been in atrial fibrillation for more than 24 h, should be treated with warfarin before cardioversion is attempted. Effective anti-coagulation (INR > 2.0) is needed for at least 1 month before the procedure.

For rate control, use one of:

- digoxin 250 µg i.v. by slow injection, repeated at 30 min intervals to a total of 1 mg
- i.v. amiodarone
- i.v. verapamil
- i.v. beta-blocker,

and remember the need for anticoagulants.

Prevention of paroxysmal atrial fibrillation

Atrial fibrillation is called 'paroxysmal' if there are attacks that revert spontaneously; 'persistent' if the rhythm is continuous but cardioversion has not been attempted; and 'permanent' if cardioversion has failed.

Digoxin will probably not prevent attacks of atrial fibrillation, but the prophylactic use of some drugs may prevent attacks for months, or possibly years:

- sotalol
- flecainide (avoid in patients with coronary disease)
- amiodarone.

These drugs can be used after DC cardioversion, but at best only about 40% of patients will still be in sinus rhythm after a year.

In very resistant cases, electrical ablation of the AV node can be used to cause complete heart block, and a permanent pacemaker inserted (see Ch. 6).

VENTRICULAR TACHYCARDIA

Ventricular tachycardia (VT) can be treated with one of:

- Lidocaine (lignocaine) 100 mg i.v., repeated twice at 5 min intervals, followed by a lidocaine infusion at 2–3 mg/min.
- Amiodarone 300 mg i.v. over 30 min then 900 mg over 24 h, followed by 200 mg t.d.s. by mouth for 1 week, 200 mg b.d. for 1 week and 200 mg daily thereafter.
- Atenolol 2.5 mg i.v., repeated at 5 min intervals to 10 mg.
- Flecainide 50–100 mg i.v., or 100 mg b.d. by mouth – but avoid in patients with coronary disease.
- Magnesium 8 mmol i.v. over 15 min, followed by 64 mmol over 24 h.

Note: When amiodarone is given i.v. a deep vein must be used. Overdose prolongs the QT interval and can cause VT. Long-term treatment may cause skin pigmentation, photosensitive rashes, abnormalities of thyroid or liver function, drug deposits in the cornea, or, occasionally, pulmonary fibrosis.

Second-line drugs for VT include disopyramide and mexiletine. Recurrent episodes, which cannot be controlled by drugs, are treated with an implanted defibrillator.

Patients with congenital long QT syndromes and paroxysmal VT are treated in the first instance with beta-blockers, or with an implanted defibrillator.

THE WOLFF–PARKINSON–WHITE SYNDROME

Adenosine, digoxin, verapamil and lidocaine (lignocaine) may increase conduction through the accessory pathway and block it in the AV node. This can be extremely dangerous if atrial fibrillation occurs, because it may lead to ventricular fibrillation. These drugs should therefore not be used for the treatment of pre-excitation tachycardias.

Drugs that slow conduction in the accessory pathway are:

- atenolol
- flecainide
- amiodarone.

These drugs can be used for prophylaxis against paroxysmal arrhythmias, but the definitive treatment is electrical ablation of the accessory pathway.

BRADYCARDIAS

Bradycardias must be treated if they are associated with hypotension, poor peripheral perfusion, or escape arrhythmias. Any bradycardia can be treated with:

- Atropine 600 μg i.v., repeated at 5 min intervals to a total 1.8 mg. Note: Overdose causes tachycardia, hallucinations and urinary retention.
- Isoprenaline 1–4 μg/min. Note: Overdose causes ventricular arrhythmias which are difficult to treat. An isoprenaline infusion should only be used while preparations are being made for pacing.

TEMPORARY PACING IN PATIENTS WITH ACUTE MYOCARDIAL INFARCTION

Pacing should be performed under the following circumstances:

- complete block with ventricular rate < 50/min
- complete block with anterior infarction
- any persistent bradycardia needing an isoprenaline infusion
- bifascicular block plus first degree block.

Pacing should be considered in:

- any complete block
- second degree block with heart rate < 50/min
- bundle branch block plus first degree block
- evidence of increasing block
- bradycardia with escape rhythms
- drug-induced tachyarrhythmias.

3 The ECG in patients with chest pain

HISTORY AND EXAMINATION

There are many causes of chest pain. All the non-cardiac conditions can mimic a myocardial infarction, and so the ECG can be extremely useful when making a diagnosis. However, the ECG is less important than the history and physical examination, because the ECG can be normal in the first few hours of a myocardial infarction.

Some causes of chest pain are listed in Box 3.1

The ECG in Figure 3.1 was recorded in an A & E department from a 44-year-old man with rather vague chest pain. He was thought to have a viral illness and his ECG was considered to be within normal limits. He was allowed home, and died later that day. The postmortem examination showed a myocardial infarction which was probably a few hours old, and corresponded with his A & E attendance.

Fig. 3.1

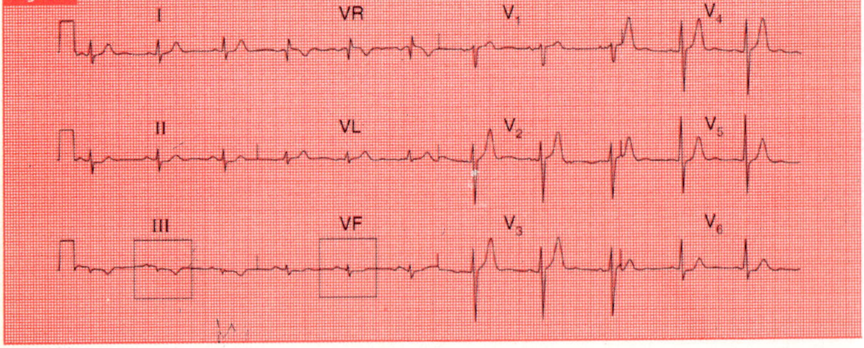

Box 3.1 Causes of chest pain

Acute chest pain
- Myocardial infarction
- Pulmonary embolism
- Pneumothorax
- Other causes of pleuritic pain
- Pericarditis
- Aortic dissection
- Ruptured oesophagus
- Oesophagitis
- Collapsed vertebra
- Herpes zoster

Chronic or recurrent chest pain
- Angina
- Nerve root pain
- Muscular pain
- Oesophageal reflux
- Nonspecific pain

Nonspecific ST segment/T wave changes

Note
- Sinus rhythm
- Normal axis
- Normal QRS complexes
- ST segments probably normal, though possibly depressed in leads III and VF
- T wave inverted in lead III (possibly a normal variant) and flattened in VF

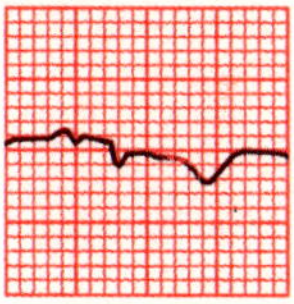

Inverted T wave in lead III

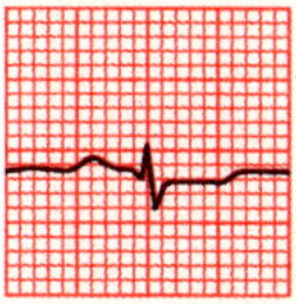

Flattened T wave in lead VF

ACUTE CHEST PAIN

The features of acute chest pain associated with different causes are summarized in Box 3.2.

The physical examination of a patient with chest pain may reveal nothing other than the signs associated with the pain itself (anxiety, sinus tachycardia, restlessness or a cold and sweaty skin), but some specific signs are worth looking for:

- Left ventricular failure suggests myocardial infarction.
- A raised jugular venous pressure suggests myocardial infarction or pulmonary embolus.
- A pleural friction rub suggests pulmonary embolism or infection.
- A pericardial friction rub suggests pericarditis (?viral,?secondary to myocardial infarction) or aortic dissection.
- Aortic regurgitation suggests aortic dissection.
- Unequal pulses or blood pressure in the arms suggests aortic dissection.
- Bony tenderness suggests musculoskeletal pain.

CHRONIC CHEST PAIN

The main differential diagnosis is between angina and the chest pain that is common in middle-aged men, but for which no clear diagnosis is usually made. This pain is sometimes called 'atypical chest pain', but this is a dangerous diagnostic label because

Box 3.2 Features of acute chest pain

Myocardial infarction
- Central
- Radiates to neck, jaw, teeth, arm(s) or back
- Severe
- Associated with nausea, vomiting and sweating
- Not all patients have typical pain, and pain can even be absent

Pulmonary embolism
- Pain similar to myocardial infarction if the embolus is central
- Pleuritic pain if the embolus is peripheral
- Associated with breathlessness or haemoptysis
- Can cause haemodynamic collapse

Other lung disease, e.g. infection or pneumothorax
- Pleuritic
  — worse on breathing
  — often associated with a cough

Pericardial pain
- Can mimic both cardiac ischaemia and pleuritic pain
- Can be recognized because it is relieved by sitting up and leaning forward

Aortic dissection
- Typically causes a 'tearing' pain (as opposed to the 'crushing' sensation of a myocardial infarction)
- Usually radiates to the back

Oesophageal rupture
- Follows vomiting

Spinal pain
- Affected by posture
- Associated root pain follows the nerve root distribution

Shingles (herpes zoster)
- Catches everyone out until the rash appears
- Tenderness of the skin may provide a clue

it implies that there is a diagnosis (by implication, cardiac ischaemia) but that the symptoms are 'atypical'. Some of these pains are musculoskeletal, Tietze's syndrome of pain from the costochondral junctions being the most obvious, but in most cases the best diagnostic label is 'chest pain of unknown cause'. This indicates a possible need for later re-evaluation.

The important features in the history that point to a diagnosis of angina are that the pain:

- is predictable
- usually occurs after a constant amount of exercise
- is worse in cold or windy weather
- is induced by emotional stress
- is induced by sexual intercourse
- is relieved by rest, and rapidly relieved by a short-acting nitrate.

The physical signs to look for are:

- evidence of risk factors (high blood pressure, cholesterol deposits, signs of smoking)
- any signs of cardiac disease (aortic stenosis, an enlarged heart, signs of heart failure)
- anaemia (which will exacerbate myocardial ischaemia)
- signs of peripheral vascular disease (which would suggest that coronary disease is also present).

THE ECG IN THE PRESENCE OF CHEST PAIN

Remember that the ECG can be normal in the early stages of a myocardial infarction. Having said that:

- An abnormal ECG is necessary to make a diagnosis of myocardial infarction before treatment is started.
- An ECG will demonstrate ischaemia in patients with angina *provided that* the patient has pain at the time the ECG is recorded.
- With pulmonary embolism there may be classical ECG changes, but these are often not present.
- With pericarditis, ECG changes, if present at all, are very nonspecific.

THE ECG IN PATIENTS WITH MYOCARDIAL ISCHAEMIA

The diagnosis of a myocardial infarction depends on the history and examination, on the measurement of biochemical markers of cardiac muscle damage (especially the troponins) and on the ECG. A rise in troponin I or troponin T levels in patients with a history suggestive of a myocardial infarction is now taken to mean that infarction has occurred, but treatment still depends on the ECG. The term 'acute coronary syndrome' is now used to include:

- myocardial infarction with ST segment elevation on the ECG (STEMI – ST segment elevation myocardial infarction)
- myocardial infarction (as shown by a troponin rise) with only T wave inversion or ST segment depression (NSTEMI – non-ST segment elevation myocardial infarction)
- chest pain with ischaemic ST segment depression but no troponin rise (what used to be called 'unstable angina')
- sudden death due to coronary disease.

Stable angina and 'chest pain of unknown cause' remain entirely proper diagnostic labels for those patients who are admitted to hospital with chest pain, but for whom the term 'acute coronary syndrome' is inappropriate.

Fig. 3.2

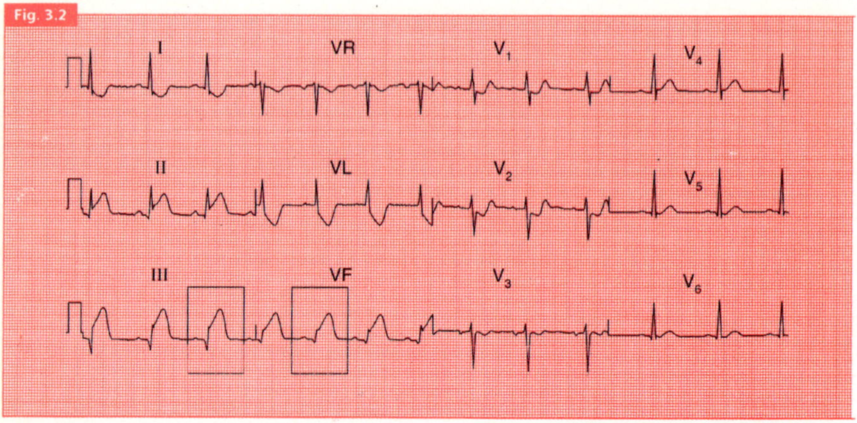

Fig. 3.3

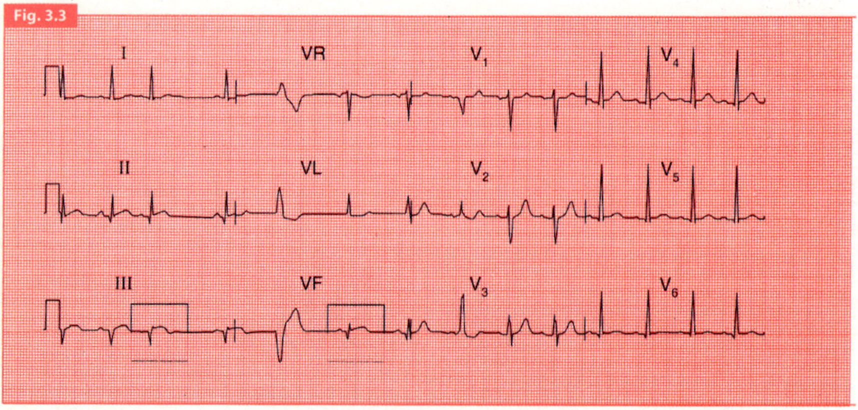

ECG CHANGES IN ST SEGMENT ELEVATION MYOCARDIAL INFARCTION (STEMI)

The sequence of features characteristic of 'full thickness', or 'ST segment elevation', myocardial infarction is:

- normal ECG
- ST segment elevation
- development of Q waves
- ST segment returns to the baseline
- T waves become inverted.

The ECG leads that show the changes typical of a myocardial infarction depend on the part of the heart affected.

INFERIOR INFARCTION

Figures 3.2, 3.3 and 3.4 show traces taken from a patient with a typical history of myocardial infarction: on admission to hospital, 3 h later, and 2 days later. The main changes are in the inferior leads II and III, and VF. Here the ST segments are initially raised, but then Q waves appear and the T waves become inverted.

Acute inferior infarction

Note

- Sinus rhythm
- Normal axis
- Small Q waves in leads II–III, VF
- Raised ST segments in leads II–III, VF
- Depressed ST segments in leads I, VL, V_2–V_3
- Inverted T waves in leads I, VL, V_3

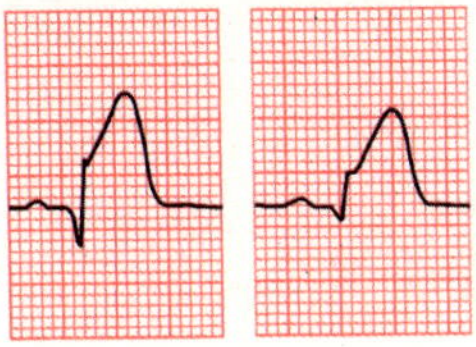

Raised ST segments in leads III and VF

Evolving inferior infarction

Note

- Same patient as in Figures 3.2 and 3.4
- Sinus rhythm with ventricular extrasystoles
- Normal axis
- Deeper Q waves in leads II–III, VF
- ST segments returning to normal, but still elevated in inferior leads
- Less ST segment depression in leads I, VL, V_3

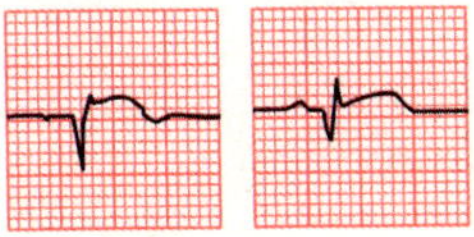

Deeper Q waves in leads III and VF

Fig. 3.4

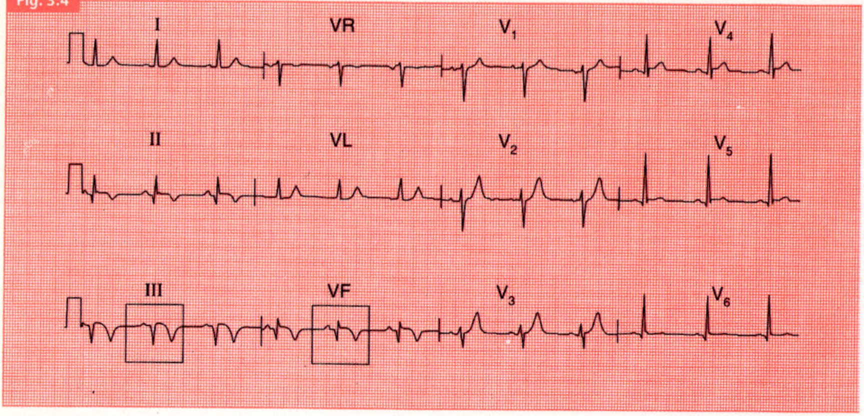

Fig. 3.5

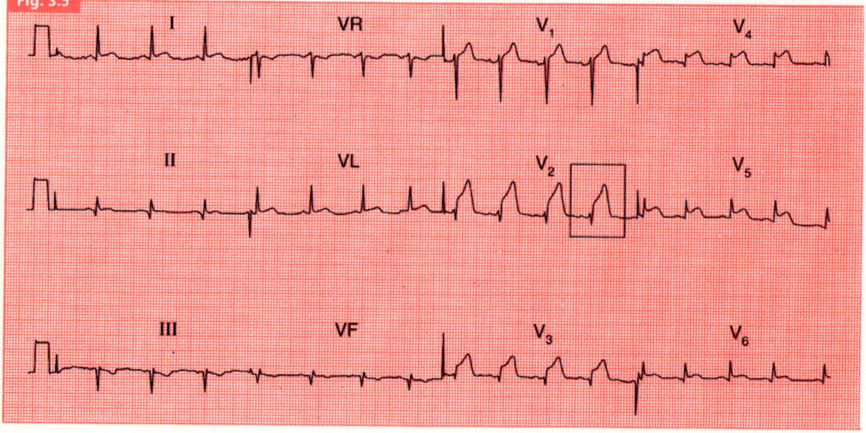

Evolving inferior infarction

Note

- Same patient as in Figures 3.2 and 3.3
- Sinus rhythm
- Normal axis
- Q waves in leads II–III, VF
- ST segments nearly back to normal
- T wave inversion in leads II–III, VF
- Lateral ischaemia has cleared (as shown by ST segments in lateral leads)

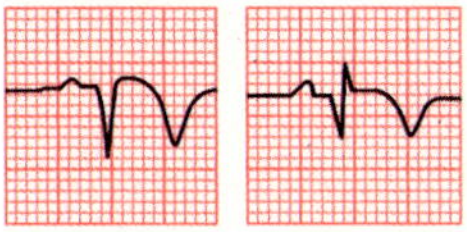

Q waves, normal ST segments, and inverted T waves in leads III and VF

Anterior infarction

Note

- Sinus rhythm
- Normal axis
- Raised ST segments in leads V_2–V_5

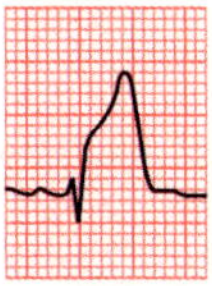

Raised ST segment in lead V_2

ANTERIOR AND LATERAL INFARCTION

The changes of anterior infarction are seen in leads V_2–V_5. Lead V_1, which lies over the right ventricle, is seldom affected (Fig. 3.5).

The lateral wall of the left ventricle is often damaged at the same time as the anterior wall, and then leads I, VL and V_6 show infarction changes. Figures 3.6 and 3.7 show the records of a patient with an acute anterolateral infarction, initially with raised ST segments and then with T wave inversion in the lateral leads. In the ECG in Figure 3.7 left axis deviation has appeared, indicating damage to the left anterior fascicle.

Figure 3.8 shows a record taken 3 days after a lateral infarction, with Q waves and inverted T waves in leads I, VL, and V_6.

The ECG in Figure 3.9 was recorded several weeks after an anterolateral myocardial infarction. Although the changes in leads I and VL appear 'old', having an isoelectric ST segment, there is still ST segment elevation in leads V_3–V_5. If the patient had just been admitted to hospital with chest pain these changes would be taken to indicate an acute infarction, but this patient had had pain more than a month previously. Persistent ST segment elevation is quite common after an anterior infarction: it sometimes indicates the development of a left ventricular aneurysm, but it is not reliable evidence of this.

Fig. 3.6

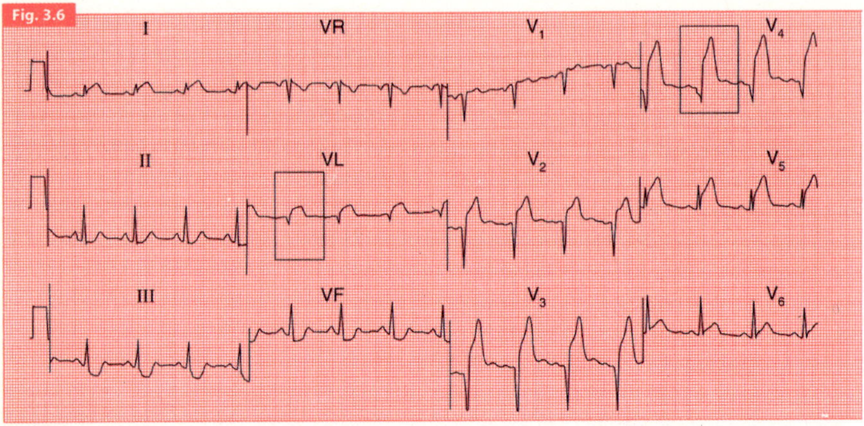

Fig. 3.7

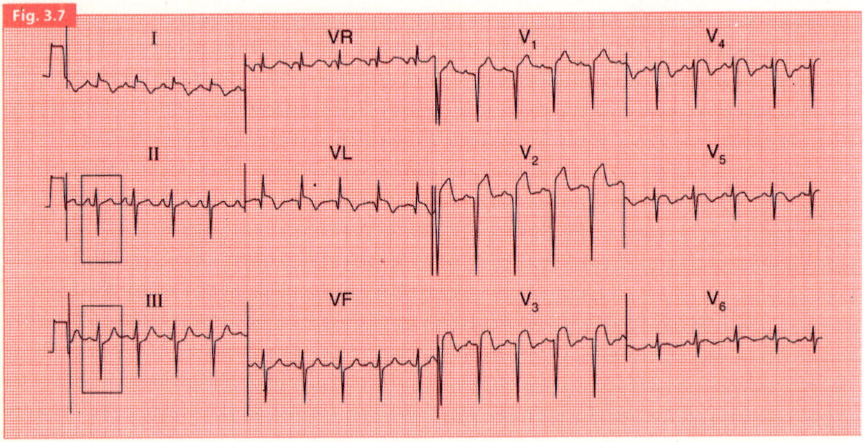

Acute anterolateral infarction

Note

- Sinus rhythm
- Normal axis
- Q waves in leads VL, V_2–V_4
- Raised ST segments in leads I, VL, V_2–V_5

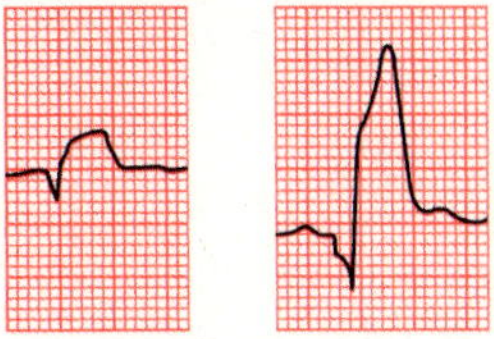

Raised ST segments in leads VL and V_4

An old anterior infarction often causes only what is called ‘poor R wave progression’. Figure 3.10 shows the record from a patient who had had an anterior infarction some years previously. A normal ECG would show progressive increase in the size of the R wave from lead V_1 to V_5 or V_6. In this case the R wave remains very small in leads V_3 and V_4, but becomes normal-sized in V_5. This loss of ‘progression’ indicates the old infarction.

The time taken for the various ECG changes of infarction to occur is extremely variable, and the ECG is an unreliable way of deciding when an infarction occurred. Serial records showing progressive changes are the only way of timing the infarction from the ECG.

Acute anterolateral infarction with left axis deviation

Note

- Same patient as in Figure 3.6
- Sinus rhythm
- Left axis deviation
- ST segments now returning to normal
- T wave inversion in leads I, VL, V_4–V_5

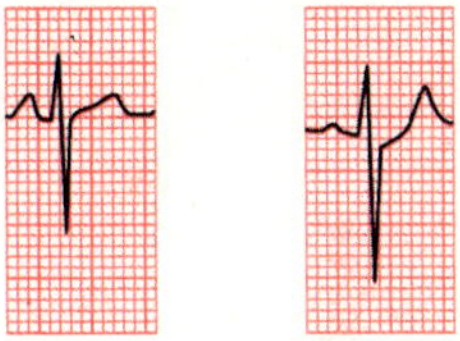

S waves in leads II and III: left axis deviation

Fig. 3.8

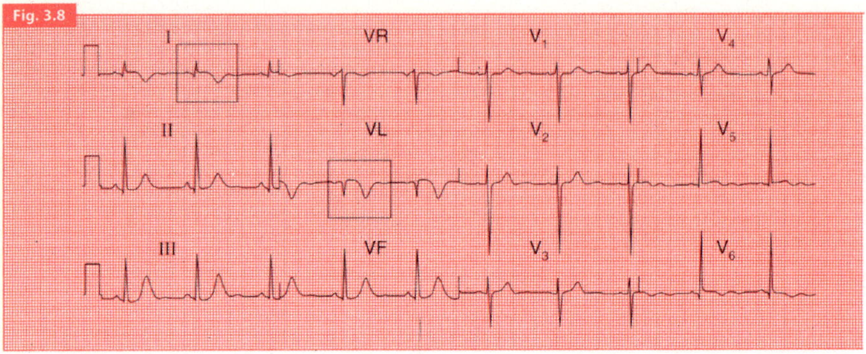

Fig. 3.9

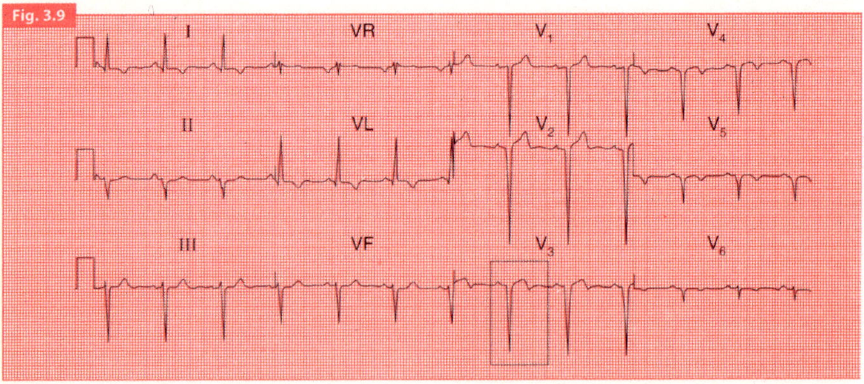

Lateral infarction (after 3 days)

Note

- Sinus rhythm
- Normal axis
- Q waves in leads I, VL, ?V_6 (could be septal)
- ST segments isoelectric
- Inverted T waves in leads I, VL, V_6

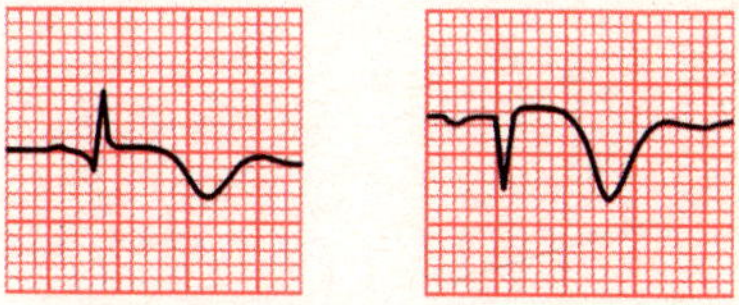

Inverted T waves in leads I and VL

Anterolateral infarction, ?age

Note

- Sinus rhythm
- Left axis deviation
- Q waves in leads I–II, V_2–V_5
- Raised ST segments in leads V_3–V_5
- Inverted T waves in leads I, VL, V_4–V_6

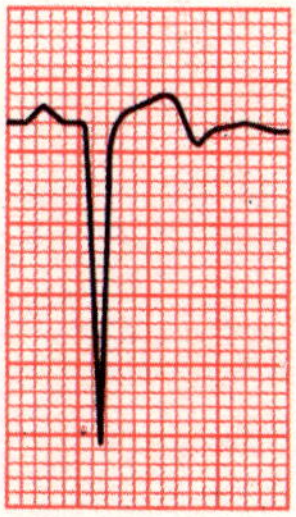

Raised ST segment in lead V_3

Fig. 3.10

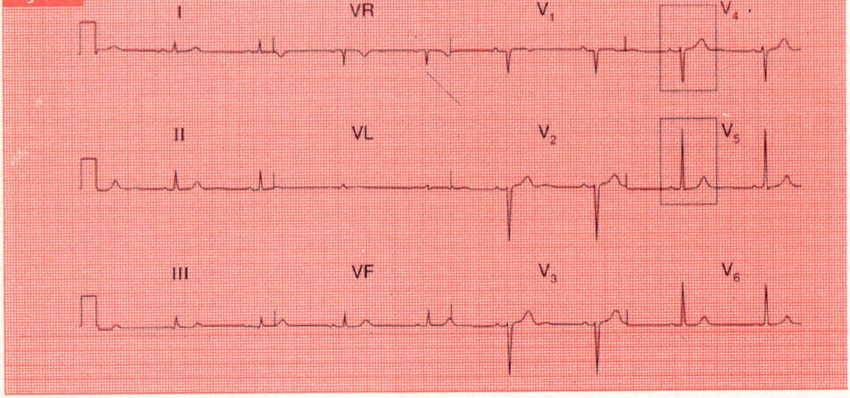

Fig. 3.11

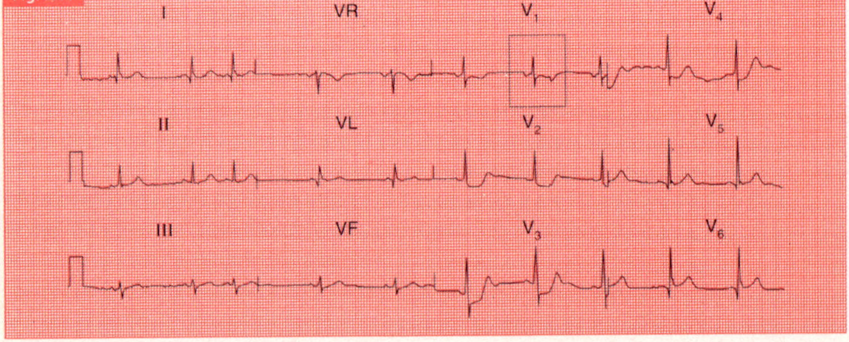

Old anterior infarction

Note

- Sinus rhythm
- Normal axis
- Small R waves in leads V_3–V_4, large R waves in V_5: this is 'poor R wave progression'

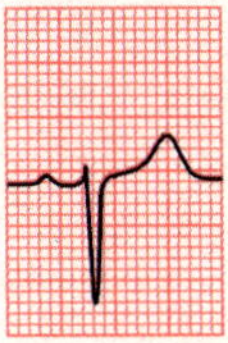

Small R wave In lead V_4

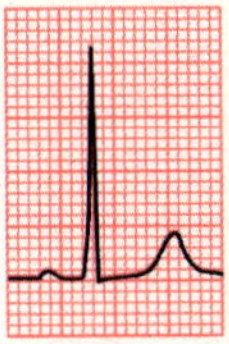

Tall R wave in lead V_5

POSTERIOR INFARCTION

It is possible to 'look at' the back of the heart by placing the V lead on the back of the left side of the chest, but this is not done routinely because it is inconvenient and the complexes recorded are often small.

An infarction of the posterior wall of the left ventricle can, however, be detected from the ordinary 12-lead ECG because it causes a dominant R wave in lead V_1. Normally the left ventricle, being more muscular than the right, exerts a greater influence on the ECG, so in lead V_1 the QRS complex is predominantly downward. With a posterior infarction, the rearward-moving electrical forces are lost so lead V_1 'sees' the unopposed forward-moving depolarization of the right ventricle, and records a predominantly upright QRS complex.

Figure 3.11 shows the first record from a patient with acute chest pain. There is a dominant R wave

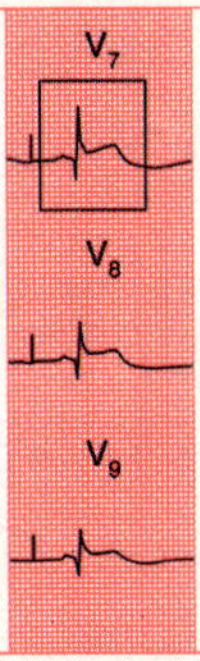

Posterior infarction

Note

- Sinus rhythm with atrial extrasystoles
- Normal axis
- Dominant R waves in lead V_1 suggest posterior infarction
- ST segment depression in leads V_2–V_4
- Q waves and ST segment elevation in leads V_7–V_9 (posterior leads)

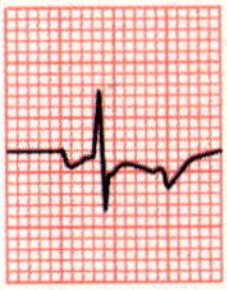

Dominant R wave in lead V_1

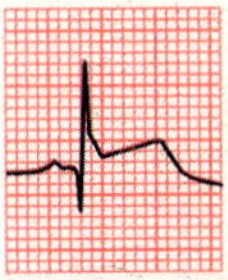

Q wave and raised ST segment in lead V_7

Fig. 3.12

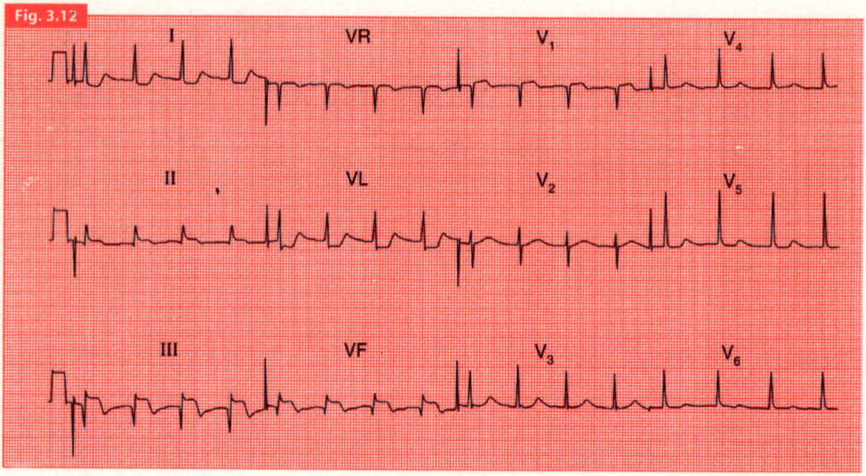

in lead V_1 and ischaemic ST segment depression (see p. 189) in leads V_2–V_4. The chest electrodes were then moved to the V_7–V_9 positions: all in the same horizontal plane as V_5, with V_7 on the posterior axillary line, V_9 at the edge of the spine, and V_8 halfway between, on the midscapular line. The ECG record then showed raised ST segments, with Q waves typical of an acute infarction.

RIGHT VENTRICULAR INFARCTION

Inferior infarction is sometimes associated with infarction of the right ventricle. Clinically, this is suspected in a patient with an inferior infarction when the lungs are clear but the jugular venous pressure is elevated. The ECG will show raised ST segments in leads recorded from the right side of the heart. The positions of the leads correspond to those on the left side as follows: V_1R is in the normal V_2 position; V_2R is in the normal V_1 position; V_3R etc. are on the right side, in positions corresponding to V_3 etc. on the left side. Figure 3.12 is from a patient with an acute right ventricular infarct.

MULTIPLE INFARCTIONS

Infarction of more than one part of the left ventricle causes changes in several different ECG territories.

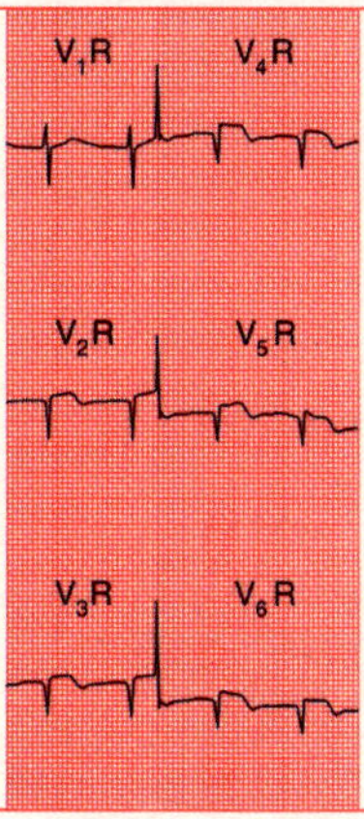

Inferior and right ventricular infarction

Note

- Sinus rhythm
- Normal axis
- Raised ST segments in leads II–III, VF
- Raised ST segments in leads V_2R–V_5R
- Q waves in leads III, VF, V_2R–V_6R

This usually implies disease in more than one of the main coronary arteries. The ECG in Figure 3.13 shows an acute inferior myocardial infarction and marked anterior ST segment depression. Later, coronary angiography showed that this patient had a significant stenosis of the left main coronary artery.

Figure 3.14 is the record from a patient with an acute inferior myocardial infarction. Poor R wave progression in leads V_2–V_4 indicates an old anterior infarction.

Figure 3.15 is an ECG showing an acute inferior infarction and anterior T wave inversion due to a STEMI (see p. 165).

Figure 3.16 is an ECG showing an acute anterior myocardial infarction. Deep Q waves in leads III and VF indicate an old inferior infarction.

Fig. 3.13

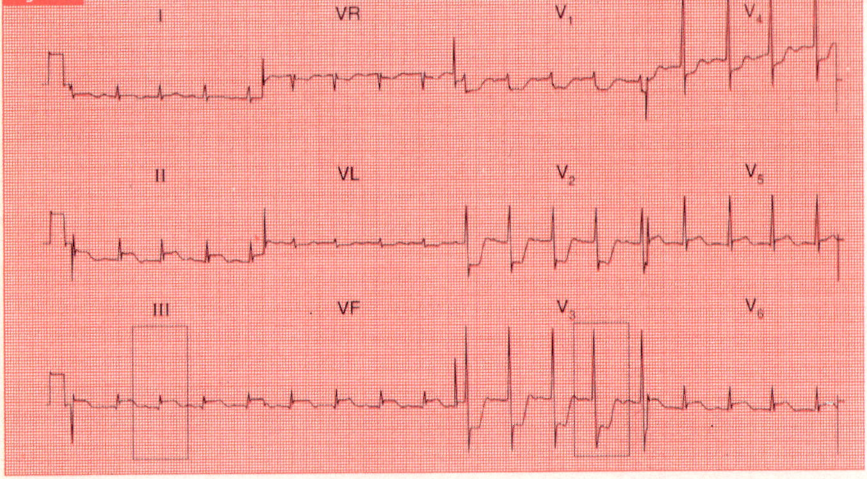

Fig. 3.14

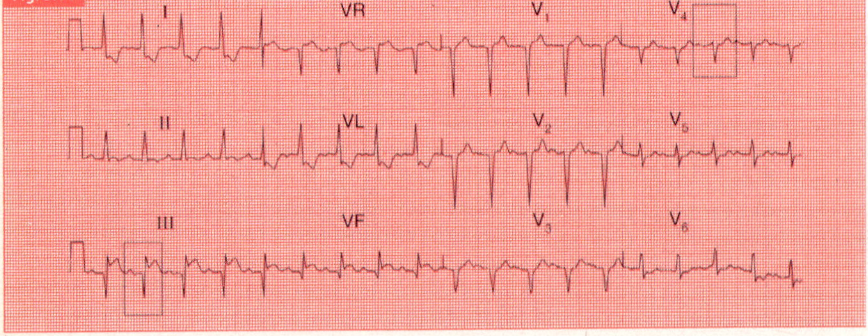

Acute inferior infarction and anterior ischaemia

Note

- Sinus rhythm
- Normal axis
- Raised ST segments in leads II–III, VF
- ST segment depression in leads V_1–V_4

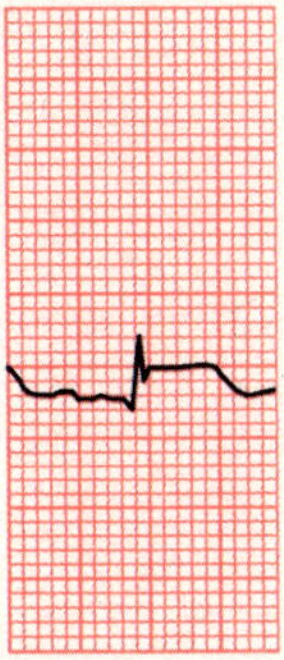

Raised ST segment in lead III

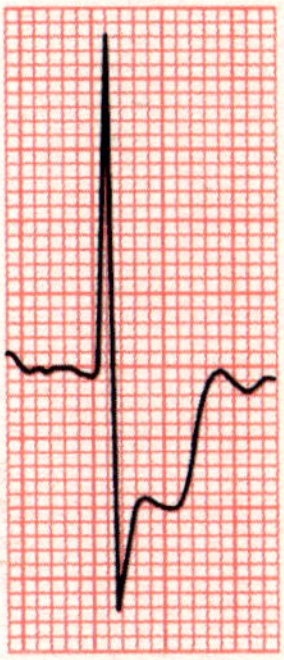

Depressed ST segment in lead V_3

Acute inferior and old anterior infarctions

Note

- Sinus rhythm
- Normal axis
- Q waves in leads III, VF
- Raised ST segments in leads III, VF
- Poor R wave progression in anterior leads

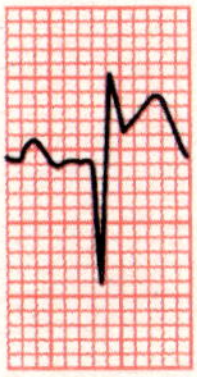

Q wave and raised ST segment in lead III

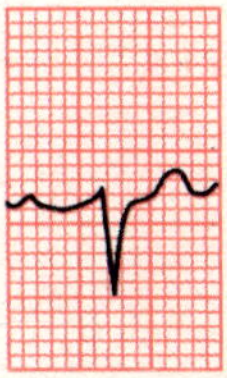

Loss of R wave in lead V_4

Fig. 3.15

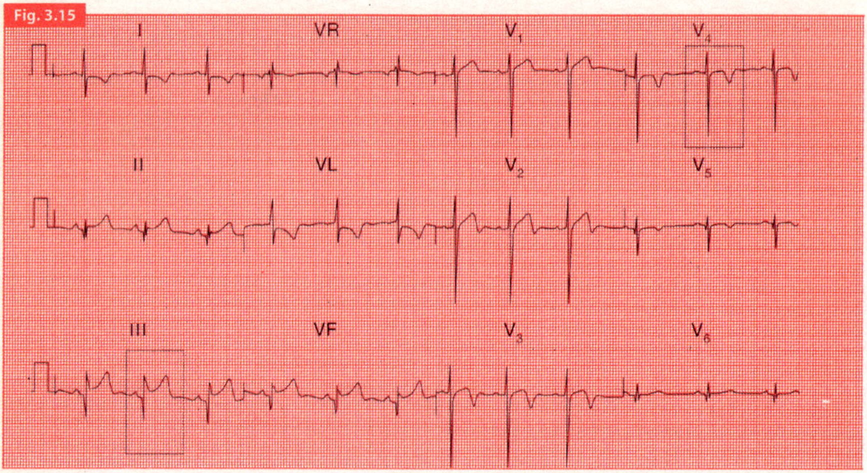

Fig. 3.16

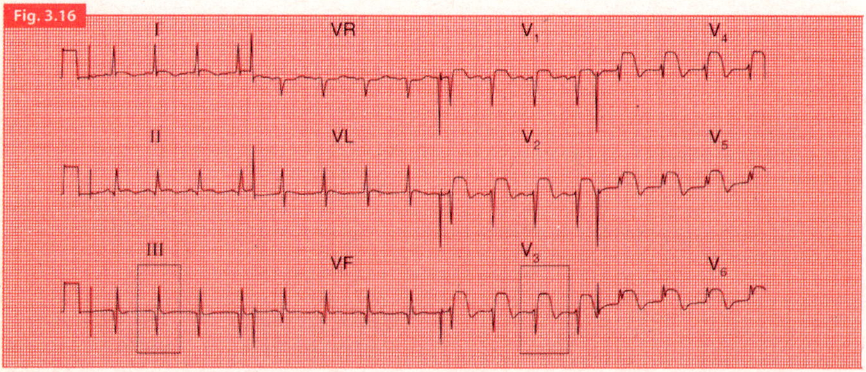

Acute inferior infarction and anterior STEMI

Note

- Sinus rhythm
- Normal axis
- Q waves in leads II–III, VF
- ST segment elevation in leads II–III, VF
- T wave inversion in leads V_3-V_5

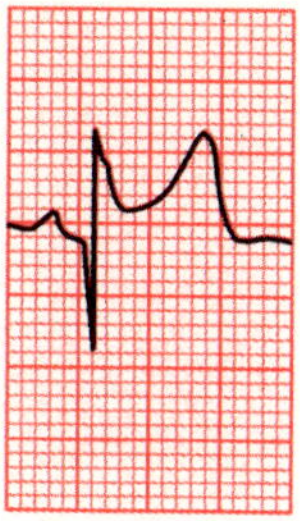

Q wave and ST segment elevation in lead III

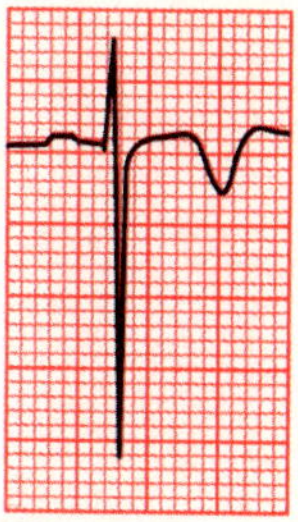

Inverted T wave in lead V_4

Acute anterior and old inferior infarctions

Note

- Sinus rhythm
- Normal axis
- Q waves in leads II–III, VF
- ST segment elevation in leads V_2–V_6

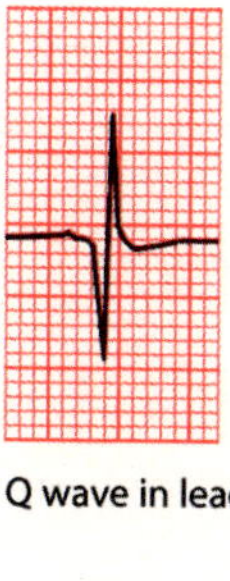

Q wave in lead III

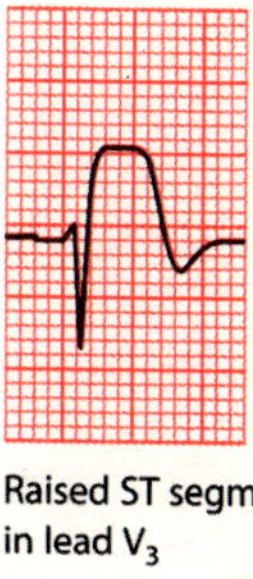

Raised ST segment in lead V_3

Fig. 3.17

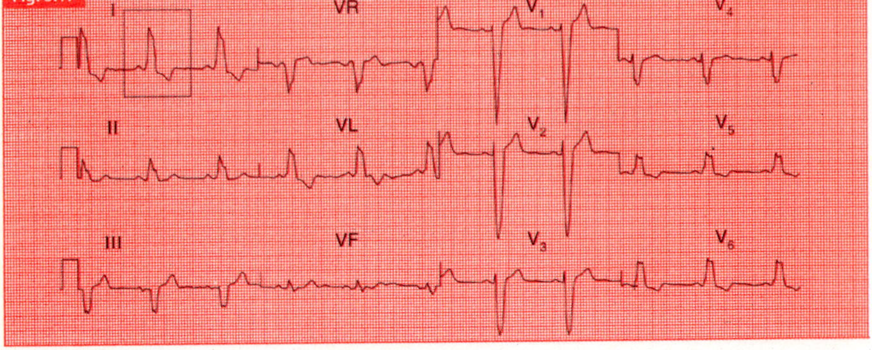

Fig. 3.18

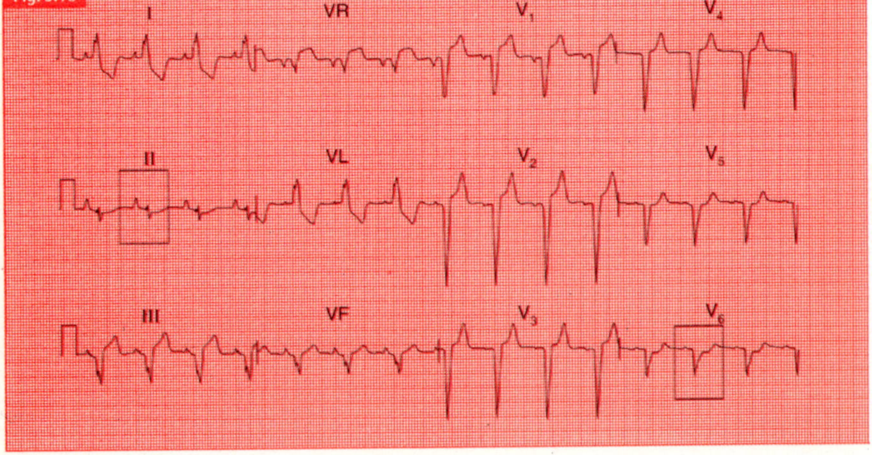

Left bundle branch block

Note

- Sinus rhythm
- Normal axis
- Wide QRS complexes with LBBB pattern
- Inverted T waves in leads I, VL, V_5–V_6

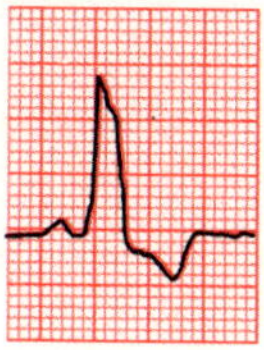

Broad QRS complex and inverted T wave in lead I

Left bundle branch block, ?right ventricular overload

Note

- Sinus rhythm
- Peaked P waves in leads I–II
- LBBB pattern, most obvious in leads I–II
- Persistent S wave in lead V_6

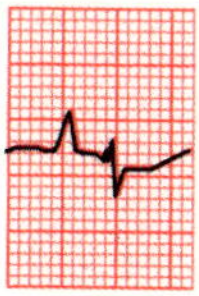

Peaked P wave in lead II

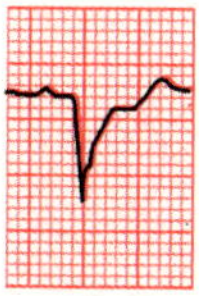

Persistent S wave in lead V_6

BUNDLE BRANCH BLOCK AND MYOCARDIAL INFARCTION

Left bundle branch block

With left bundle branch block (LBBB) (Fig. 3.17), no changes due to myocardial infarction can be seen. However, this does not mean that the ECG can be totally disregarded. If a patient has chest pain that could be ischaemic and the ECG shows LBBB that is known to be new, it can be assumed that an acute infarction has occurred and appropriate treatment should be given.

Figure 3.18 is the record from another patient presenting with chest pain who had LBBB, but there are important differences compared to Figure 3.17. Peaked P waves suggest right atrial hypertrophy. 'Clockwise rotation' with no left ventricular QRS complex pattern in lead V_6 raises the possibility of either a pulmonary embolus (see p. 211) or chronic lung disease.

Right bundle branch block

Right bundle branch block (RBBB) will not necessarily obscure the pattern of inferior infarction (Fig. 3.19).

Anterior infarction is more difficult to detect, but RBBB does not affect the ST segment and when this is raised in a patient who clinically has had an infarction, the change is probably significant (Fig. 3.20).

ST segment depression associated with RBBB indicates ischaemia (Fig. 3.21). However, T wave inversion in the anterior leads (Fig. 3.22) is more difficult to interpret because it is a common feature of RBBB itself.

Fig. 3.19

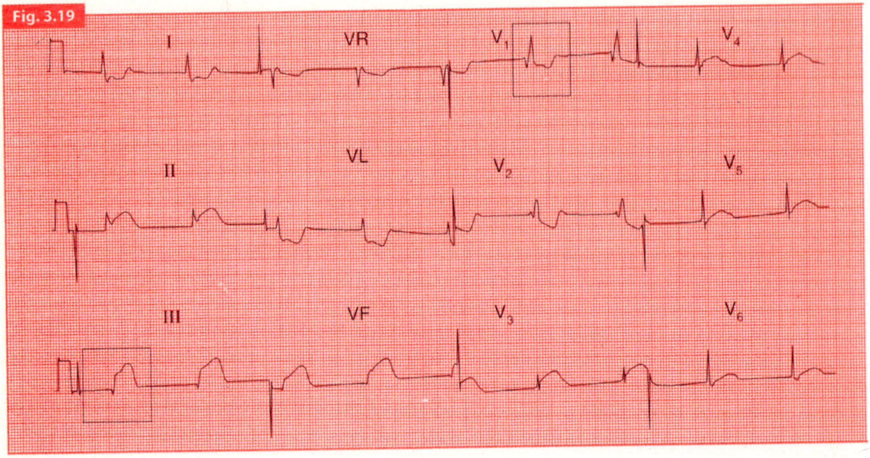

Fig. 3.20

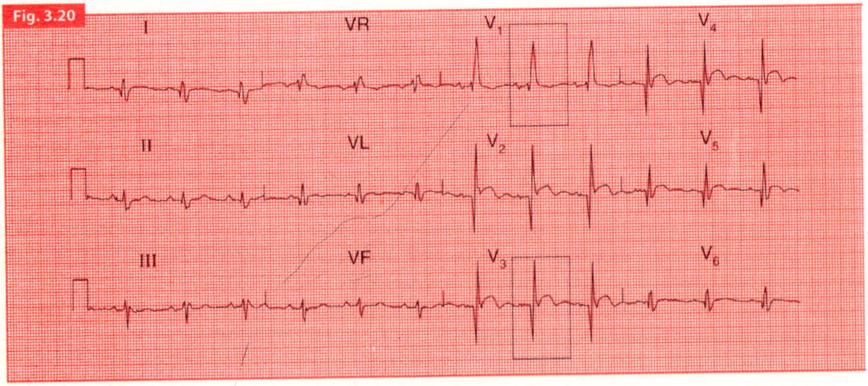

Right bundle branch block and acute inferior infarction

Note

- Sinus rhythm
- Normal axis
- Wide QRS complex with RSR[1] pattern in lead V_1
- Raised ST segments in leads II–III, VF

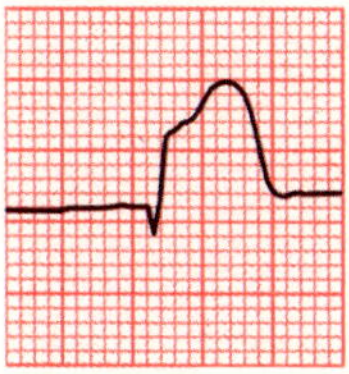

Raised ST segments in lead III

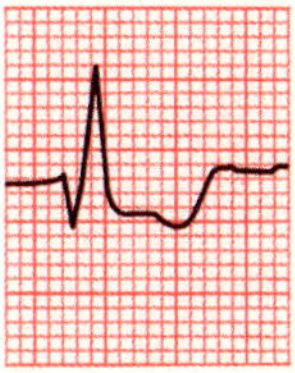

RSR[1] pattern in lead V_1

Right bundle branch block and anterior infarction

Note

- Sinus rhythm
- Normal axis
- RBBB pattern
- Raised ST segments in leads V_2–V_5

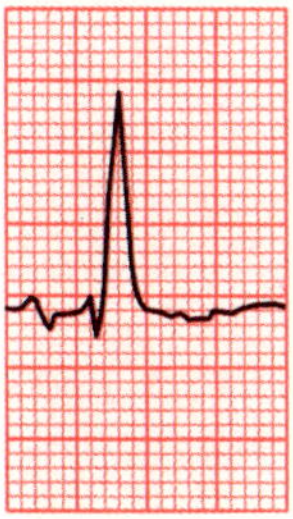

RSR[1] pattern in lead V_1

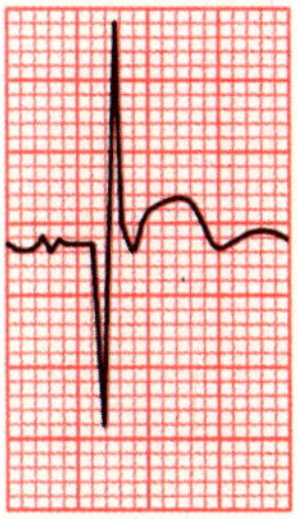

Raised ST segment in lead V_3

Fig. 3.21

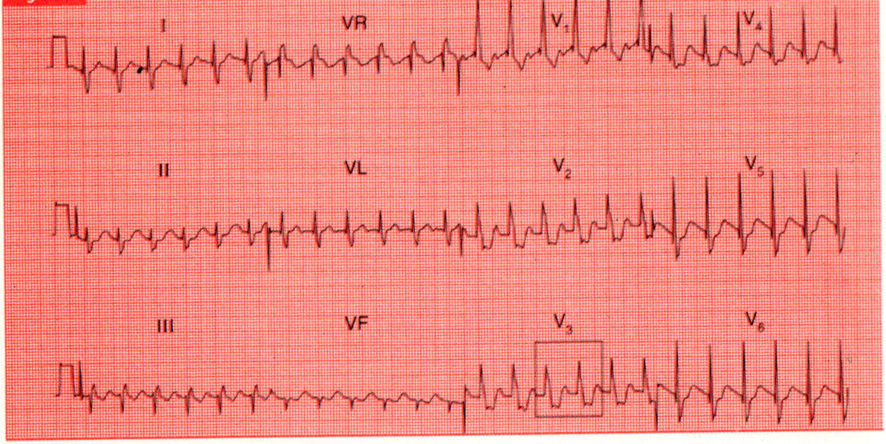

Fig. 3.22

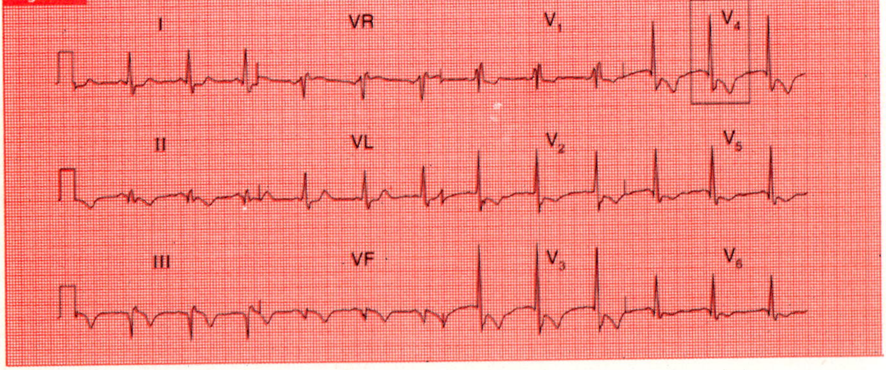

Right bundle branch block and anterior ischaemia

Note

- Sinus rhythm
- RBBB pattern
- ST segment depression in leads V_2–V_4

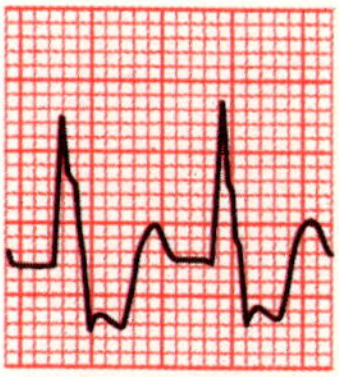

ST segment depression in lead V_3

Inferior infarction, right bundle branch block, ?anterior ischaemia

Note

- Sinus rhythm
- Q waves with inverted T waves in leads II–III, VF
- RBBB pattern
- Deep T wave inversion in leads V_3–V_4

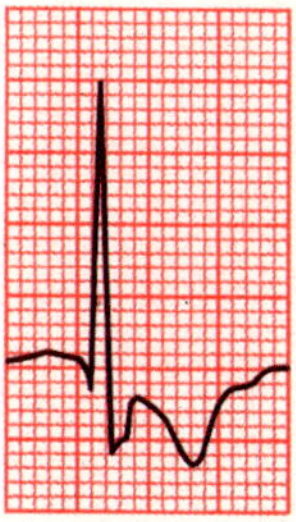

T wave inversion in lead V_4

Fig. 3.23

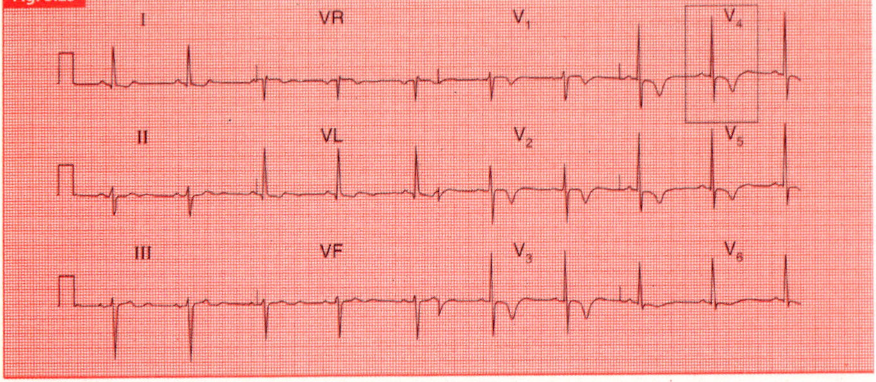

Fig. 3.24

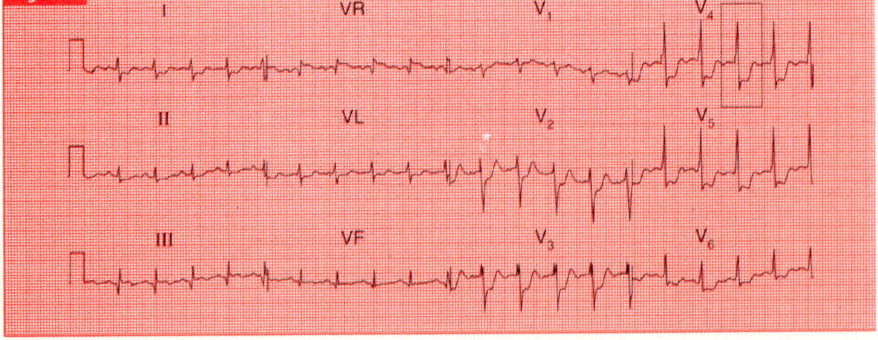

Anterior non-ST segment elevation myocardial infarction (NSTEMI)

Note

- Sinus rhythm
- Left axis deviation
- Normal QRS complexes
- Inverted T waves in all chest leads

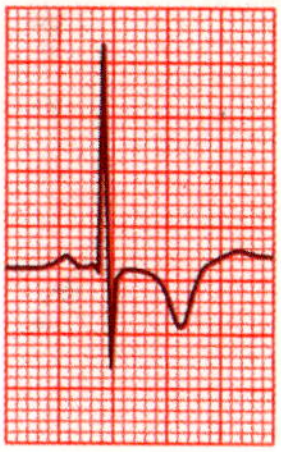

Inverted T wave in lead V_4

Anterior ischaemia, possible old inferior infarction

Note

- Sinus rhythm
- Normal axis
- Small Q waves in leads III, VF
- Inverted T waves in lead III
- Marked ST segment depression in leads V_2–V_6

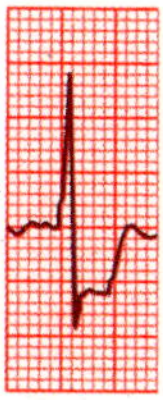

ST segment depression in lead V_4

ECG CHANGES IN NON-ST SEGMENT ELEVATION MYOCARDIAL INFARCTION (NSTEMI)

When the infarction does not involve the whole thickness of the ventricular wall, no electrical 'window' will be formed so there will be no Q waves: hence the term 'non-Q wave infarction', although this has now been superseded by the term 'NSTEMI'. The infarction will cause an abnormality of repolarization that leads to T wave inversion. This pattern is most commonly seen in the anterior and lateral leads (Fig. 3.23).

This ECG pattern is sometimes called 'subendocardial infarction', but the pathological changes seen in heart muscle after myocardial infarction often do not fit neatly into 'subendocardial' or 'full thickness' patterns. Acute NSTEMI is usually associated with a rise in the blood troponin level. Compared to patients with STEMIs, those with NSTEMIs have a high incidence of reinfarction during the following 3 months, but thereafter their fatality rates are similar.

ISCHAEMIA WITHOUT MYOCARDIAL INFARCTION

Cardiac ischaemia causes horizontal ST segment depression. This appears and disappears with the pain of stable angina. Persistent pain and ST segment depression (Fig. 3.24) may be associated with a rise in troponin level. When this occurs the prognosis is essentially the same as that following an NSTEMI.

Fig. 3.25

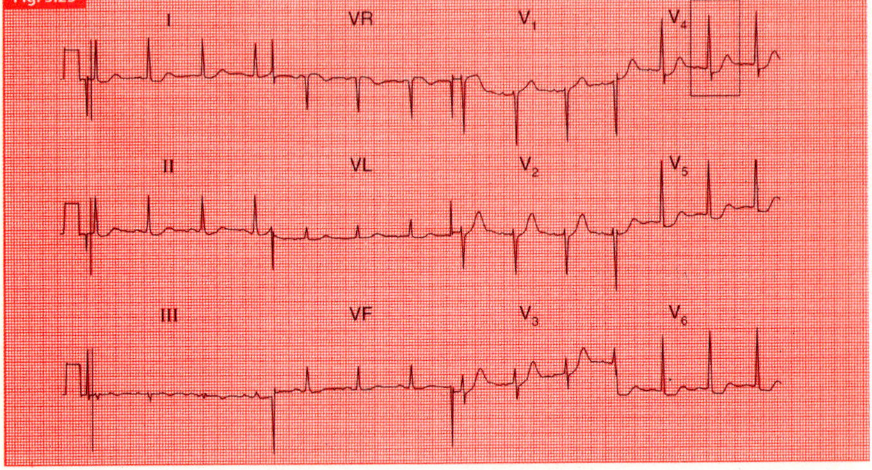

Fig. 3.26

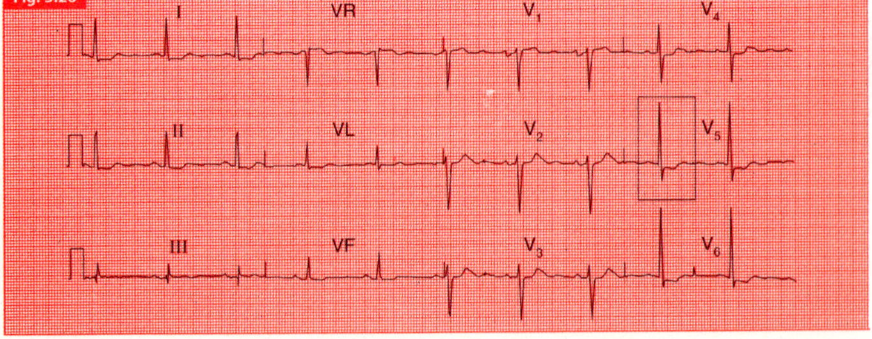

Anterior ischaemia

Note

- Sinus rhythm
- Normal axis
- Normal QRS complexes
- ST segment depression in leads V_4–V_6

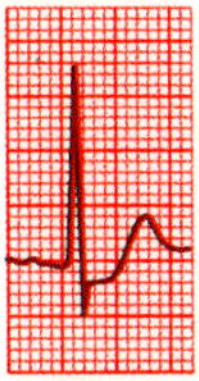

ST segment depression in lead V_4

If a patient has chest pain that persists long enough for him or her to seek hospital admission, and the ECG shows ST segment depression, the outlook is relatively poor – even when the ST segment depression is not marked (Figs 3.25 and 3.26) and there is no rise in troponin level. These patients usually need further investigation, though on the whole they can be managed as outpatients.

Ischaemia may be precipitated by an arrhythmia, and will be resolved when either the heart rate is controlled or the arrhythmia is corrected. The ECG in Figure 3.27 shows ischaemia during atrial fibrillation with a rapid ventricular rate (this patient had not been treated with digoxin). The ECG in Figure 3.28 shows ischaemic ST segment depression in a patient with an AV nodal re-entry tachycardia and a ventricular rate of over 200/min.

Anterolateral ischaemia

Note

- Sinus rhythm
- Possible left atrial hypertrophy (bifid P wave in lead I)
- Normal axis
- Normal QRS complexes
- ST segment depression in leads I, II, V_4–V_6

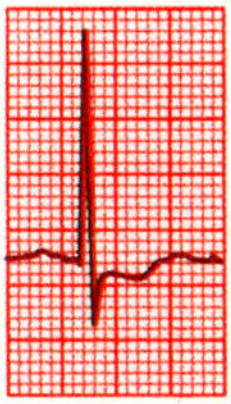

ST segment depression in lead V_5

Fig. 3.27

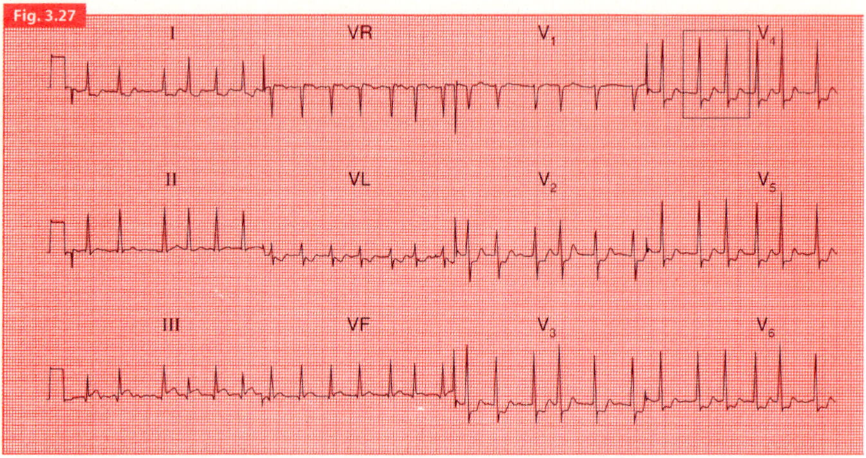

Fig. 3.28

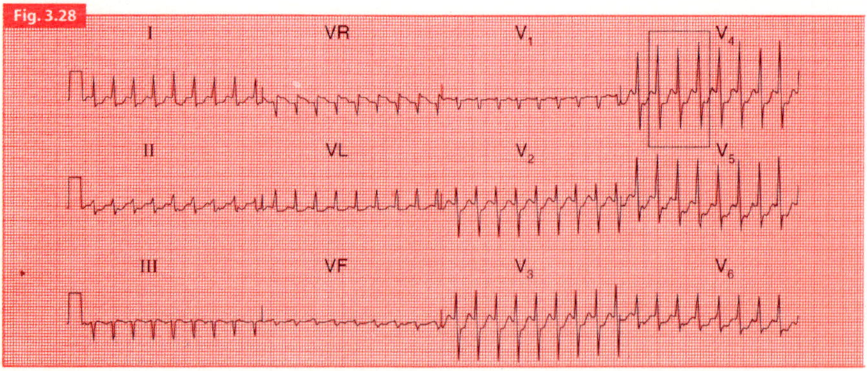

Atrial fibrillation and anterior ischaemia

Note

- Atrial fibrillation, ventricular rate about 130/min
- Normal axis
- Normal QRS complexes
- ST segment depression in leads V_2–V_6

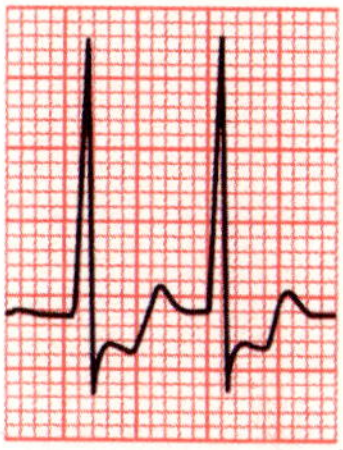

ST segment depression in lead V_4

AV nodal re-entry tachycardia with anterior ischaemia

Note

- Regular narrow complex tachycardia, rate 215/min
- No P waves
- ST segment depression in leads V_2–V_6

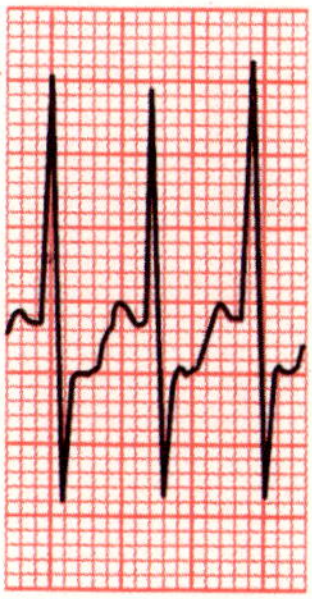

Narrow complexes and ST segment depression in lead V_4

PRINZMETAL'S 'VARIANT' ANGINA

Angina can occur at rest due to spasm of the coronary arteries. This is accompanied by elevation rather than depression of the ST segments. The ECG appearance is similar to that of an acute myocardial infarction, but the ST segment returns to normal as the pain settles (Fig. 3.29). This ECG appearance was first described by Prinzmetal, and it is sometimes called 'variant' angina.

EXERCISE TESTING

Although any form of exercise that induces pain should produce ischaemic changes in the ECG, it is best to use a reproducible test that patients find reasonably easy to perform, and to use carefully graded increments of exercise. The use of non-standard tests means that the results may be difficult to interpret, and that repeated tests in the same patient cannot be compared meaningfully. It is important to remember that exercise testing provides much useful information in addition to causing changes in the ST segment of the ECG. Things to look for during an exercise test include:

- the patient's attitude to exercise
- the reasons for exercise limitation
  - chest pain
  - breathlessness
  - claudication
  - fatigue
  - musculoskeletal problems
- the pumping capability of the heart
  - maximum heart rate achieved
  - maximum rise in blood pressure
- physical fitness
  - workload at which maximum heart rate is achieved
  - duration of tachycardia following exercise
- ischaemic changes in the ECG
- exercise-induced arrhythmias.

Fig. 3.29

Prinzmetal's variant angina

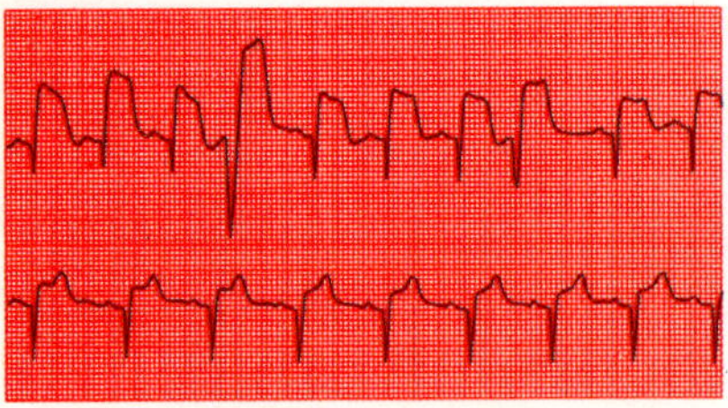

Note

- Continuous record
- Initially the patient had pain and the ST segment was raised
- The fourth beat is probably a ventricular extrasystole
- As the patient's pain settled the ST segment returned to normal

PRACTICAL ASPECTS OF EXERCISE TESTING

Reproducible exercise testing needs either a bicycle ergometer or a treadmill. In either case, the exercise should begin at a low level that the patient finds easy, and should be made progressively more difficult. On a bicycle, the pedal speed should be kept constant and the workload increased in steps of 25 watts. On a treadmill, both the slope and the speed can be changed and the protocol evolved by Bruce (Table 3.1) is the one most commonly used.

The workload achieved by a patient on a treadmill is sometimes expressed as metabolic equivalents (METS). The rate at which oxygen is used by an average person at rest is 1 MET, and it equals 3.5 ml/kg/min. However, few people are average and oxygen consumption is dependant on weight, age and gender, so METS are not particularly useful. Box 3.3 shows the estimated workloads imposed by various activities, and hence how exercise tolerance (as measured on the treadmill) indicates what a patient might be expected to achieve.

Box 3.3 Average workloads, expressed in metabolic equivalents

Activity	METS
Cleaning floors	4.0
Gardening	4.0
Sexual intercourse	5.0
Bedmaking	5.0–6.0
Carrying a medium suitcase	7.0

Table 3.1 Bruce protocol for exercise testing using a treadmill, 3 min at each stage

Stage	Speed		Slope		METS (metabolic equivalents)
	Miles per hour	Kilometres per hour	Grade (%)	Degrees to horizontal	
Low level					
01	1.7	2.7	0	0	2.9
02	1.7	2.7	5	2.9	3.7
Standard Bruce protocol					
1	1.7	2.7	10	5.7	5.0
2	2.5	4.0	12	6.8	7.0
3	3.4	5.5	14	8.0	9.5
4	4.2	6.8	16	9.1	13.5
5	5.0	8.0	18	10.2	17.0

A 12-lead ECG, the heart rate and the blood pressure should be recorded at the end of each exercise period. The maximum heart rate and blood pressure are in some ways more important than the maximum workload achieved, because the latter is markedly influenced by physical fitness. However, the ECG recorded during exercise testing is unreliable in cases of:

- bundle branch block
- ventricular hypertrophy
- the Wolff–Parkinson–White syndrome
- digoxin therapy
- beta-blocker therapy.

REASONS FOR DISCONTINUING AN EXERCISE TEST

1. At the request of the patient – because of pain, breathlessness, fatigue or dizziness.
2. If the systolic blood pressure begins to fall. Normally, systolic pressure will rise progressively with increasing exercise level, but in any subject a point will be reached at which systolic pressure reaches a plateau and then starts to fall. A fall of 10 mmHg is an indication that the heart is not pumping effectively and the test should be stopped – if it is continued, the patient will become dizzy and may fall. In healthy subjects, a fall in systolic pressure is seen only at high workloads, but in patients with severe heart disease the systolic pressure may fail to rise on exercise. The amount of exercise the patient can carry out before the systolic pressure falls is thus a useful indicator of the severity of any heart disease.
3. It is conventional to discontinue the test if the heart rate increases to 80% of the predicted maximum for the patient's age. This maximum can be calculated in beats/min by subtracting the patient's age in years from 220. Patients with severe heart disease will usually fail to attain 80% of their predicted maximum heart rate, and the peak rate is another useful indicator of the state of the patient's heart. It is, of course, important to take note of any treatment the patient may be receiving, because a beta-blocker will prevent the normal increase in heart rate.
4. Exercise should be discontinued immediately if an arrhythmia occurs. Many patients will have ventricular extrasystoles during exercise. These can be ignored unless their frequency begins to rise, or a couplet of extrasystoles occurs.
5. The test should be stopped if the ST segment in any lead becomes depressed by 4 mm. 2 mm of horizontal depression in any lead is usually taken as indicating that a diagnosis of ischaemia can be made (a 'positive' test), and if the aim of the test is to confirm or refute a diagnosis of angina there is no point in continuing once this has occurred. It may, however, be useful to find out just how much a patient can do, and if this is the aim of the test it is not unreasonable to continue, if the patient's symptoms are not severe.

INTERPRETATION OF ECG CHANGES DURING EXERCISE TESTING

The final report of the test should indicate the duration of exercise, the workload achieved, the maximum heart rate and systolic pressure, the reason for discontinuing the test, and a description of any arrhythmias or ST segment changes.

An exercise test is usually considered 'positive' for ischaemia if horizontal or downward-sloping ST segment depression of 2 mm or more develops during exercise, and resolves on resting. A diagnosis of ischaemia becomes almost certain if these changes are accompanied by the appearance and then disappearance of angina. Figures 3.30 and 3.31 show an ECG that was normal when the patient was at rest, but which demonstrated clear ischaemia during exercise.

There are, however, other ECG changes that may be seen during an exercise test. Figures 3.32 and 3.33 show the records of tests in a patient who had had an anterior myocardial infarction some weeks previously. At rest, some ST segment elevation persisted in the anterior leads. During exercise the ST elevation became more marked. The reasons for this are uncertain. It has been suggested that the change is due to the development of an abnormality of left ventricular contraction, but other evidence suggests that it is simply another ECG manifestation of ischaemia. There is, however, no doubt that this is an abnormal result.

When the resting ECG shows T wave inversion and on exercise the T waves become upright, this is called 'pseudonormalization', and it is a sign of ischaemia (Fig. 3.34).

When the ST segment becomes depressed during exercise, but slopes upwards, the change is not an indication of ischaemia (Figs 3.35 and 3.36). Deciding whether ST segment depression slopes upwards or is horizontal can be quite difficult.

'False positive' changes also occur when exercise testing is performed in patients taking digoxin. Figures 3.37 and 3.38 show the results of an exercise test in a patient being treated with digoxin, whose coronary angiogram was normal.

In a patient suspected of having coronary disease, exercise testing gives the 'right' answer in about 75% of patients tested – to be more precise, exercise testing has a sensitivity of 78% and a specificity of 70%. All tests at times give 'false positive' and 'false negative' results, reflecting their sensitivity and specificity, and false positive tests are particularly common in middle-aged women. In an asymptomatic subject in whom the likelihood of coronary disease is low, the chance of a 'false positive' result may be higher than the chance of a 'true positive'. Also, the greater the likelihood that the patient has coronary disease, the more likely it is that a positive test is 'true' rather than 'false'. The statistics (Bayes' theorem) may seem complex, but the important thing is to remember that exercise testing is not infallible.

Exercise testing thus has to be used and interpreted with care.

Fig. 3.30

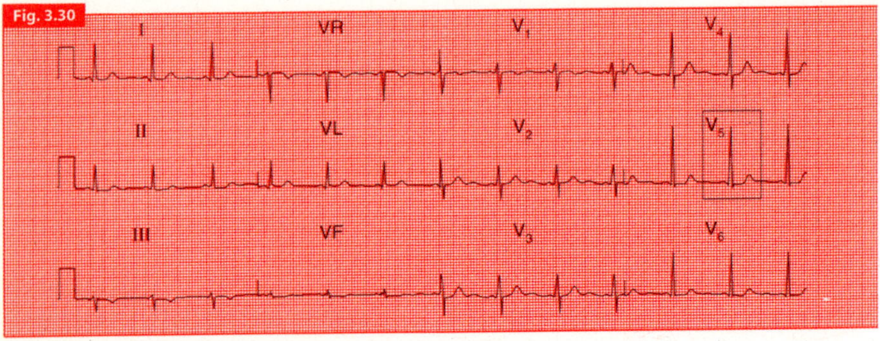

Fig. 3.31

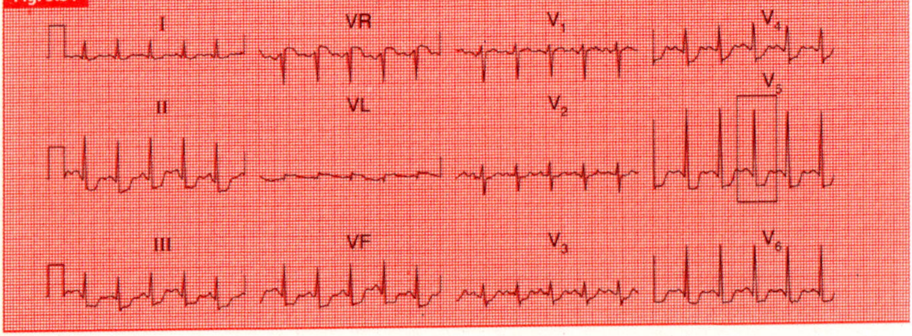

Probably normal record

Note

- Sinus rhythm
- Normal axis
- Normal QRS complexes
- Some nonspecific T wave change in leads III, VF

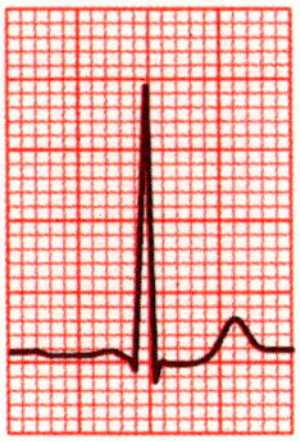

Normal ST segment in lead V_5

Exercise-induced ischaemia

Note

- Same patient as in Figure 3.30
- Sinus rhythm, 138/min
- Horizontal ST segment depression in leads II-III, VF, V_4–V_6

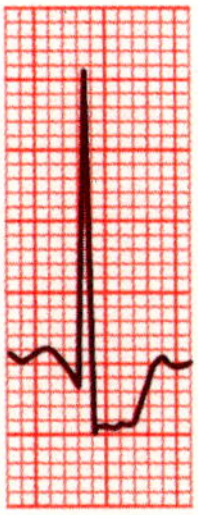

Horizontal ST segment depression in lead V_5

Fig. 3.32

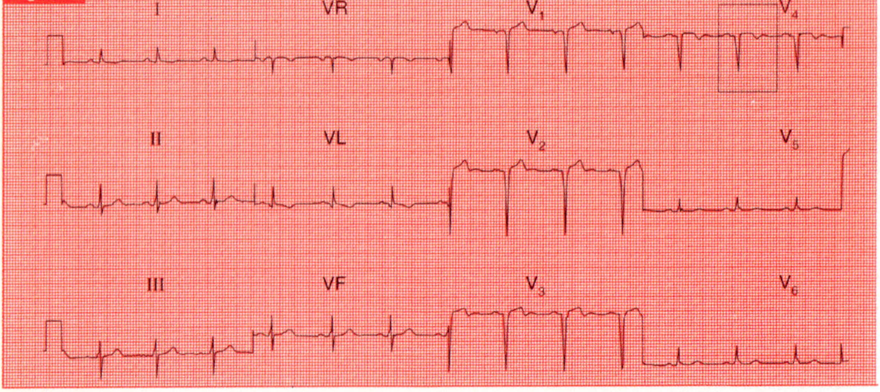

Fig. 3.33

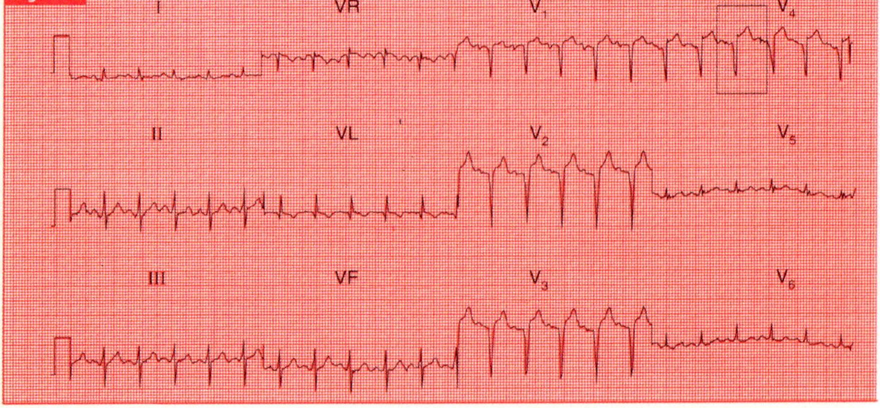

Anterior infarction, ?age

Note

- Sinus rhythm
- Normal axis
- Q waves in leads V_2–V_4
- Slight ST segment elevation in leads V_2–V_4

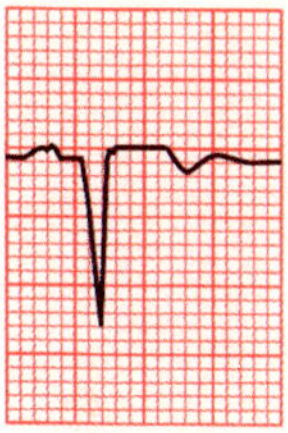

Q wave, slight ST segment elevation and inverted T wave in lead V_4

Exercise-induced ST segment elevation

Note

- Same patient as in Figure 3.32
- The ST segments are now higher in leads V_3–V_4

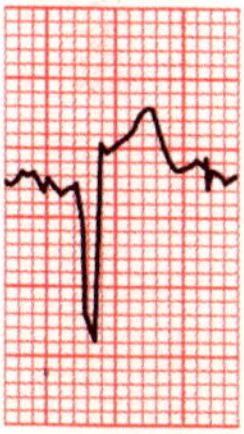

More ST segment elevation in lead V_4

Fig. 3.34

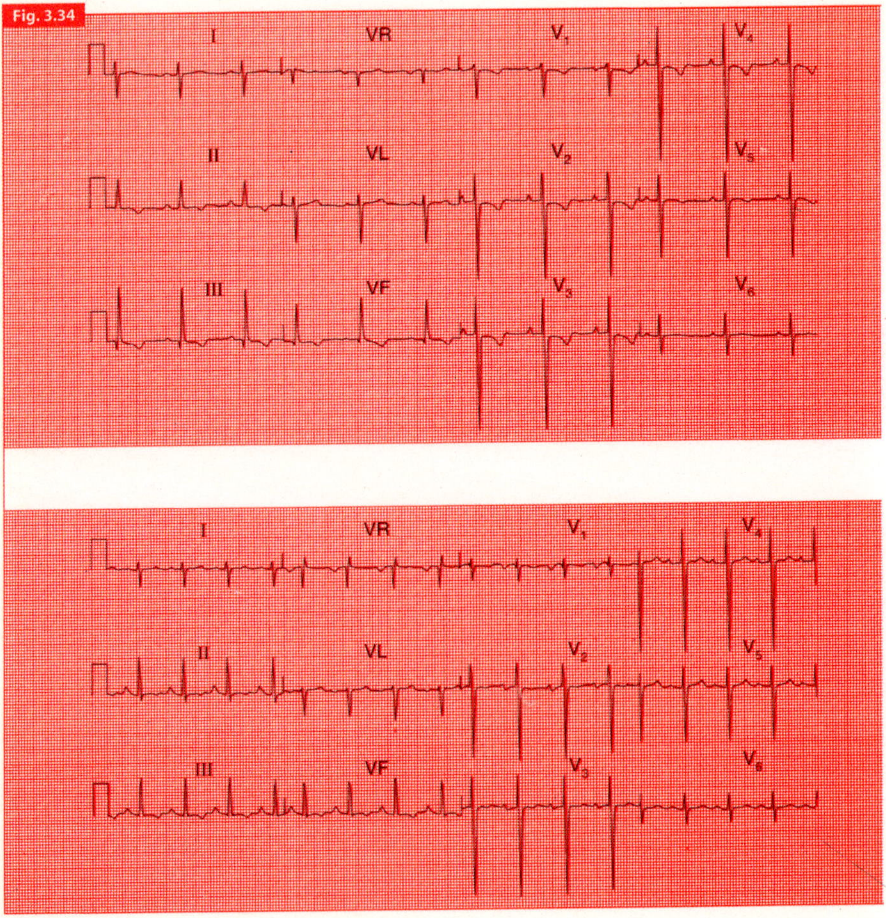

Pseudonormalization

Note

At rest (upper trace):

- Right axis deviation
- Small Q waves with inverted T waves in leads III and VF suggest an old inferior infarction
- T wave inversion in leads II and V_2–V_4 suggests ischaemia (T wave inversion in lead V_1 is normal)

On exercise (lower trace):

- Q waves disappear
- T wave inversion partly 'normalizes' in lead II and completely 'normalizes' in the chest leads, but persists in lead VF

This pattern suggests the pseudonormalization of an ECG showing ischaemia at rest

Fig. 3.35

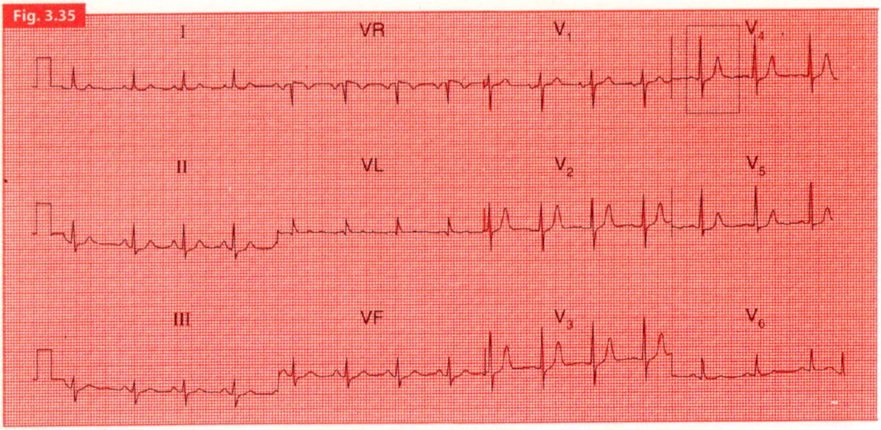

Fig. 3.36

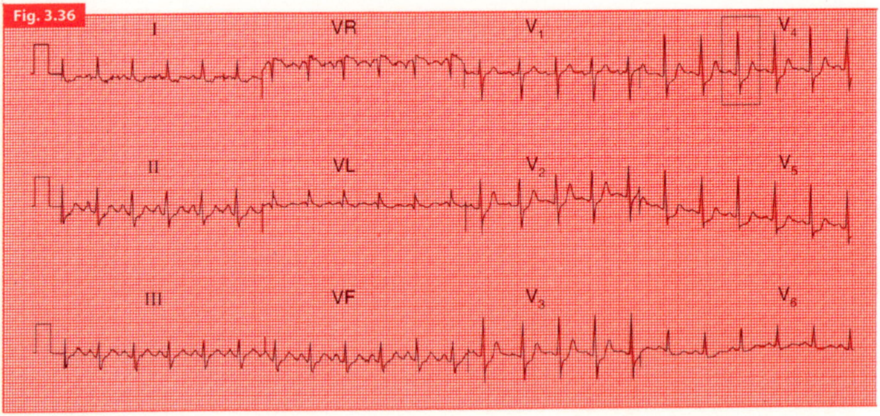

Normal ECG

Note

- Sinus rhythm
- Normal axis
- Normal QRS complexes
- Possible minimal ST segment depression in lead V_5

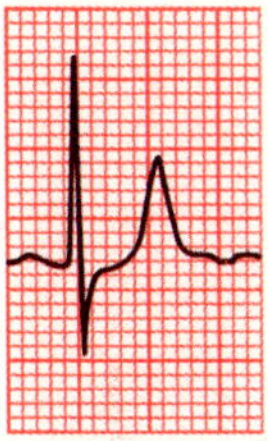

Normal ST segment in lead V_4

Exercise-induced ST segment depression

Note

- Same patient as Figure 3.35
- On exercise there is ST segment depression which slopes upwards
- This is not diagnostic of ischaemia, but the change in lead V_5 is suspicious

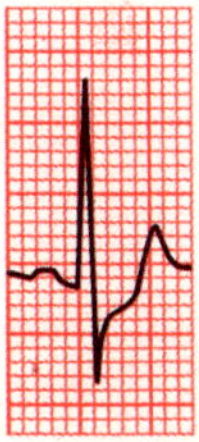

Upward-sloping ST segment depression in lead V_4

Fig. 3.37

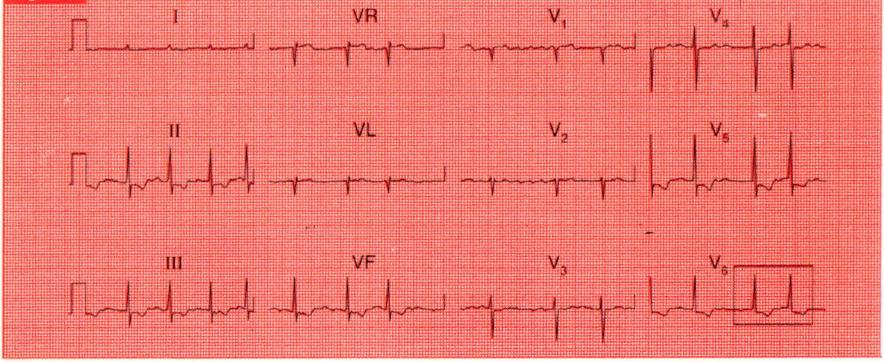

Fig. 3.38

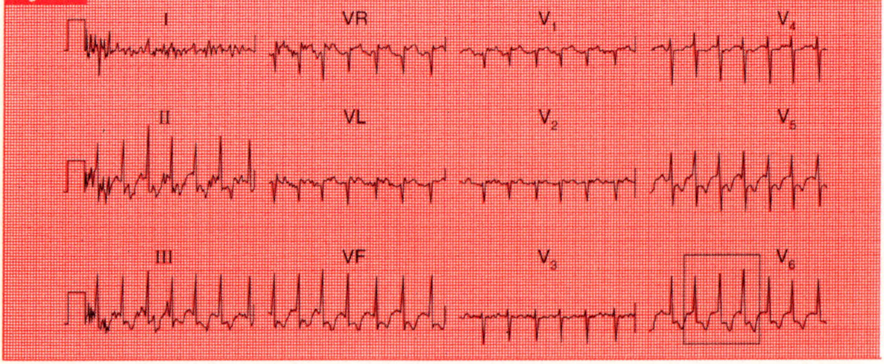

Atrial fibrillation: digoxin effect at rest

Note

- Atrial fibrillation
- ST segments slope downwards and T waves are inverted in leads V_5–V_6: typical of digoxin effect

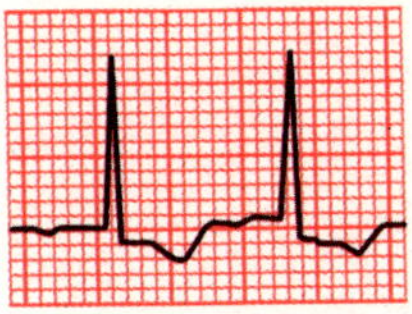

Downward-sloping ST segment and inverted T wave in lead V_6

Atrial fibrillation: digoxin effect on exercise

Note

- Same patient as Figure 3.37
- Heart rate 165/min
- ST segment depression in lead V_6 could be ischaemic but could be a 'false positive' due to digoxin

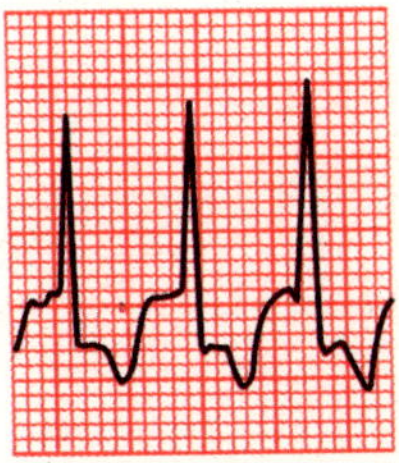

Further ST segment depression in lead V_6

Fig. 3.39

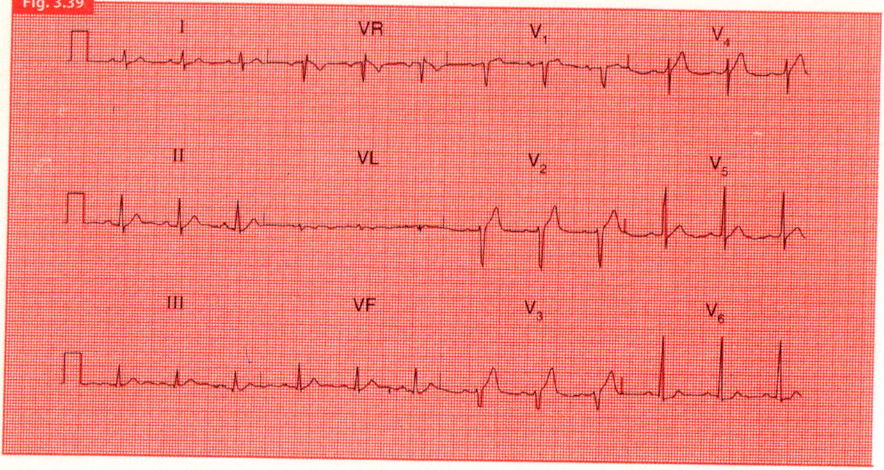

Fig. 3.40

Exercise-induced ventricular extrasystoles

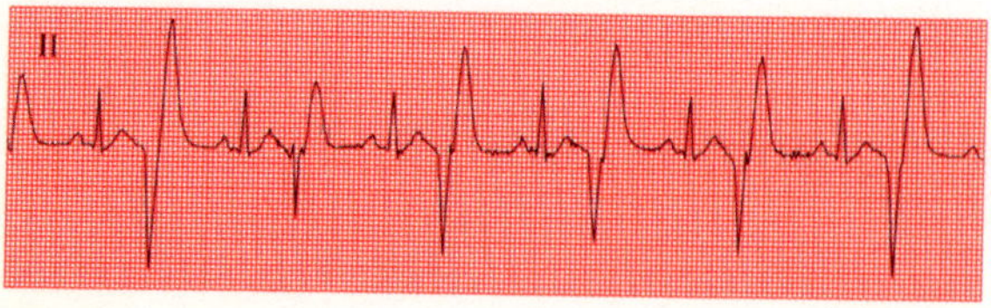

Note

- Same patient as in Figures 3.39 and 3.41
- Sinus rhythm with coupled ventricular extrasystoles

Pre-exercise: normal ECG

Note

- Sinus rhythm
- Heart rate 75/min
- Possible nonspecific ST segment depression in lead V_6

RISKS OF EXERCISE TESTING

Exercise testing involves a risk of about 1 in 5000 of the development of ventricular tachycardia or ventricular fibrillation, and a risk of about 1 in 10 000 tests of myocardial infarction or death. There is also a risk of injury if the patient falls, or jumps, off the treadmill.

The ECGs in Figures 3.39, 3.40 and 3.41 are from a patient whose resting ECG was normal, but as the test proceeded he began to develop ventricular extrasystoles and then suddenly developed ventricular fibrillation. This demonstrates the need for full resuscitation facilities to be available at the time of exercise testing.

Fig. 3.41

Exercise-induced ventricular fibrillation

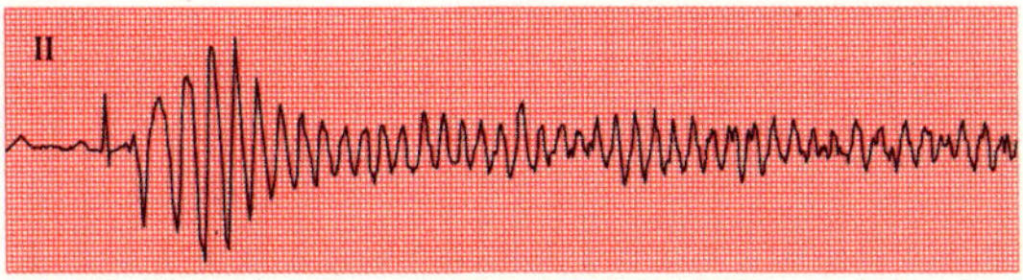

Note

- Same patient as in Figures 3.39 and 3.40
- One sinus beat is followed by an extrasystole with the R on T phenomenon
- A few beats of ventricular tachycardia decay into ventricular fibrillation

Fig. 3.42

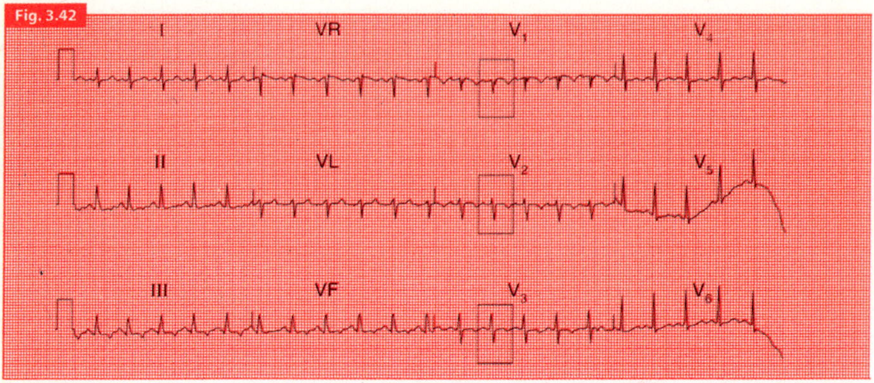

Fig. 3.43

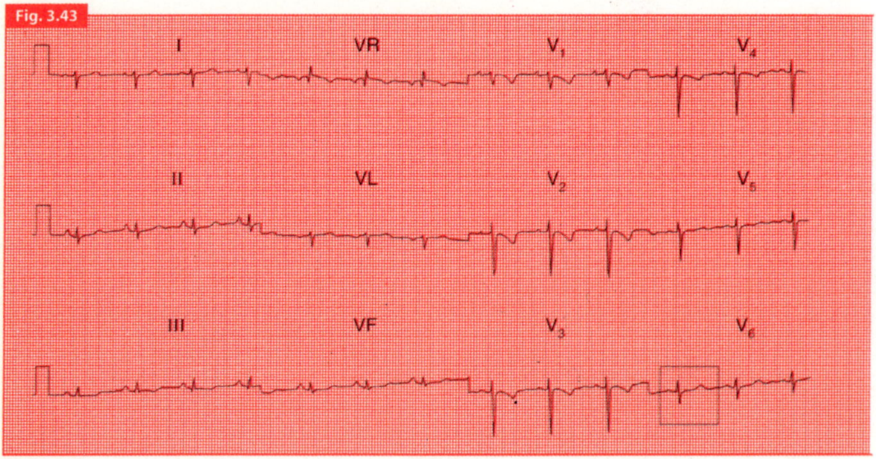

Pulmonary embolus

Note

- Sinus rhythm, 130/min
- Normal axis
- Normal QRS complexes
- Inverted T wave in leads V_1–V_3, VF

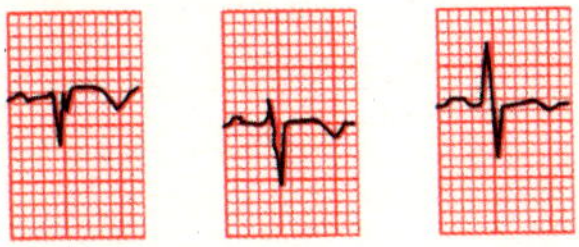

Inverted T wave in leads V_1–V_3

Pulmonary embolus

Note

- Sinus rhythm
- Right axis deviation
- Persistent S wave in lead V_6
- T wave inversion in leads V_1–V_4

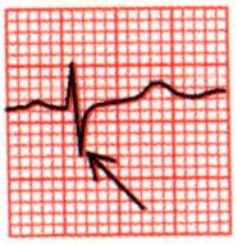

Persistent S wave in lead V_6

THE ECG IN PULMONARY EMBOLISM

Most patients with a pulmonary embolus will have sinus tachycardia, but an otherwise normal ECG.

The ECG abnormalities that may occur in pulmonary embolism are those associated with right ventricular problems:

- right axis deviation
- dominant R wave in lead V_1
- inverted T waves in leads V_1–V_3, and sometimes V_4
- right bundle branch block pattern
- Q wave and inverted T wave in lead III.

Supraventricular arrhythmias, especially atrial fibrillation, may also occur. There is no particular sequence in which these changes develop, and they can be seen in any combination. The full ECG pattern of right ventricular hypertrophy (right axis deviation, dominant R waves in lead V_1, inverted T waves in leads V_1–V_4, and persistent S waves in lead V_6) is usually only seen in patients with long-standing thromboembolic pulmonary hypertension.

Figures 3.42, 3.43, 3.44 and 3.45 show the records from four patients with a pulmonary embolus – but remember, in most patients the ECG is normal.

Fig. 3.44

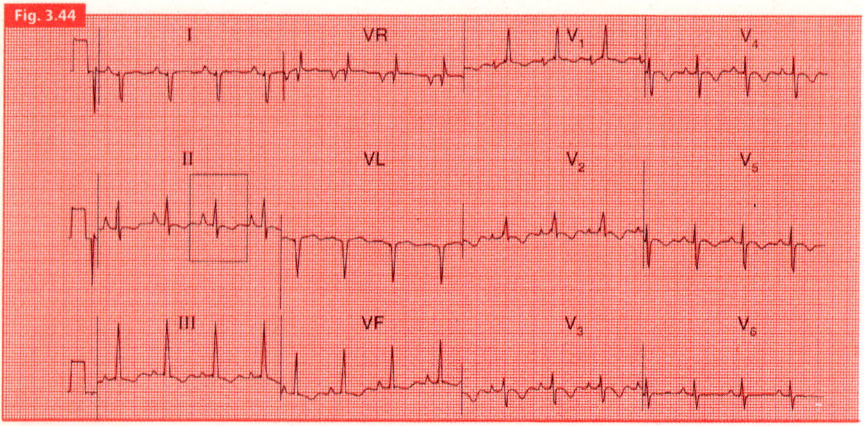

Fig. 3.45

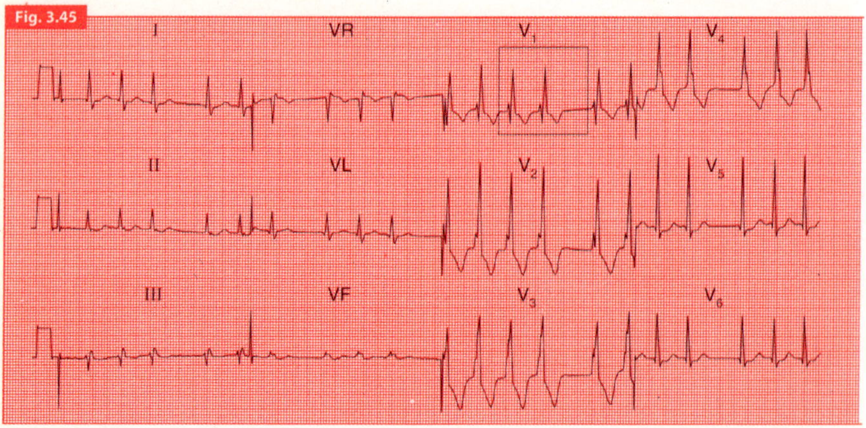

Pulmonary embolus

Note

- Sinus rhythm
- Peaked P wave suggests right atrial hypertrophy
- Right axis deviation
- Right bundle branch block pattern
- Persistent S wave in lead V_6
- T wave inversion in leads V_1–V_4

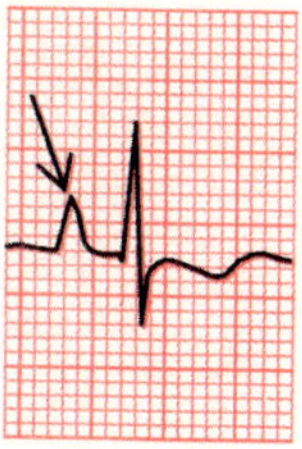

Peaked P wave in lead II

Pulmonary embolus

Note

- Atrial fibrillation
- Right bundle branch block pattern

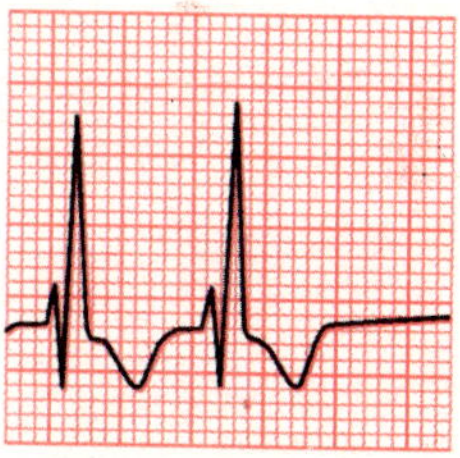

RSR[1] pattern in lead V_1

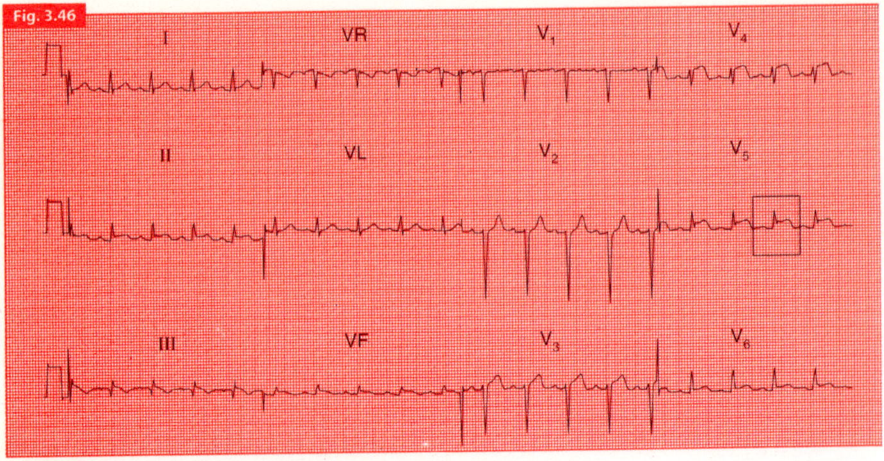
Fig. 3.46
I
VR
V1
V4
II
VL
V2
V5
III
VF
V3
V6

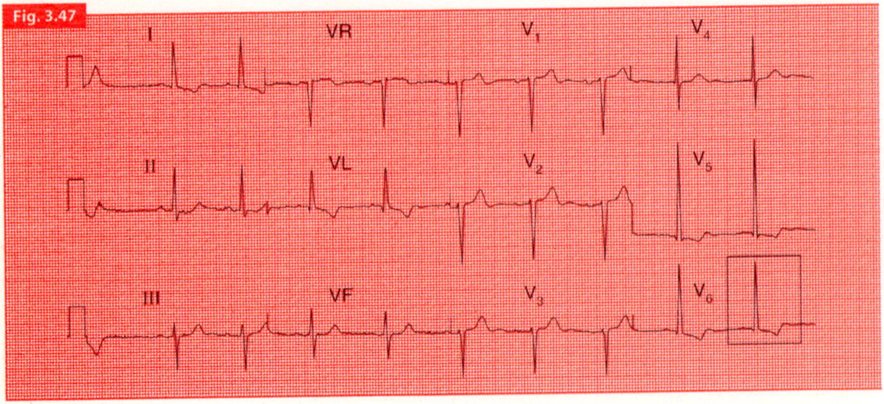
Fig. 3.47
I
VR
V1
V4
II
VL
V2
V5
III
VF
V3
V6

Pericarditis

Note
- Sinus rhythm
- Normal axis
- Normal QRS complexes
- ST segment elevation in leads I–III, VF, V_3–V_6

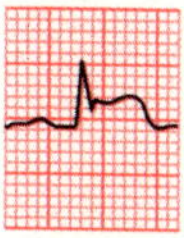

ST segment elevation in lead V_5

Left ventricular hypertrophy

Note
- Sinus rhythm
- Tall R waves in leads V_5–V_6
- Inverted T waves in lateral leads

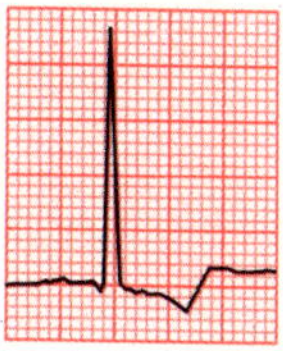

Tall R wave and inverted T wave in lead V_6

THE ECG IN OTHER CAUSES OF CHEST PAIN

PERICARDITIS

Pericarditis classically causes raised ST segments in most leads (Fig. 3.46). This may suggest a widespread acute infarction, but in pericarditis the ST segment remains elevated and Q waves do not develop. This pattern is actually very rare: most patients with pericarditis have either a normal ECG, or a variety of nonspecific ST segment/T wave changes.

AORTIC STENOSIS AND AORTIC DISSECTION

Aortic stenosis is an important cause of angina. The ECG should show left ventricular hypertrophy (Fig. 3.47). However, the ECG is an unreliable guide to left ventricular hypertrophy and the difficulty of distinguishing it from ischaemia is discussed in Chapter 4.

The presence of left ventricular hypertrophy in the ECG of a patient with chest pain also raises the possibility of aortic dissection.

احمر

Fig. 3.48

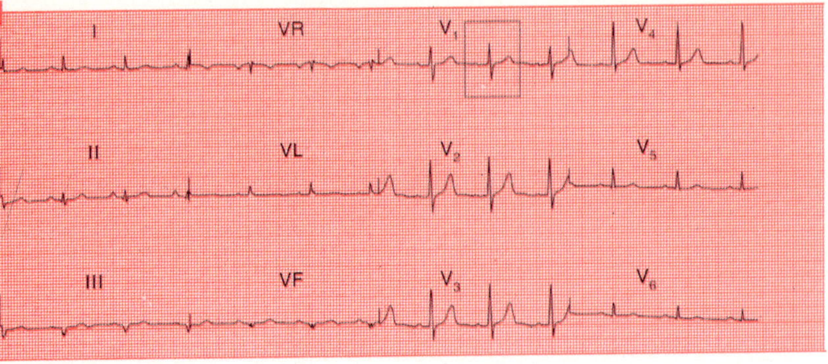

Fig. 3.49

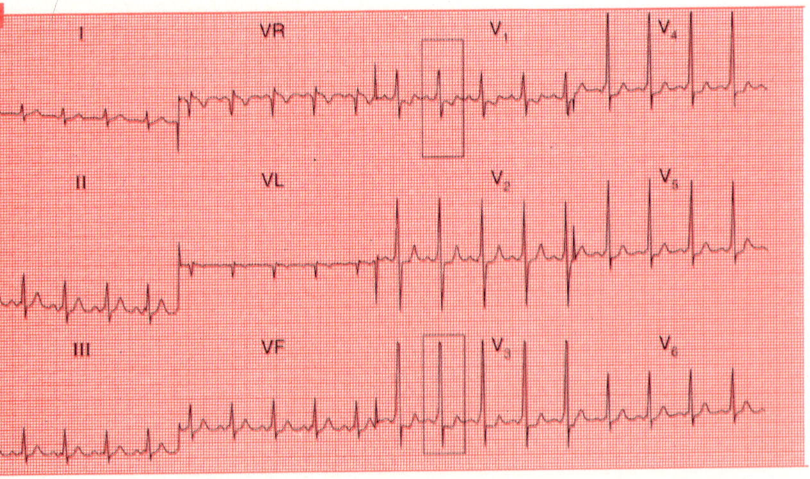

Old posterior infarction

Note

- Sinus rhythm
- Normal axis
- Dominant R waves in leads V_1–V_2
- No other abnormalities

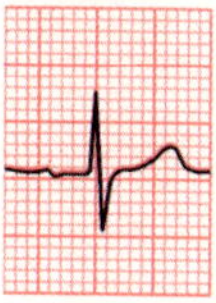

Dominant R wave in lead V_1

The Wolff–Parkinson–White syndrome type A

Note

- Sinus rhythm
- Short PR interval
- Slurred upstroke to QRS complexes
- Dominant R wave in lead V_1: the WPW syndrome type A

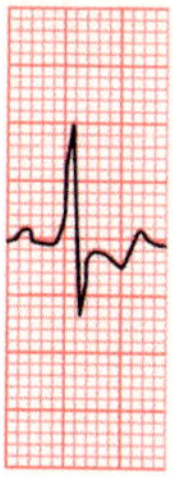

Dominant R wave in lead V_1

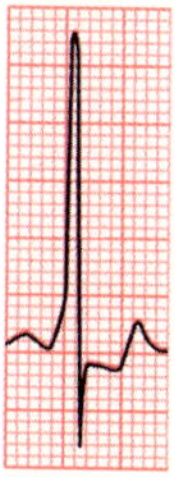

Delta wave in lead V_3

ECG PITFALLS IN THE DIAGNOSIS OF CHEST PAIN

The normal variants of the ECG have been described in Chapter 1. The important features that may cause confusion with ischaemia are:

- septal Q waves (mainly in leads II, VL, V_6)
- Q waves in lead III but not VF
- anterior T wave inversion (not uncommon in lead V_2, common in black people in leads V_2, V_3 and sometimes V_4)
- 'high take-off' ST segments.

Several abnormal ECG patterns may cause difficulty in making a diagnosis in patients with chest pain, which was the presenting problem in the following examples. These are summarized in Table 3.2 (p. 224).

R WAVE CHANGES

The ECG in Figure 3.48 shows a dominant R wave in lead V_1. This might be due to right ventricular hypertrophy or to a posterior infarction. Occasionally it could be a normal variant. Here, the normal axis goes against a diagnosis of right ventricular hypertrophy, and a review of previous ECGs from the patient showed that the dominant R wave was due to a posterior infarction.

The ECG in Figure 3.49 also shows a dominant R wave in lead V_1. In a patient with chest pain, a posterior infarction might again be considered. However, the PR interval is short and there is a delta wave, so this shows the Wolff–Parkinson–White (WPW) syndrome.

Fig. 3.50

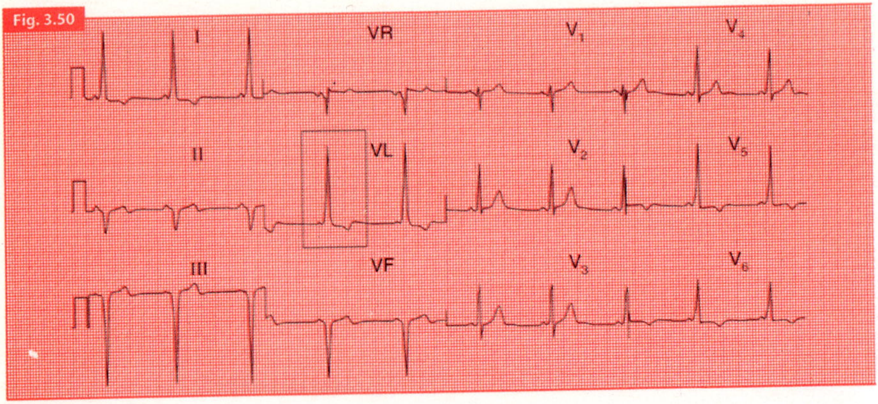

Fig. 3.51

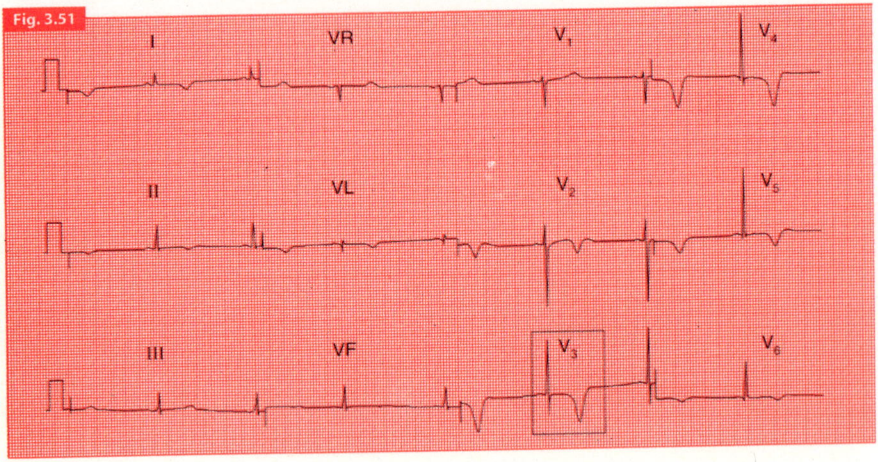

The Wolff–Parkinson–White syndrome type B

Note

- Sinus rhythm
- Short PR interval
- Left axis deviation
- Delta wave
- Inverted T waves in leads I, VL, V_5–V_6
- No dominant R wave in lead V_1 (the WPW syndrome type B)

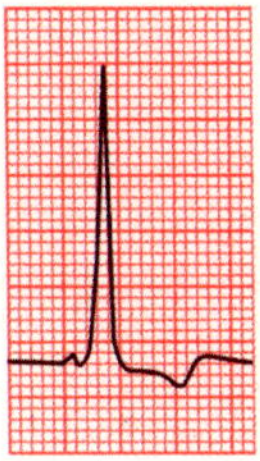

Short PR interval and delta wave in lead VL

Unexplained T wave abnormality

Note

- Sinus rhythm
- Normal axis
- Normal QRS complexes
- QT interval 600 ms
- T wave inversion in leads I–II, VL, V_2–V_6

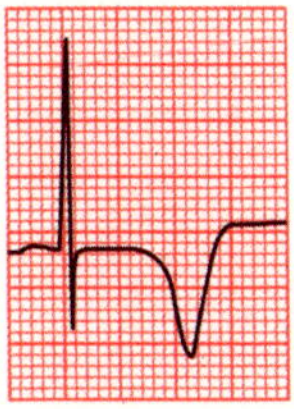

Long QT interval and inverted T wave in lead V_3

ST SEGMENT AND T WAVE CHANGES

It is, however, repolarization (T wave) changes that cause most problems. The lateral T wave inversion in the ECG in Figure 3.50 might suggest ischaemia, but again this is the WPW syndrome, in which repolarization abnormalities are common.

The anterior and lateral T wave inversion in the ECG in Figure 3.51 suggests either an NSTEMI or hypertrophic cardiomyopathy. This particular patient was white, asymptomatic and had no family history of arrhythmias or any cardiac disease. There was no echocardiographic evidence of cardiomyopathy, and coronary angiography was normal. The ECG reverted to normal on exercise, and the T wave inversion and the long QT interval remained unexplained.

Differentiation between lateral ischaemia and left ventricular hypertrophy on the ECG is extremely difficult. The ECG in Figure 3.52 shows lateral T wave inversion. There are small Q waves in leads III and VF, suggesting a possible old inferior infarction, and the QRS complexes in the chest leads are not particularly tall. Nevertheless, in this patient the lateral T wave inversion was due to left ventricular hypertrophy.

The patient whose ECG is shown in Figure 3.53 had mild hypertension. The QRS complexes are tall (see Ch. 4) and there is lateral T wave inversion, suggesting left ventricular hypertrophy. However, there is also T wave inversion in leads V_3 and V_4, which is unusual in left ventricular hypertrophy. This patient had severe narrowing of the left main coronary artery.

Fig. 3.52

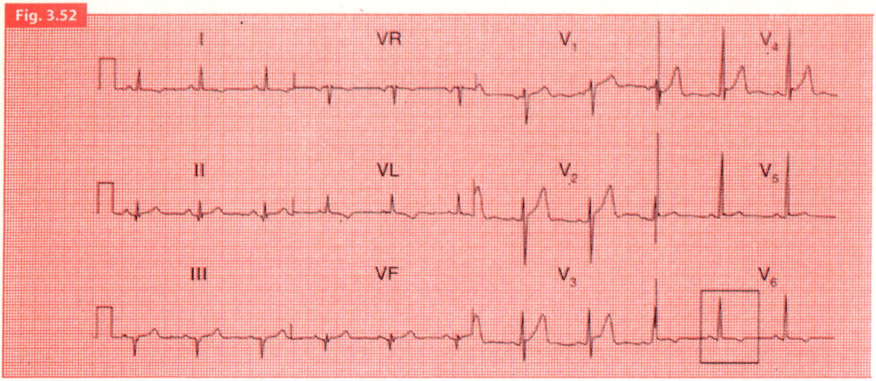

Fig. 3.53

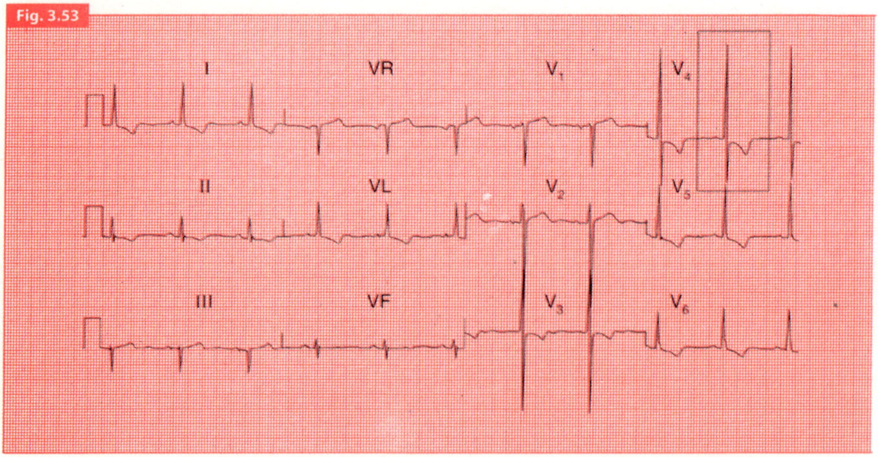

Left ventricular hypertrophy

Note

- Sinus rhythm
- Normal axis
- Height of R wave in lead V_5 + depth of S wave in lead V_2 = 37 mm
- High take-off ST segment in lead V_4
- T wave inversion in leads I, VL, V_6

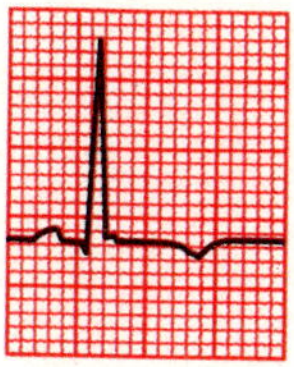

Inverted T wave in lead V_6

Old anterolateral NSTEMI

Note

- Sinus rhythm
- Normal axis
- Tall QRS complexes
- T wave inversion in leads I, VL, V_3–V_6, but this is more marked in lead V_4 than in V_6

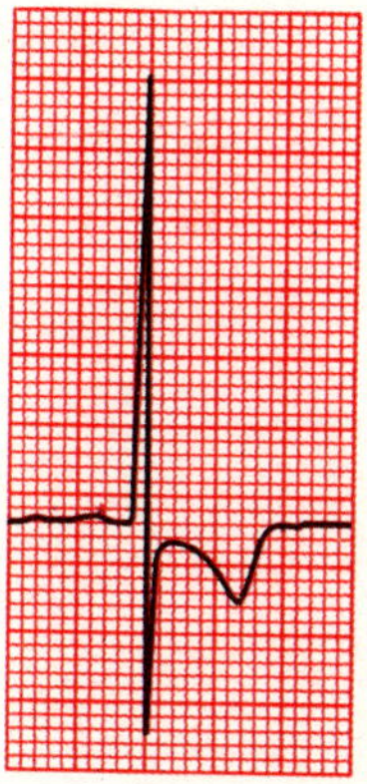

Inverted T wave in lead V_4

Fig. 3.54

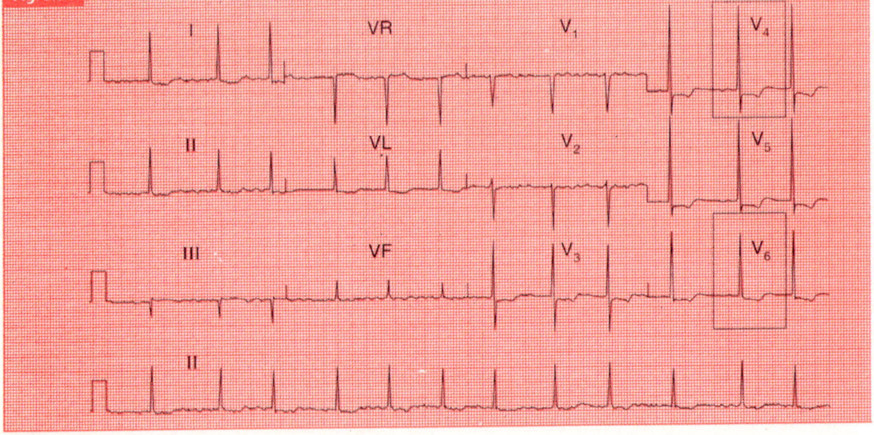

Fig. 3.55

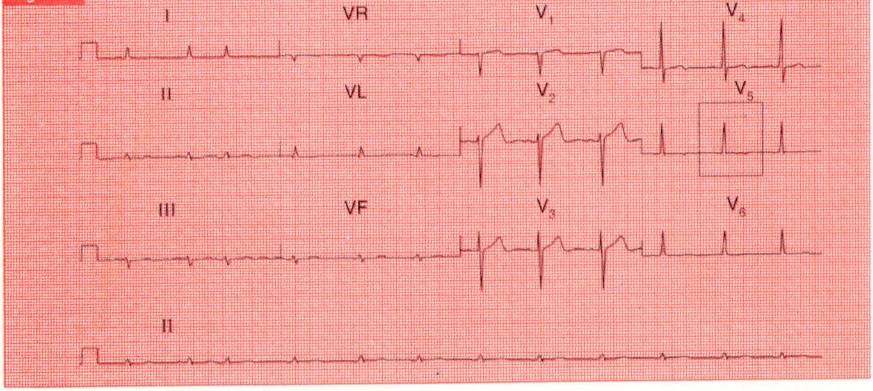

Digoxin effect and ischaemia

Note

- Atrial fibrillation
- Normal axis
- Normal QRS complexes
- Horizontal ST segment depression in lead V_4
- Downward-sloping ST segment in lead V_6
- Inverted T waves in leads V_3–V_4

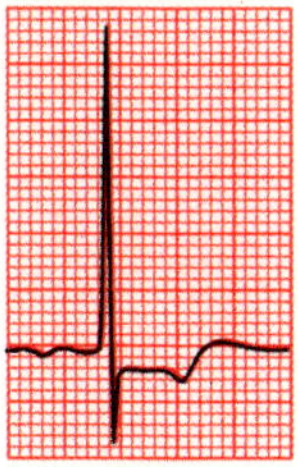

Horizontal ST segment in lead V_4

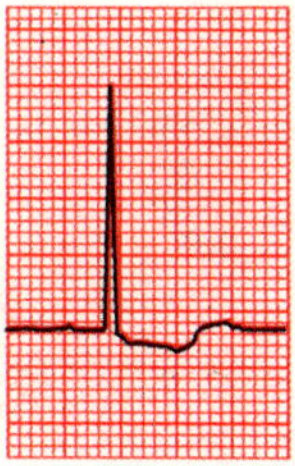

Downward-sloping ST segment in lead V_6

Nonspecific T wave flattening

Note

- Recorded at half sensitivity
- Sinus rhythm with supraventricular extrasystoles
- Normal QRS complexes
- Flat T waves in leads I, VL, V_5–V_6

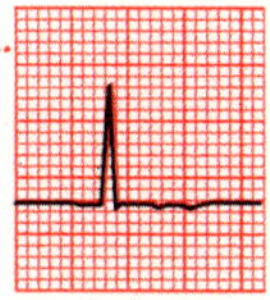

Flat T wave in lead V_5

Digoxin therapy causes downward-sloping ST segment depression and T wave inversion (see Ch. 5), particularly in the lateral leads, as is seen in Figure 3.54. The fact that the rhythm is atrial fibrillation with a controlled ventricular rate suggests that the patient is being treated with digoxin. However, T wave inversion in leads V_3 and V_4 is much more likely to be due to ischaemia, as was the case here.

An extremely common finding on the ECG is 'nonspecific T wave flattening' (Fig. 3.55). When a patient is completely well and the heart is clinically normal, this is of no importance. However, in a patient with chest pain that appears to be cardiac, 'nonspecific' ST segment/T wave changes may indicate ischaemia.

Table 3.2 ECG pitfalls in the diagnosis of chest pain

Condition	ECG pattern	May be confused with
Normal record	Q waves in lead III but not VF	Inferior infarction
	T wave inversion in leads V_1–V_3 (especially in black people)	Anterior infarction
Left ventricular hypertrophy	T wave inversion in lateral leads	Ischaemia
Right ventricular hypertrophy	Dominant R waves in lead V_1	Posterior infarction
	Inverted T waves in leads V_1–V_3	Anterior infarction
The Wolff–Parkinson–White syndrome	Inverted T waves in leads V_2–V_5	Anterior infarction
Hypertrophic cardiomyopathy	T wave inversion in leads V_2–V_5	Anterior infarction
Subarachnoid haemorrhage	T wave inversion in any leads	Ischaemia
Digoxin effect	Downward-sloping ST segment depression or T wave inversion, especially in leads V_5–V_6	Ischaemia

WHAT TO DO

It is essential to remember that while the ECG can on occasions be extremely helpful in the diagnosis of chest pain, frequently it is not. The history, and to a lesser extent the physical examination, are far more important.

ACUTE CHEST PAIN SUGGESTING MYOCARDIAL INFARCTION

The treatment of patients with chest pain differs, depending on whether the ECG shows ST segment elevation (STEMI) or not (NSTEMI). Both patient categories can be said to have an 'acute coronary syndrome', though this is often used as if it were synonymous with NSTEMI.

The ECG can be normal in the first hour or two of a STEMI, so in order to differentiate between a STEMI and an NSTEMI it is essential that 12-lead ECGs should be repeated at least hourly until the diagnosis is clear. Blood samples should be taken immediately to identify troponin (T or I) and CK-MB levels. However, it is important to remember that the plasma troponin levels may not rise for up to 12 h, so the test should not be considered negative until 12 h after the onset of chest pain.

STEMI

Patients with STEMI require immediate coronary recanalization by means of either percutaneous coronary intervention (PCI) or thrombolysis.

NSTEMI

Patients with NSTEMI should be treated immediately with aspirin, low-molecular-weight heparin, clopidogrel, beta-blockers (provided there are no contraindications), a statin and nitrates.

Two risk categories of NSTEMI can be identified, which require different subsequent treatments.

Patients at high risk have any of:

- persistent or recurrent chest pain
- ST segment depression
- diabetes
- elevated troponin levels
- haemodynamic instability
- rhythm instability.

In addition to the baseline treatment above, these patients require an infusion of a glycoprotein IIb/IIIa inhibitor followed by coronary angiography before discharge from hospital. Angiography is urgent in unstable patients. Most high-risk patients will need angioplasty or bypass surgery, often as a matter of urgency.

Low-risk patients include those with all of:

- no recurrent chest pain
- an ECG showing T wave inversion, flat T waves or no ECG changes at all
- normal troponin levels after 12 h.

Heparin can be discontinued but aspirin, beta-blockers, nitrates, a statin and clopidogrel are continued. As soon as possible, an exercise test should be performed to assess the probability and severity of coronary disease. On the basis of the test results and the clinical picture, a decision can be made about the need for, and urgency of, coronary angiography.

LONG-TERM TREATMENT

In all patients it is important to manage risk factors aggressively, with the cessation of smoking, weight control and regular exercise. Aspirin, beta-blockers and statins are needed indefinitely, and clopidogrel for 9 months.

OTHER INVESTIGATIONS FOR PATIENTS WITH ACUTE CHEST PAIN

Chest X-rays are seldom helpful. Unless a pneumothorax or some other cause of pleurisy, or a dissecting aneurysm, seem possible the patient should not be detained waiting for an X-ray examination. Chest X-rays taken using portable equipment are rarely useful.

Echocardiography is the investigation of choice if pericarditis is suspected, because most patients will have a pericardial effusion which is easily detected. Subsequent treatment will depend on the underlying cause of the pericarditis. Possible causes are listed in Box 3.4

Echocardiography may also help in the diagnosis of an aortic dissection, but not reliably – CT scanning is probably the investigation of choice in such cases. Echocardiography may also be helpful in suspected pulmonary embolism, because it may show right ventricular dilatation.

Box 3.4 Causes of pericarditis

- Viral
- Bacterial (including tuberculosis)
- Dressler's syndrome after myocardial infarction
- Malignancy
- Uraemia
- Acute rheumatic fever
- Myxoedema
- Connective tissue disease
- Radiotherapy

CHRONIC CHEST PAIN

Chronic or intermittent chest pain must be investigated and treated as the history dictates. If angina seems likely but the resting ECG is normal, an exercise test may be useful in establishing the diagnosis and giving a rough indication of the severity of the angina.

A trial of sublingual glyceryl trinitrate 0.5 mg may help make the diagnosis of angina, and in such cases patients should then be encouraged to use the drug liberally and prophylactically. Beta-blockers are the first-line agents for preventing angina. If the patient is unable to take a beta-blocker (e.g. because of asthma), treatment should start with a calcium-channel blocker such as amlodipine. Nicorandil and ivabradine may also be useful, especially in patients intolerant of other drugs. All these drugs can be combined, or a long-acting nitrate such as isosorbide mononitrate can be substituted for one of these classes of drug. A combination of two of these drug classes is sometimes helpful; the addition of the third seldom provides much further benefit. Secondary prophylactic measures, including aspirin and a statin, are essential.

Coronary angiography is essential if coronary artery bypass grafting or percutaneous transluminal coronary angioplasty is being considered, so patients still symptomatic despite maximum medical therapy need to be investigated. Angiography is also necessary in young people with a strongly positive exercise test at a low workload (say, 3 mm depression at Bruce Stage 2 or less).

The ECG in patients with breathlessness

4

HISTORY AND EXAMINATION

There are many causes of breathlessness (see Box 4.1). Everyone is breathless at times, and people who are physically unfit or who are overweight will be more breathless than others. Breathlessness can also result from anxiety, but when it is due to physical illness the important causes are anaemia, heart disease and lung disease; a combination of causes is common. The most important function of the history is to help to determine whether the patient does indeed have a physical illness and if so, which system is affected.

Breathlessness in heart disease is due to either increased lung stiffness, as a result of pulmonary congestion, or pulmonary oedema. Pulmonary congestion occurs when the left atrial pressure is high. A high left atrial pressure occurs either in mitral

Box 4.1 Causes of breathlessness

	Underlying cause
Physiological and psychological	• Lack of fitness • Obesity • Pregnancy • Locomotor diseases (including ankylosing spondylitis and neurological diseases) • Anxiety
Heart disease	
Left ventricular failure	• Ischaemia • Mitral regurgitation • Aortic stenosis • Aortic regurgitation • Congenital disease • Cardiomyopathy • Myocarditis • Arrhythmias
High left atrial pressure	• Mitral stenosis • Atrial myxoma
Lung disease	• Chronic obstructive pulmonary disease • Any interstitial lung disease (e.g. infection, tumour, infiltration) • Pulmonary embolism • Pleural effusion • Pneumothorax
Pericardial disease	• Constrictive pericarditis
Anaemia	

stenosis or in left ventricular failure. Pulmonary oedema occurs when the left atrial pressure exceeds the oncotic pressure exerted by the plasma proteins.

Congestive cardiac failure (right heart failure secondary to left heart failure) can be difficult to distinguish from cor pulmonale (right heart failure due to lung disease). With both, the patient is breathless. Both are associated with pulmonary crackles – in left heart failure due to pulmonary oedema, and in cor pulmonale due to the lung disease. Also in both, the patient may complain of orthopnoea. In heart failure, this is due to the return to the effective circulation of blood that was pooled in the legs. In patients with chest disease (especially chronic obstructive airways disease) orthopnoea results from a need to use diaphragmatic respiration. Both pulmonary congestion and lung disease can cause a diffuse wheeze. The diagnosis therefore depends on a positive identification, either in the history or on examination, of heart or lung disease.

The main value of the ECG in patients with breathlessness is to indicate whether heart disease of any sort is present, and whether the left or the right side of the heart is affected. The ECG is best at identifying rhythm abnormalities (which may lead to left ventricular impairment and so to breathlessness) and conditions affecting the left ventricle – particularly ischaemia. The patient with a completely normal ECG is unlikely to have left ventricular failure, though of course there are exceptions. Lung disease eventually affects the right side of the heart, and may cause ECG changes suggesting that significant lung disease is present.

RHYTHM PROBLEMS

A sudden rhythm change is a common cause of breathlessness, and even of frank pulmonary oedema. Arrhythmias can be paroxysmal, so the patient may be in sinus rhythm when examined, and a patient who is suddenly breathless may not be aware of an arrhythmia. When sudden breathlessness is associated with palpitations it is important to establish whether the breathlessness or the palpitations came first – palpitations following breathlessness may be due to the sinus tachycardia of anxiety. The ECG in Figure 4.1 is from a patient who developed pulmonary oedema due to the onset of uncontrolled atrial fibrillation.

Less dramatic rhythm abnormalities can also contribute to breathlessness, especially to breathlessness on exertion. This is true of both fast and slow rhythms. The ECG in Figure 4.2 is from a patient who was breathless on exercise, partly because of coupled ventricular extrasystoles, which markedly reduced cardiac output as a result of an effective rate of half of the 76/min recorded on the ECG.

Fig. 4.1

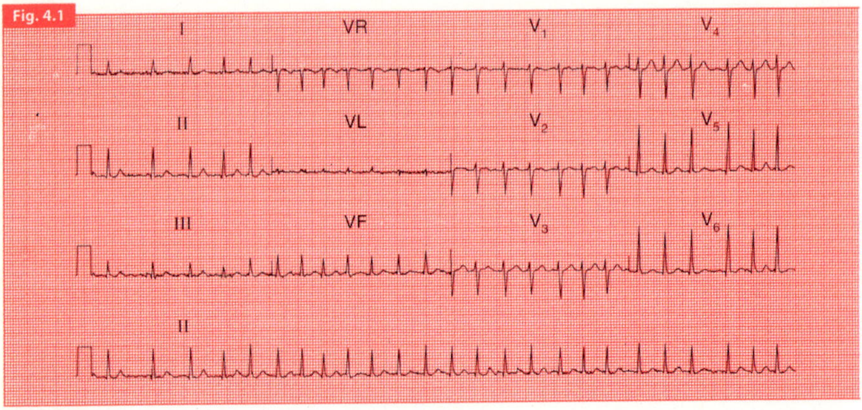
I
VR
V_1
V_4
II
VL
V_2
V_5
III
VF
V_3
V_6
II

Fig. 4.2

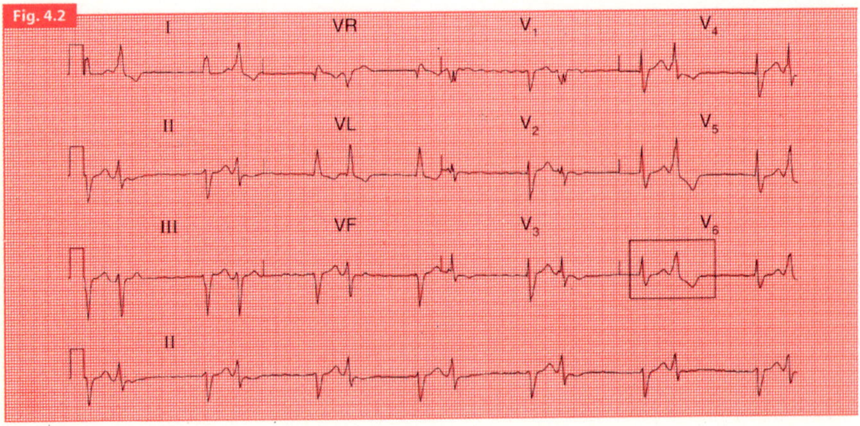
I
VR
V_1
V_4
II
VL
V_2
V_5
III
VF
V_3
V_6
II

Uncontrolled atrial fibrillation

Note

- Atrial fibrillation, with ventricular rate 170/min
- No other abnormalities
- No evidence of digoxin effect

Atrial fibrillation with coupled ventricular extrasystoles

Note

- Atrial fibrillation, with slow and regular ventricular response
- Coupled ventricular extrasystoles
- In supraventricular beats, leads V_5–V_6 show a deep wide S wave, suggesting right bundle branch block
- ?Digoxin toxicity

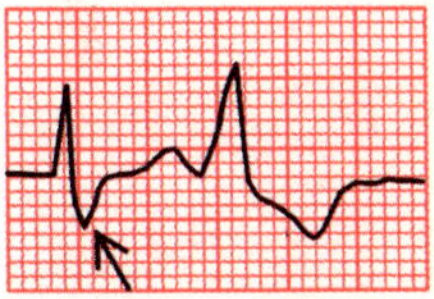

Deep wide S wave in supraventricular beat in lead V_6

Fig. 4.3

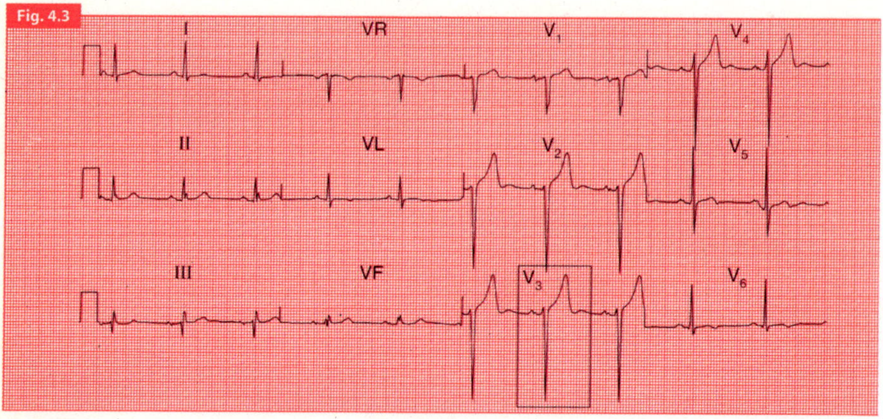

Fig. 4.4

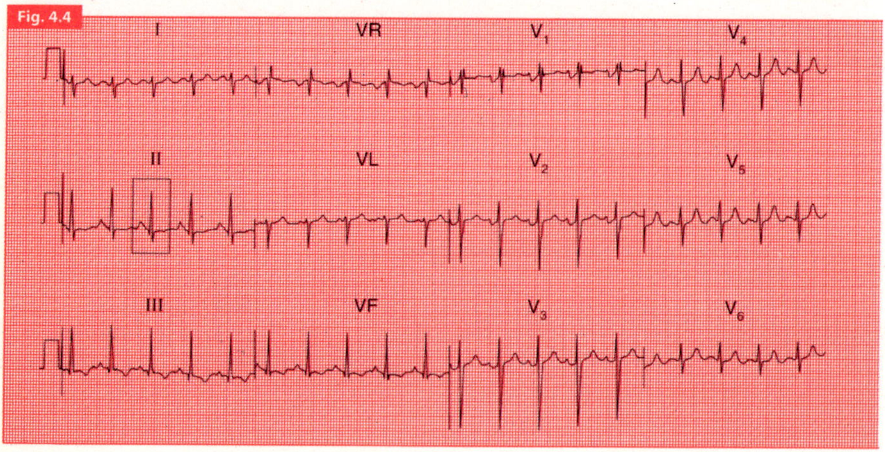

Left atrial hypertrophy and left ventricular hypertrophy

Note

- Sinus rhythm
- Bifid P waves
- Normal axis
- Tall QRS complexes
- Inverted T waves in lead V_6, suggesting left ventricular hypertrophy

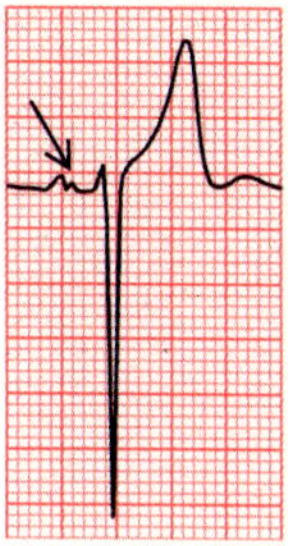

Bifid P wave in lead V_3

Mitral stenosis and pulmonary hypertension

Note

- Sinus rhythm
- Bifid P wave (best seen in lead II)
- Right axis deviation
- Partial right bundle branch block pattern
- Persistent S wave in lead V_6

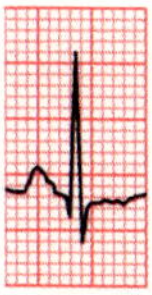

Bifid P wave in lead II

THE ECG IN DISORDERS AFFECTING THE LEFT SIDE OF THE HEART

THE ECG IN LEFT ATRIAL HYPERTROPHY

Left atrial hypertrophy causes a double (bifid) P wave. Left atrial hypertrophy without left ventricular hypertrophy is classically due to mitral stenosis, so the bifid P wave is sometimes called 'P mitrale'. This is misleading, because most patients whose ECGs have bifid P waves either have left ventricular hypertrophy that is not obvious on the ECG or – and perhaps this is more common – have a perfectly normal heart. The bifid P wave is thus not a useful measure of left atrial hypertrophy.

Figure 4.3 shows an ECG with a bifid P wave indicating left atrial hypertrophy. This was confirmed by echocardiography in the patient, who also had concentric left ventricular hypertrophy due to hypertension.

Significant mitral stenosis usually – but not always – leads to atrial fibrillation, in which no P waves, bifid or otherwise, can be seen. Occasional patients, such as the one whose ECG is shown in Figure 4.4, develop pulmonary hypertension and remain in sinus rhythm. There is then a combination of a bifid P wave with evidence of right ventricular hypertrophy. This combination does allow a confident diagnosis of severe mitral stenosis.

Fig. 4.5

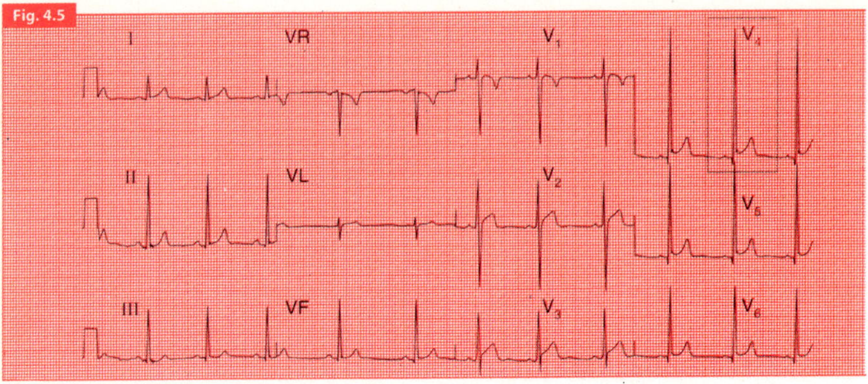

Fig. 4.6

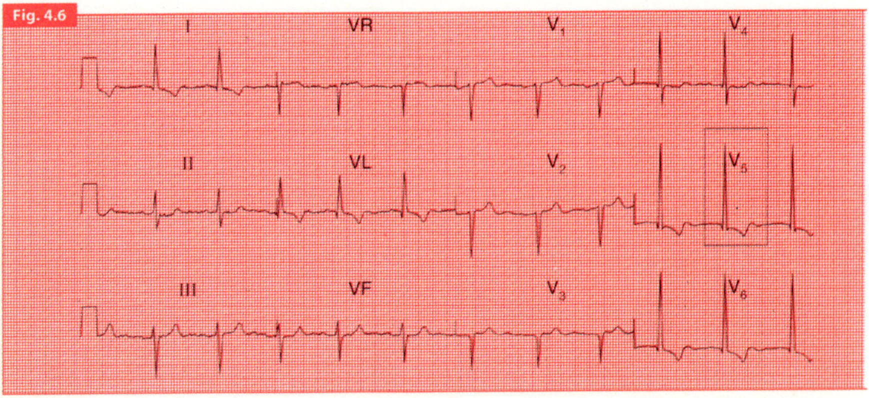

Probably normal ECG

Note

- Sinus rhythm
- Normal axis
- Very tall R waves (meeting 'voltage criteria' for left ventricular hypertrophy)
- No other evidence of left ventricular hypertrophy

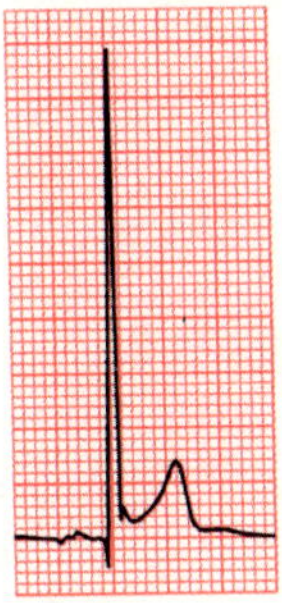

Tall R wave in lead V_4

Left ventricular hypertrophy

Note

- Sinus rhythm
- Voltage criteria for left ventricular hypertrophy
- Inverted T waves in leads I, VL, V_5–V_6

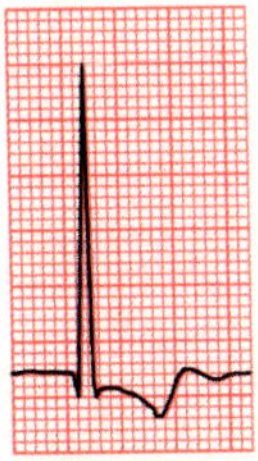

Tall R wave and inverted T wave in lead V_5

THE ECG IN LEFT VENTRICULAR HYPERTROPHY

Left ventricular hypertrophy may be caused by hypertension, aortic stenosis or incompetence, or mitral incompetence.

The ECG features of left ventricular hypertrophy are:

- an increased height of the QRS complex
- inverted T waves in the leads that 'look at' the left ventricle: I, VL, and V_5–V_6.

Left axis deviation is not uncommon, but is due more to fibrosis causing left anterior hemiblock than to the left ventricular hypertrophy itself. The ECG is, in fact, a poor guide to the severity of left ventricular hypertrophy.

Numerous criteria have been proposed that claim to detect the presence of left ventricular hypertrophy from ECG measurements. Most depend on measuring R or S waves in different leads, and some take the width of QRS complexes into account. The most commonly used indicator is the Sokolov–Lyon voltage criterion. This defines left ventricular hypertrophy as being present when the depth of the S wave in lead V_1 plus the height of the R wave in lead V_5 or V_6 (whichever is the greater) exceeds 35 mm.

Unfortunately, voltage criteria have a low sensitivity as detectors of left ventricular hypertrophy and are essentially useless. They would frequently lead to a diagnosis of left ventricular hypertrophy in perfectly healthy young men, even in those who are not athletic (Fig. 4.5).

The complete ECG picture of left ventricular hypertrophy is easy to recognize. The ECG in Figure 4.6 is from a patient with severe and untreated hypertension. It shows the 'voltage criteria' which,

Fig. 4.7

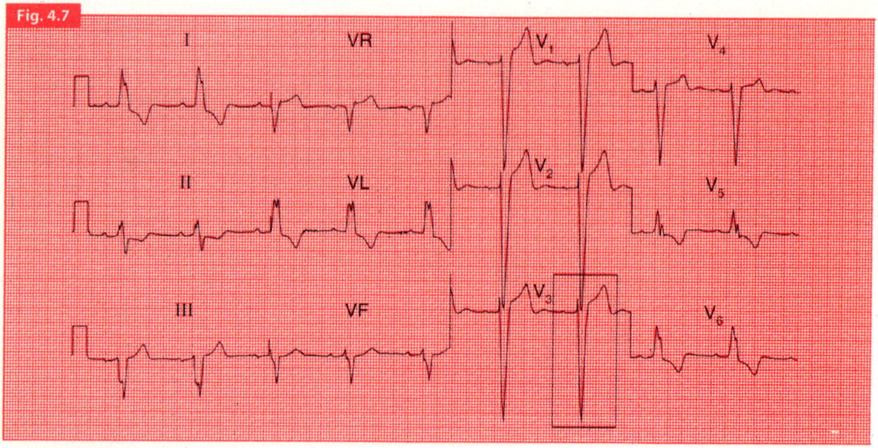

Fig. 4.8

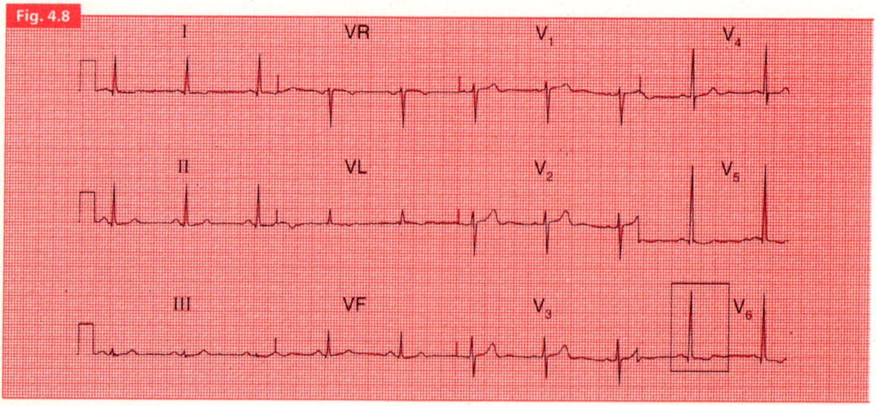

Left bundle branch block with aortic stenosis

Note

- Sinus rhythm
- Normal axis
- Broad QRS complexes with LBBB pattern
- Very deep S waves in lead V_3
- Inverted T waves in leads I, VL, V_5–V_6

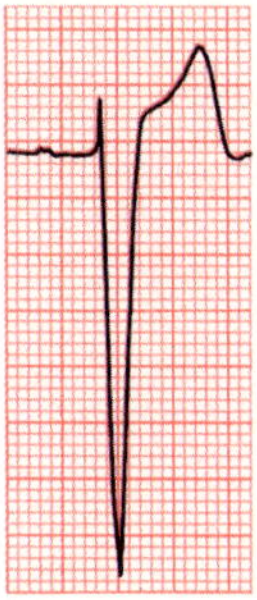

Broad QRS complex and deep S wave in lead V_3

Left ventricular hypertrophy

Note

- Sinus rhythm
- Normal axis
- Voltage criteria for left ventricular hypertrophy not met
- Inverted T waves in leads I, VL, V_6

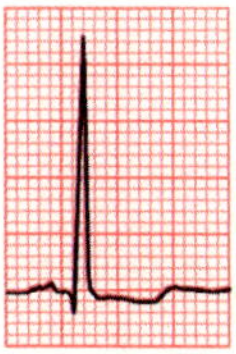

Normal R wave and inverted T wave in lead V_6

when combined with the T wave inversion, probably are significant. In this case, the small Q waves in the lateral leads are septal and do not indicate a previous infarction. Note that the T wave inversion is most prominent in lead V_6, and becomes progressively less so in leads V_5 and V_4. This pattern of T wave inversion is sometimes referred to as 'left ventricular strain', but this is an old-fashioned and essentially meaningless term.

The most important cause of severe left ventricular hypertrophy is aortic valve disease: when aortic stenosis or incompetence causes left ventricular hypertrophy, aortic valve replacement must be considered. Aortic valve disease is frequently associated with left bundle branch block (LBBB) (Fig. 4.7), which completely masks any evidence of left ventricular hypertrophy. The patient who is breathless, or who has chest pain or dizziness, and has signs of aortic valve disease and an ECG showing LBBB, needs urgent investigation.

Unfortunately the severity of ECG changes is an unreliable guide to the importance of the underlying cardiac problem. The ECG in Figure 4.8 shows lateral T wave inversion, but does not meet the 'voltage criteria', in a patient with moderate aortic stenosis (aortic valve gradient 60 mmHg).

In contrast, the ECG in Figure 4.9 is from a patient with severe aortic stenosis and an aortic valve gradient > 120 mmHg, yet it shows little to suggest severe left ventricular hypertrophy.

Fig. 4.9

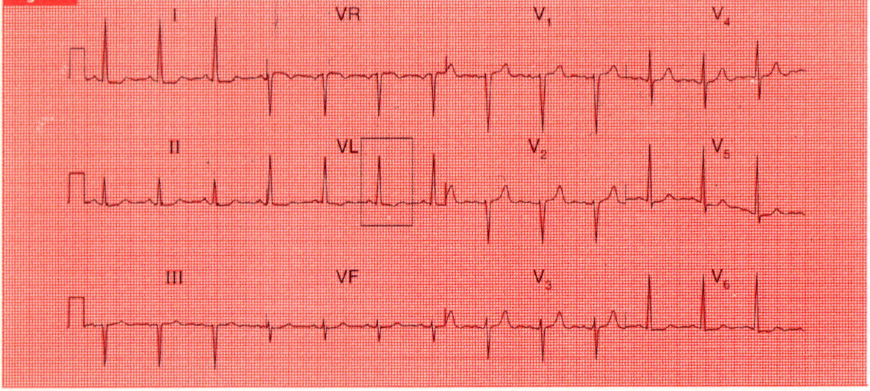

Fig. 4.10

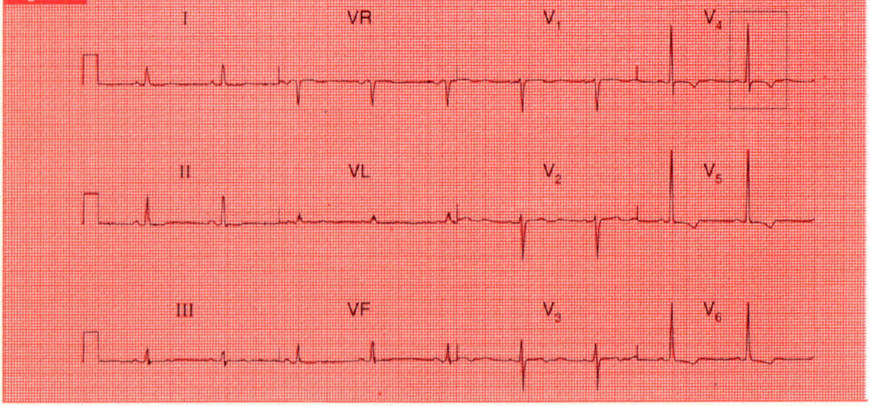

?Left ventricular hypertrophy with severe aortic stenosis

Note

- Sinus rhythm
- Normal axis
- Voltage criteria for left ventricular hypertrophy not met
- Minor ST segment/T wave changes in leads I, VL, V_6

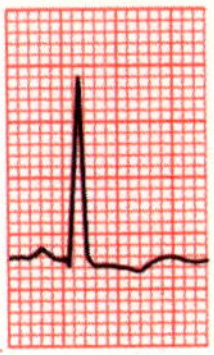

Minor ST segment/T wave changes in lead VL

Probable ischaemia

Note

- Sinus rhythm
- Normal axis
- T wave inversion in leads II, V_3–V_6, but most prominent in V_4–V_5

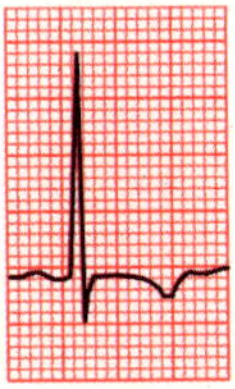

Inverted T wave in lead V_4

ECGS THAT CAN MIMIC LEFT VENTRICULAR HYPERTROPHY

The main problem is differentiating lateral T wave changes due to left ventricular hypertrophy from those due to ischaemia; this has been discussed in Chapter 3. The history and physical examination become extremely important, and the ECG must not be viewed in isolation. The ECG in Figure 4.10 is from a patient with chest pain that was compatible with, but not diagnostic of, angina and who had physical signs suggesting mild aortic stenosis. The T wave inversion is more prominent in leads V_4 and V_5 than in V_6, and is present in V_3. The T waves are upright in leads I and VL. These changes point to ischaemia rather than left ventricular hypertrophy, and ischaemia proved to be present in this patient.

The ECG in Figure 4.11 is from a patient with hypertension and breathlessness. He was shown to have left ventricular hypertrophy and coronary disease, but all the changes here could have been due to left ventricular hypertrophy alone.

When a breathless patient has an ECG with gross lateral T wave changes (Fig. 4.12), hypertrophic cardiomyopathy is a possibility.

Lateral T wave changes associated with left anterior hemiblock often accompany left ventricular hypertrophy. However, there was no echocardiographic evidence of this in the patient whose ECG is shown in Figure 4.13. Here the changes must be due to conducting system disease.

Another example of a conducting tissue abnormality that could be mistaken for left ventricular hypertrophy is the Wolff–Parkinson–White (WPW) syndrome. The ECG in Figure 4.14 is from a young man with the WPW syndrome type B. There is left ventricular hypertrophy according to 'voltage criteria', and there is also lateral T wave inversion,

Fig. 4.11

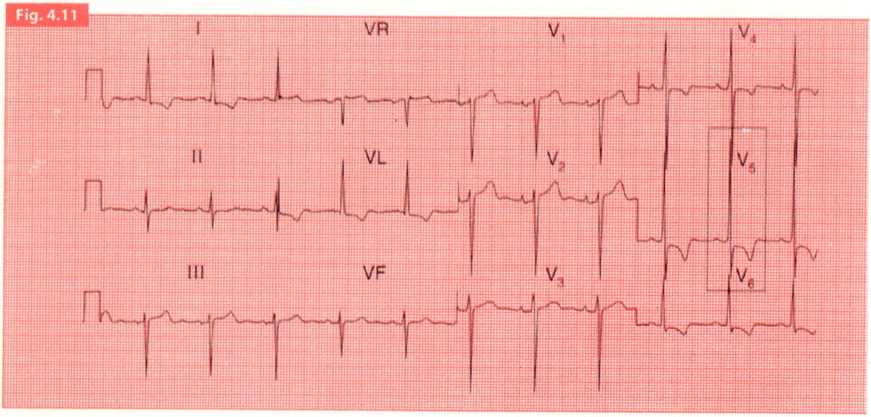

Fig. 4.12

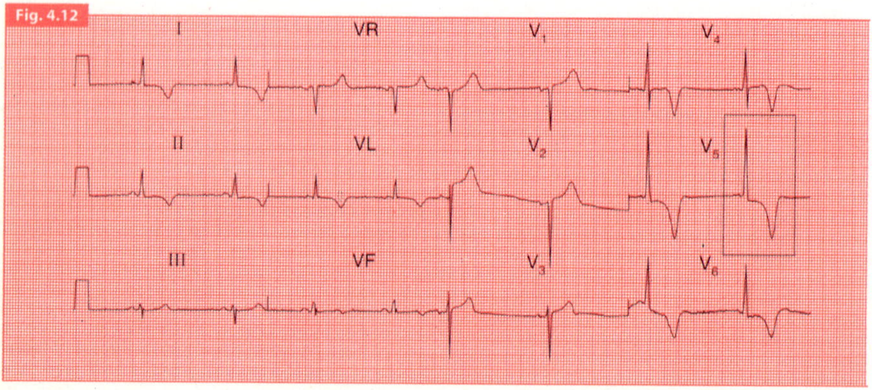

?Left ventricular hypertrophy, ?ischaemia

Note

- Sinus rhythm
- Bifid P waves, best seen in lead I
- Normal axis
- T wave inversion in leads I, VL, V_3–V_6, but most prominent in V_5

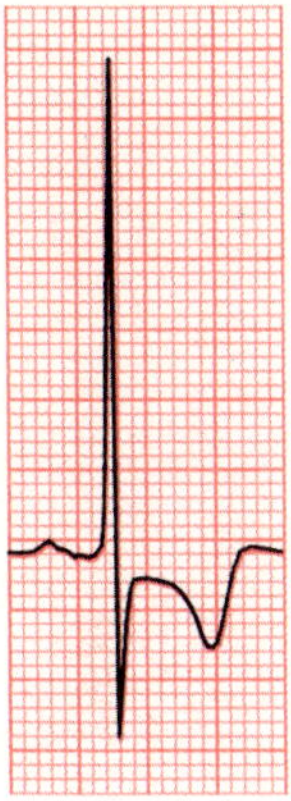

Maximal T wave inversion in lead V_5

Hypertrophic cardiomyopathy

Note

- Sinus rhythm
- Bifid P wave, best seen in lead V_4
- Voltage criteria for left ventricular hypertrophy not met
- Gross T wave inversion in leads V_4–V_6

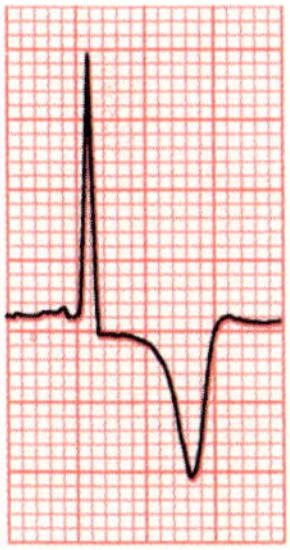

Normal R wave and dramatic T wave inversion in lead V_5

Fig. 4.13

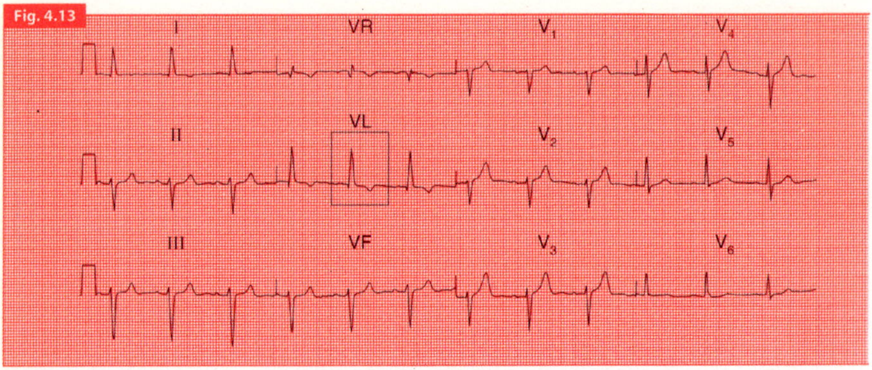

Fig. 4.14

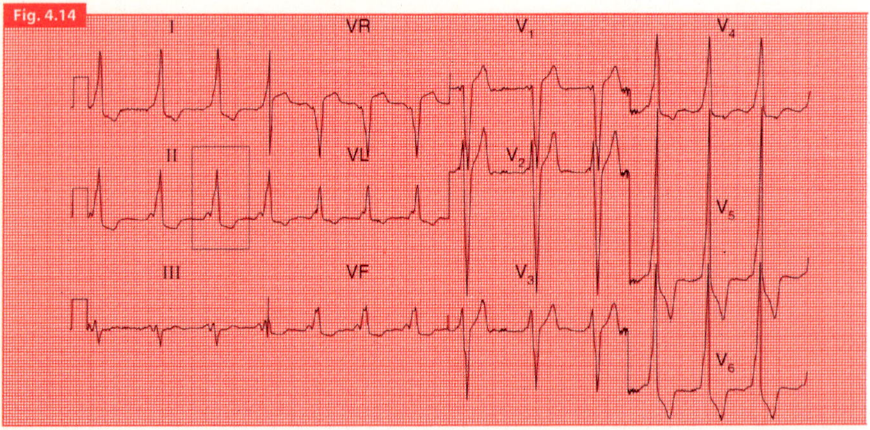

Left anterior hemiblock

Note

- Sinus rhythm
- Left axis deviation
- Inverted T waves in leads I, VL

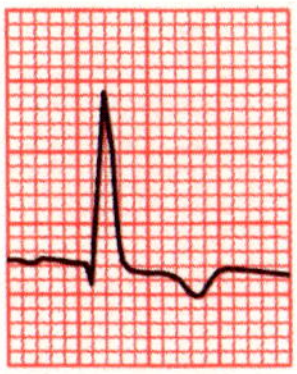

Inverted T wave in lead VL

The Wolff–Parkinson–White syndrome (no left ventricular hypertrophy)

Note

- Short PR interval
- Broad QRS complexes with delta waves
- Very tall R waves
- Inverted T waves in leads I, II, VL, V_4–V_6

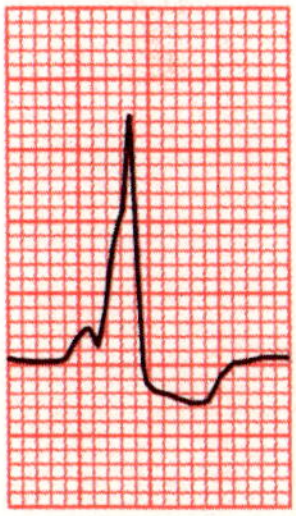

Short PR interval and delta wave in lead II

Fig. 4.15

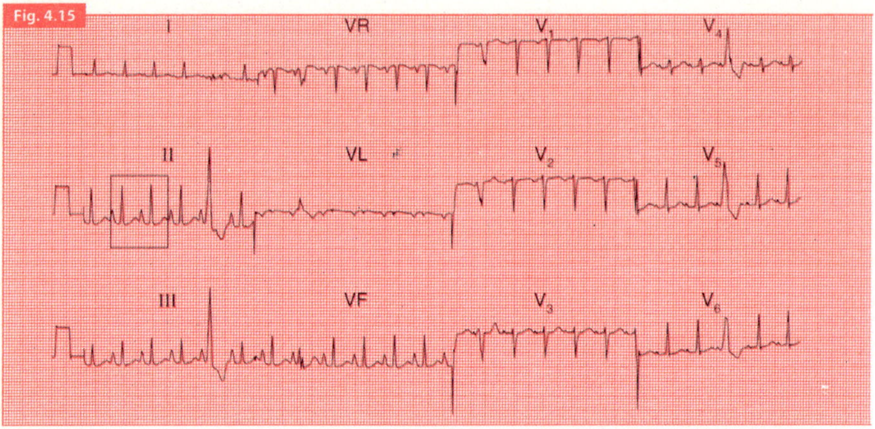

Fig. 4.16

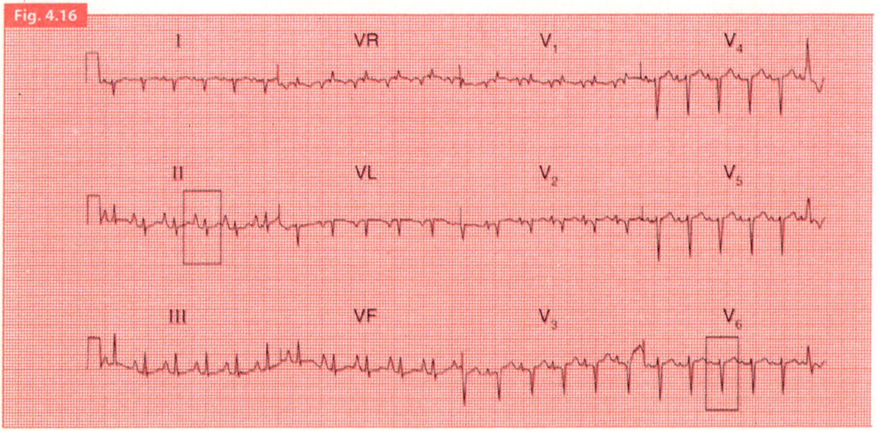

Right atrial hypertrophy

Note

- Sinus rhythm with occasional aberrant conduction
- Tall and peaked P waves
- No other abnormality

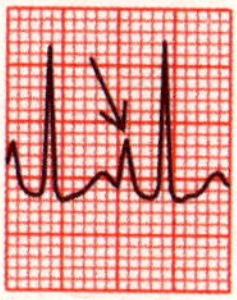

Peaked P wave in lead II

Right atrial and right ventricular hypertrophy

Note

- Peaked P waves, especially in lead II
- Right axis deviation
- Persistent S waves in lead V_6 (clockwise rotation) suggest chronic lung disease

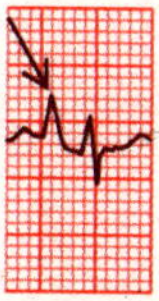

Peaked P wave in lead II

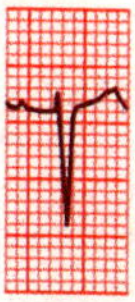

Persistent S wave in lead V_6

but the diagnosis is made from the short PR intervals and the delta waves. The height of the QRS complexes and the T wave inversion in this situation do not indicate left ventricular hypertrophy.

THE ECG IN DISORDERS AFFECTING THE RIGHT SIDE OF THE HEART

THE ECG IN RIGHT ATRIAL HYPERTROPHY

Right atrial hypertrophy causes tall and peaked P waves. There is, in fact, such variation within the normal range of P waves that the diagnosis of right atrial hypertrophy is difficult to make. Its presence can be inferred when peaked P waves are associated with the ECG changes of right ventricular hypertrophy. Evidence of right atrial hypertrophy without right ventricular hypertrophy will usually only be seen in patients with tricuspid stenosis (Fig. 4.15).

The ECG in Figure 4.16 is from a patient with right atrial and right ventricular hypertrophy due to severe chronic obstructive pulmonary disease.

THE ECG IN RIGHT VENTRICULAR HYPERTROPHY

Right ventricular hypertrophy can be the result of chronic lung disease (e.g. chronic obstructive airways disease, bronchiectasis), pulmonary embolism (especially when repeated episodes cause thromboembolic pulmonary hypertension), idiopathic pulmonary hypertension, or congenital heart disease. None of these has a specific ECG abnormality.

Fig. 4.17

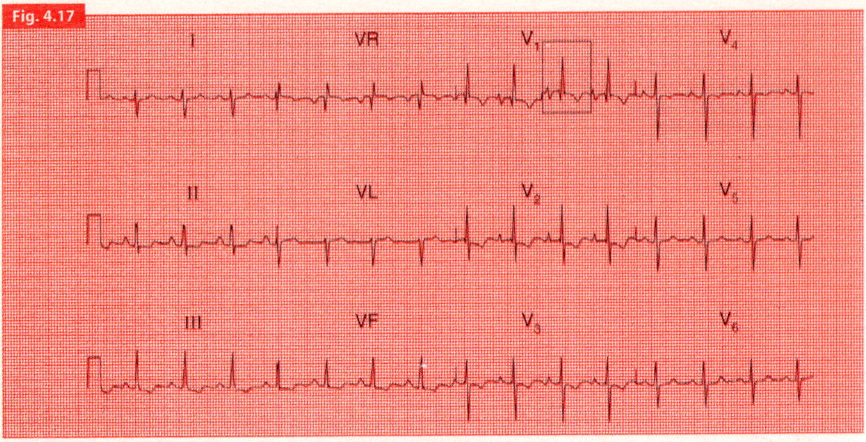

Table 4.1 Possible alternative causes of the ECG appearance of right ventricular hypertrophy

ECG feature	Cause
Right axis deviation	Normal in tall thin people
Dominant R wave in lead V_1	Normal variant Posterior infarction The Wolff–Parkinson–White syndrome Right bundle branch block of any cause
Inverted T waves in leads V_1–V_2	Normal variant, especially in black people Anterior non-ST segment elevation myocardial infarction The Wolff–Parkinson–White syndrome Right bundle branch block of any cause Cardiomyopathy
Apparent clockwise rotation	Dextrocardia

> **Marked right ventricular hypertrophy**
>
> **Note**
>
> - Sinus rhythm
> - Peaked P waves
> - Right axis deviation
> - Dominant R waves in lead V_1
> - Persistent S waves in lead V_6
>
> 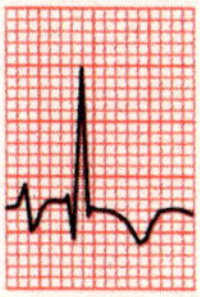
>
> Dominant R wave in lead V_1

The ECG changes associated with right ventricular hypertrophy are:

- right axis deviation
- a dominant R wave in lead V_1
- clockwise rotation of the heart: as the septum is displaced laterally, the transition of the QRS complex in the chest leads from a right to a left ventricular configuration occurs between leads V_4 and V_6 instead of in V_2–V_4. There is thus a persistent S wave in lead V_6, which normally does not show an S wave at all.
- inversion of the T wave in leads that 'look at' the right ventricle: V_1, V_2, and occasionally V_3.

In extreme cases it is easy to diagnose right ventricular hypertrophy from the ECG. The ECG in Figure 4.17 came from a patient incapacitated by breathlessness due to primary pulmonary hypertension.

As with the ECG in left ventricular hypertrophy, none of the ECG changes of right ventricular hypertrophy individually provide unequivocal evidence of right ventricular hypertrophy (see Table 4.1). Conversely, it is possible to have marked right ventricular hypertrophy without all the ECG features being present. Minor degrees of right axis deviation are seen in normal people, and a dominant R wave in lead V_1 is occasionally seen in normal people, although it is never more than 3 or 4 mm tall. A dominant R wave in lead V_1 may also indicate a 'true posterior' myocardial infarction (see Ch. 3). There may be variation in the T wave inversion in leads V_1 and V_2 in normal subjects (see Ch. 1); and, particularly in black people, the T wave can be inverted in leads V_2 and V_3.

The ECG in Figure 4.18 shows a dominant R wave in lead V_1 but no other evidence of right ventricular hypertrophy. This could indicate a posterior myocardial infarction (see Ch. 3), but this trace was from a young man who was asymptomatic, who had no abnormalities on examination, and whose echocardiogram was normal. This is a normal variant.

The ECG in Figure 4.19 is from a young woman who had become progressively more breathless since the birth of her baby 4 months previously. She had had no chest pain. No previous ECGs were available. The anterior T wave changes could be a normal variant in a black woman. T wave inversion in leads V_3–V_4 could indicate anterior ischaemia, but the important point here is that the T wave inversion is most prominent in leads V_1 and V_2, and becomes progressively less in V_3 and V_4. This is

Fig. 4.18

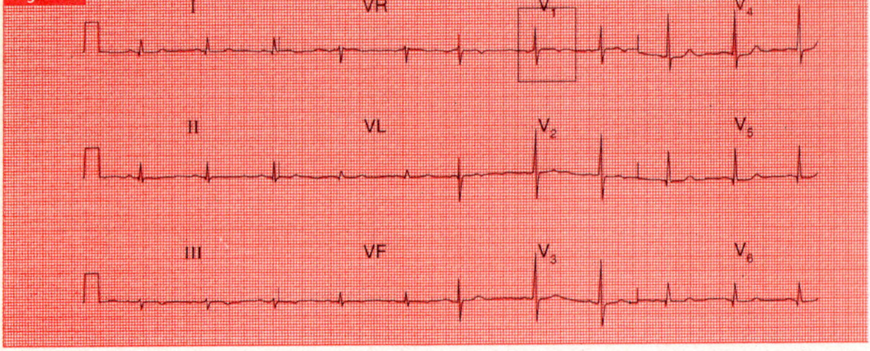

Fig. 4.19

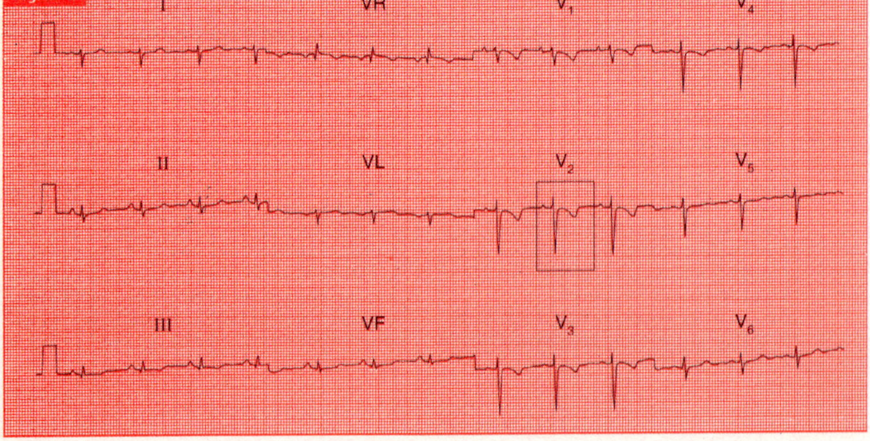

Probable normal variant

Note

- Sinus rhythm
- Normal axis
- Dominant R waves in lead V_1
- Inverted T waves in lead III

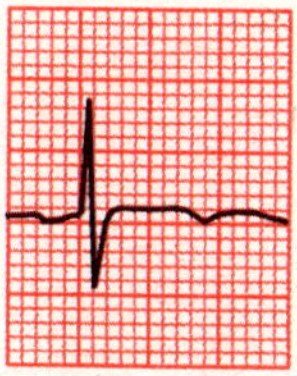

Dominant R wave in lead V_1

Right ventricular hypertrophy

Note

- Sinus rhythm
- Right axis deviation
- No dominant R waves in lead V_1
- Inverted T waves in leads V_1–V_4, maximal in lead V_1
- Persistent S waves in lead V_6

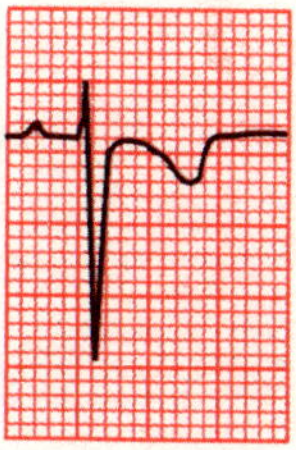

Inverted T wave in lead V_2

Fig. 4.20

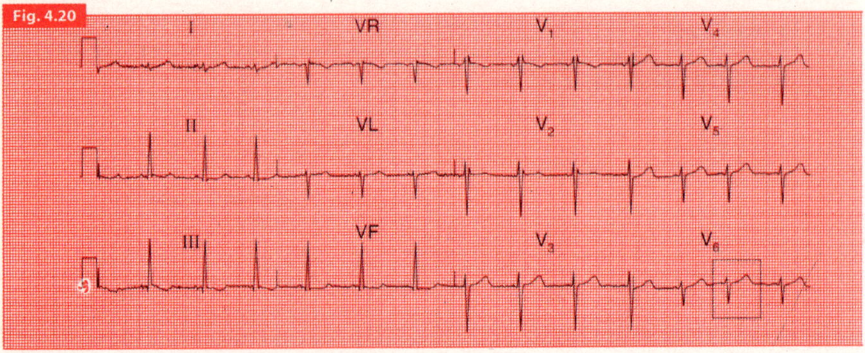

Fig. 4.21

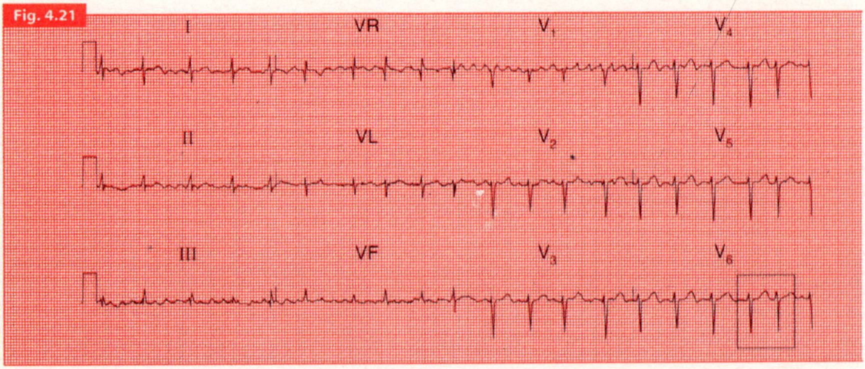

Chronic lung disease

Note

- Sinus rhythm
- Right axis deviation
- Prominent S waves in lead V_6
- Nonspecific T wave changes in leads III and VF

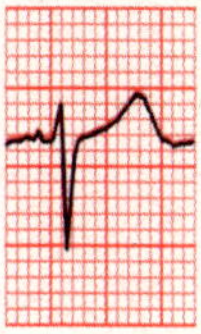

Persistent S wave in lead V_6

?Pulmonary embolus

Note

- Atrial fibrillation, ventricular rate 114/min
- Dominant S wave in lead V_6
- No other evidence of right ventricular hypertrophy

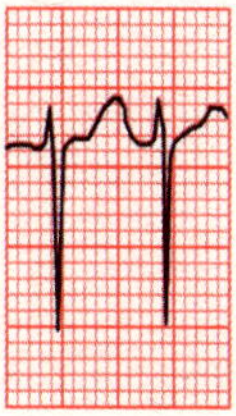

Persistent S wave in lead V_6

characteristic of T wave inversion due to right ventricular hypertrophy. In this case the T wave inversion, combined with right axis deviation and a persistent S wave in lead V_6, suggests right ventricular hypertrophy. The patient was shown to have had recurrent small pulmonary emboli.

A prominent S wave in lead V_6 is sometimes called 'persistent' because this lead should show a pure left ventricular type of complex with a dominant R wave and no S wave. The 'transition point', when the R and S waves are equal, indicates the position of the interventricular septum and this is normally under the position of lead V_3 or V_4. In the ECG in Figure 4.20 a 'transition point' is not present at all, and lead V_6 shows a small R wave and a dominant S wave. This is due to the right ventricle underlying more of the precordium than usual. This change is characteristic of chronic lung disease.

When breathlessness is accompanied by a sudden change in rotation, a pulmonary embolus is likely. The ECG in Figure 4.21 is from a patient who had had a normal preoperative ECG but who developed breathlessness with atrial fibrillation a week after cholecystectomy. The deep S wave in lead V_6 is the pointer towards a pulmonary embolus being the cause of the atrial fibrillation.

As with the ECG in left ventricular hypertrophy, it is the appearance of changes in serial recordings that provides the best evidence of minor or moderate degrees of right ventricular hypertrophy. In the majority of cases in which the ECG suggests right ventricular hypertrophy, it is not possible to diagnose the underlying disease process with certainty.

WHAT TO DO

The possible effects of various types of cardiac disease on the heart and the ECG are summarized in Boxes 4.2–4.8. However, in most patients with breathlessness, the ECG does not contribute very much to diagnosis and management and the important thing is to treat the patient and not the ECG.

The ECG cannot diagnose heart failure, although heart failure is unlikely if the ECG is totally normal. By demonstrating ischaemia or enlargement of one or more of the cardiac chambers, the ECG may help to identify the underlying disease that requires treatment. However, the symptoms of acute heart failure need empirical treatment whatever the ECG shows, and this should not be delayed while an ECG is being recorded.

The ECG can provide confirmatory evidence that breathlessness is due to a pulmonary embolus or chronic lung disease, but it is an unreliable way of making this diagnosis and treatment cannot depend on the ECG. Similarly, the ECG will not help in the diagnosis of anaemia, though it may show ischaemic changes.

In general then, the management of the breathless patient does not depend on the ECG unless breathlessness is due to heart failure which is secondary to an arrhythmia. In that case, the ECG is essential both for diagnosis and for monitoring the response to therapy.

Box 4.2 The ECG in valve disease

Mitral stenosis
- Atrial fibrillation
- Left atrial hypertrophy, if in sinus rhythm
- Right ventricular hypertrophy

Mitral regurgitation
- Atrial fibrillation
- Left atrial hypertrophy, if in sinus rhythm
- Left ventricular hypertrophy

Aortic stenosis
- Left ventricular hypertrophy
- Incomplete left bundle branch block (i.e. loss of Q waves in leads V_5–V_6)
- Left bundle branch block

Aortic regurgitation
- Left ventricular hypertrophy
- Prominent but narrow Q wave in lead V_6
- Left anterior hemiblock
- Occasionally, left bundle branch block

Mitral valve prolapse
- Sinus rhythm, or wide variety of arrhythmias
- Inverted T waves in leads II–III, VF
- T wave inversion in precordial leads
- ST segment depression
- Exercise-induced ventricular arrhythmias
- Note: abnormalities can vary in different records from the same individual

Biventricular hypertrophy
- Left ventricular hypertrophy plus right axis deviation
- Left ventricular hypertrophy plus clockwise rotation
- Left ventricular hypertrophy with tall R waves in lead V_1

Box 4.3 The ECG in congestive cardiomyopathy

- Arrhythmias, especially atrial fibrillation and ventricular tachycardia
- First degree block
- Right or left atrial enlargement
- Low amplitude QRS complexes
- Left anterior hemiblock
- Left bundle branch block
- Right bundle branch block
- Left ventricular hypertrophy
- Nonspecific ST segment and T wave changes

Box 4.4 The ECG in hypertrophic cardiomyopathy

- Short PR interval
- Various rhythm disturbances, including ventricular tachycardia and ventricular fibrillation
- Left atrial hypertrophy
- Left anterior hemiblock or left bundle branch block
- Left ventricular hypertrophy
- Prolonged QT interval
- Deep T wave inversion anteriorly

Box 4.5 The ECG in myocarditis

- Sinus tachycardias and other arrhythmias
- First, second or third degree block
- Widened QRS complexes
- Irregularity of QRS waveform
- Q waves
- Prolonged QT interval
- ST segment elevation or depression
- T wave inversion in any lead

Box 4.6 The ECG in acute rheumatic fever

- Sinus tachycardia
- First degree block
- ST segment/T wave changes of acute myocarditis
- Changes associated with pericarditis

Box 4.7 The ECG in pulmonary embolism

- Sinus tachycardia
- Atrial arrhythmias
- Right atrial hypertrophy
- Right ventricular hypertrophy
- Right axis deviation
- Clockwise rotation with persistent S wave in lead V_6
- Right bundle branch block
- Combination of S wave in lead I with Q wave and inverted T wave in lead III

Box 4.8 The ECG in chronic obstructive pulmonary disease

- Small complexes
- Right atrial hypertrophy (P pulmonale)
- Right axis deviation
- Right ventricular hypertrophy
- Clockwise rotation (deep S waves in lead V_6)
- Right bundle branch block

5 The effect of other conditions on the ECG

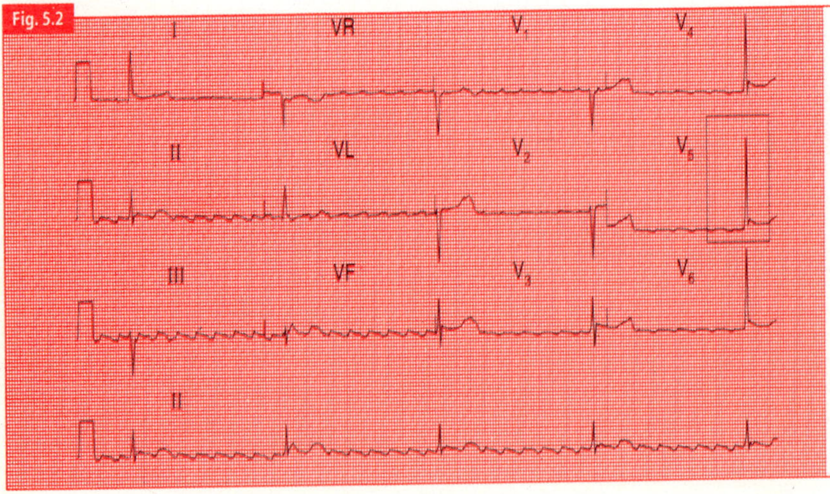

Fig. 5.2

Fig. 5.1

Parkinsonism

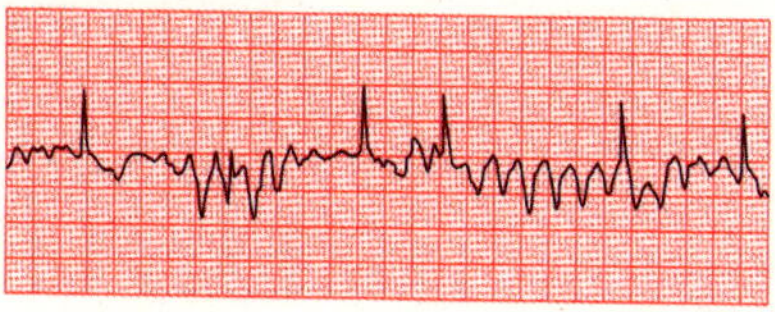

Note

- Muscle tremor at 5/s gives an appearance resembling atrial flutter
- The irregular QRS complexes may indicate that the rhythm is actually atrial fibrillation
- This record demonstrates the importance of looking at the patient as well as the ECG

The ECG is not a good method for investigating or diagnosing any condition that is not primarily cardiac. However, some generalized diseases do affect the ECG – it is important to recognize this, and not assume that a patient has heart disease simply because their ECG seems abnormal.

Atrial flutter, hypothermia

Note

- Atrial flutter with ventricular rate 26/min
- J waves visible in leads V_4–V_6

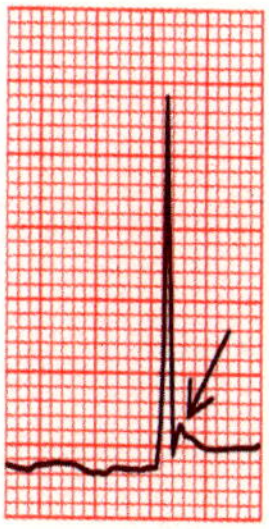

J wave in lead V_5

ARTEFACTS IN ECG RECORDINGS

THE EFFECTS OF ABNORMAL MUSCLE MOVEMENT

Although ECG recorders are designed to be especially sensitive to the electrical frequencies of cardiac muscle contraction, the ECG will also record the contraction of skeletal muscles. The most common pattern of 'ECG abnormality' is a high-frequency oscillation due to general muscular tension in a patient who is not properly relaxed.

Sustained involuntary tremors, such as those associated with Parkinsonism (Fig. 5.1) cause rhythmic ECG abnormalities that may be confused with cardiac arrhythmias.

HYPOTHERMIA

Hypothermia causes shivering, and therefore artefacts due to muscular activity. However, there can be other changes in the ECG and the characteristic ECG feature of hypothermia is the 'J wave'. This is a small hump seen at the end of the QRS complex (see Fig. 5.2).

Fig. 5.3

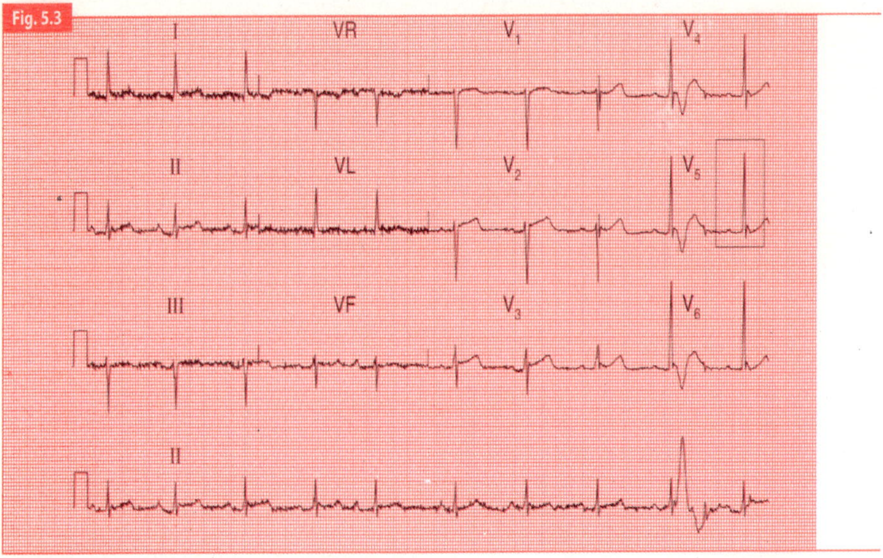
I
VR
V1
V4
II
VL
V2
V5
III
VF
V3
V6
II

Fig. 5.4

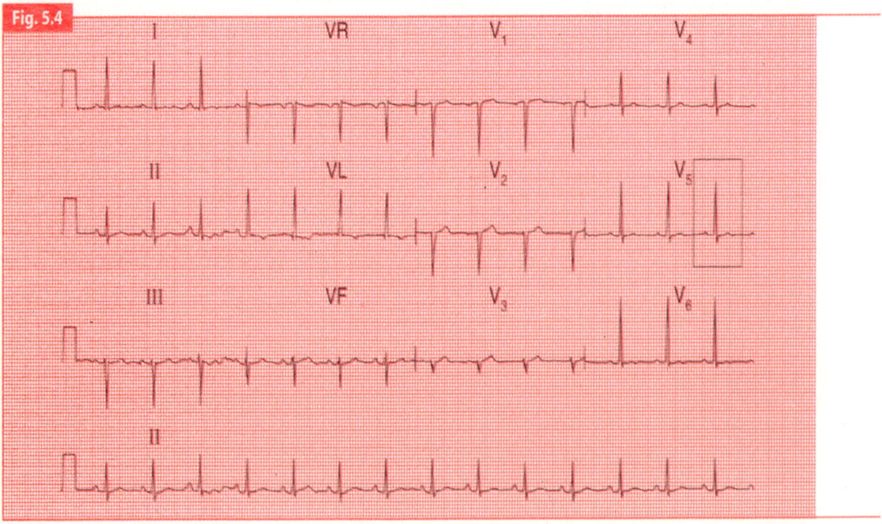
I
VR
V1
V4
II
VL
V2
V5
III
VF
V3
V6
II

Hypothermia

Note

- Same patient as in Figures 5.2 and 5.4
- Sinus rhythm is restored
- Patient has begun to shiver (muscle artefact in the limb leads, with a further artefact in the penultimate complex of the rhythm strip)
- First degree block
- J waves still visible

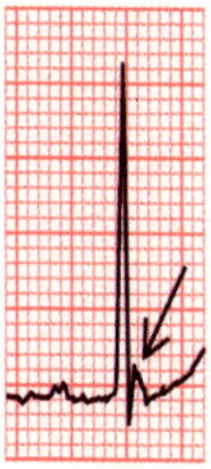

J wave in lead V_5

Re-warming after hypothermia

Note

- Same patient as in Figures 5.2 and 5.3
- Patient is now in sinus rhythm with a normal PR interval
- J waves have disappeared
- There are some nonspecific ST segment and T wave changes in leads I–II, VL, V_6

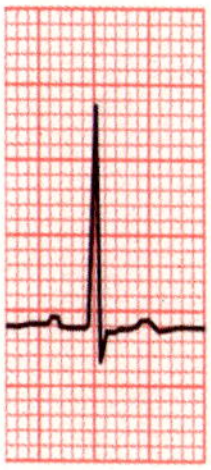

No J wave in lead V_5

The ECG in Figure 5.2 was recorded from a 76-year-old woman who was admitted to hospital with a temperature of 30°C after lying for a prolonged period in a freezing house, after a fall. She initially had a heart rate of 26/min and the rhythm was atrial flutter. J waves can be seen in the lateral chest leads. On re-warming she began to shiver, and despite the muscle artefact can be seen to have reverted to sinus rhythm with first degree block. J waves are still visible (Fig. 5.3). When her temperature had returned to normal, the PR interval normalized and the J waves disappeared (Fig. 5.4).

THE ECG IN CONGENITAL HEART DISEASE

The ECG provides a limited amount of help in the diagnosis of congenital heart disease by showing which chambers of the heart are enlarged. It is important to remember (see Ch. 1) that at birth the ECG of a normal infant shows a pattern of 'right ventricular hypertrophy' and this gradually disappears during the first 2 years of life.

If the infant pattern persists beyond the age of 2 years, right ventricular hypertrophy is indeed present. If there is a left ventricular, or normal adult, pattern before this age, then left ventricular hypertrophy is probably present. In older children the same criteria for left and right ventricular hypertrophy as in adults apply.

Table 5.1 lists some common congenital disorders and the associated ECG appearance.

The ECG in Figure 5.5 shows all the features of severe right ventricular hypertrophy: it came from a boy with severe pulmonary stenosis.

The ECG in Figure 5.6 shows left ventricular hypertrophy, and was recorded in an 8-year-old with severe aortic stenosis.

The ECG in Figure 5.7 shows right ventricular hypertrophy, and came from a young woman who had had a partial correction of Fallot's tetralogy 20 years previously.

The ECG in Figure 5.8 suggests right atrial hypertrophy and shows right bundle branch block. It came from a teenager with Ebstein's anomaly and an atrial septal defect.

It is usually fairly obvious that a patient has congenital heart disease of some sort, but the condition that may be missed is an atrial septal defect. The ECG in Figure 5.9 is from a 50-year-old woman who complained of mild but increasing breathlessness. She had a rather nonspecific systolic murmur at the left sternal edge. Her GP recorded an ECG which showed right bundle branch block, and as a result she had an echocardiogram which showed an atrial septal defect.

Fig. 5.5

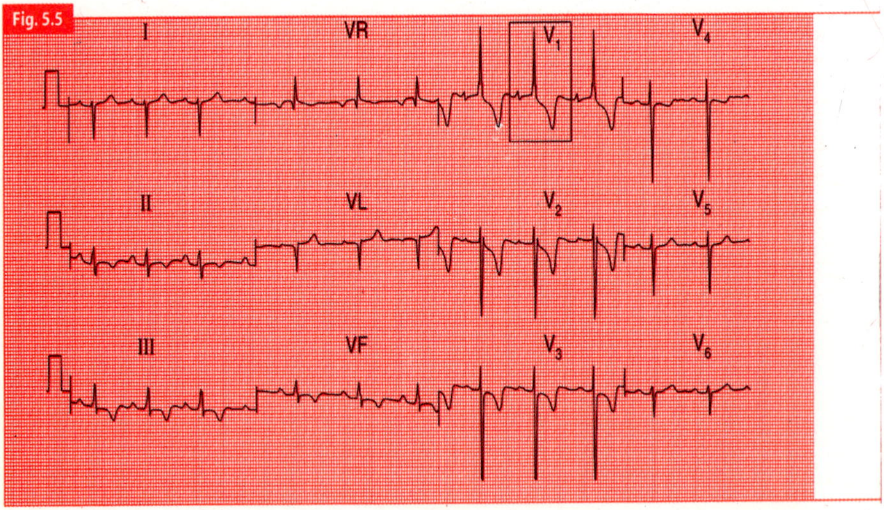

Table 5.1 ECG appearance in common congenital disorders

ECG appearance	Congenital disorder
Right ventricular hypertrophy	Pulmonary hypertension of any cause (e.g. Eisenmenger's syndrome) Severe pulmonary stenosis Fallot's tetralogy Transposition of the great arteries
Left ventricular hypertrophy	Aortic stenosis Coarctation of the aorta Mitral regurgitation Obstructive cardiomyopathy
Biventricular hypertrophy	Ventricular septal defect
Right atrial hypertrophy	Tricuspid stenosis
Right bundle branch block	Atrial septal defect Complex defects
Left axis deviation	Endocardial cushion defects Corrected transposition

Pulmonary stenosis

Note

- Sinus rhythm
- Right axis deviation
- Dominant R waves in lead V_1
- Persistent S waves in lead V_6
- Inverted T waves in leads V_1–V_4

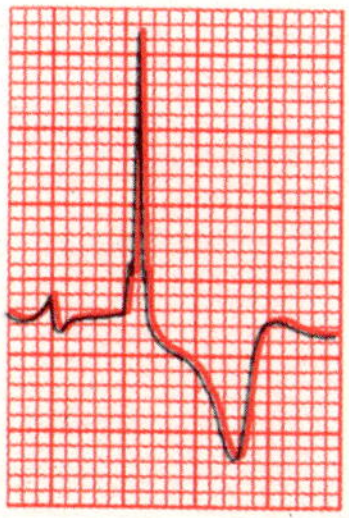

Dominant R wave in lead V_1

Fig. 5.6

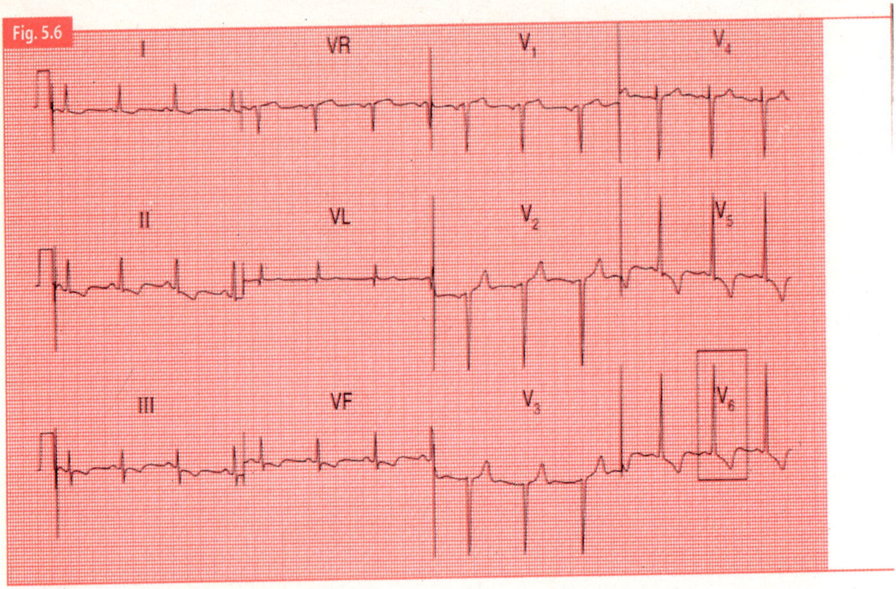

Fig. 5.7

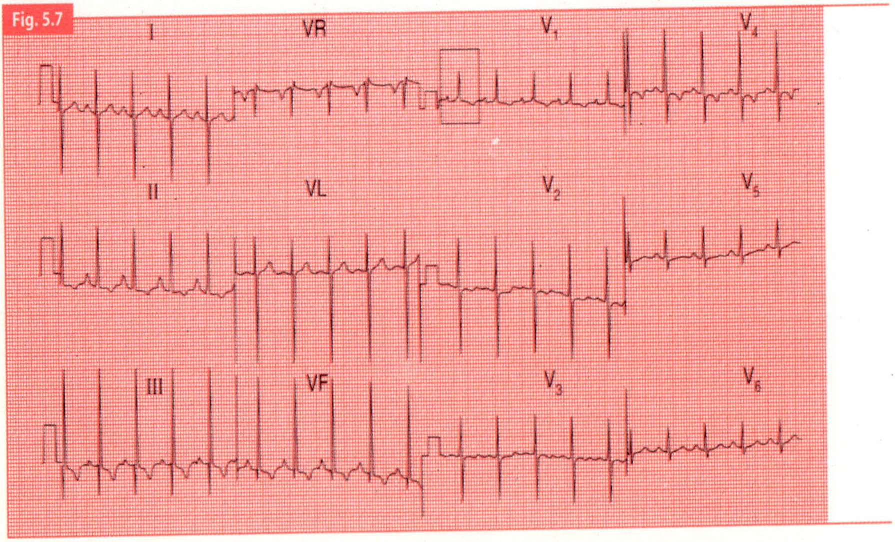

Left ventricular hypertrophy

Note

- Sinus rhythm
- Normal axis
- Left ventricular hypertrophy according to voltage criteria
- T wave inversion in leads I, V_5–V_6

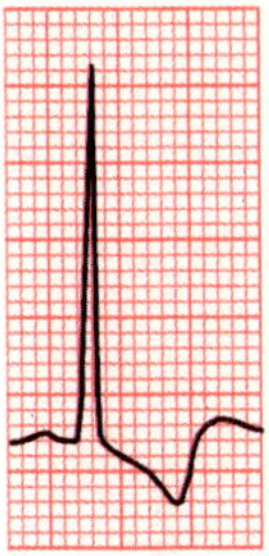

Tall R wave and inverted T wave in lead V_6

Right ventricular hypertrophy in Fallot's tetralogy

Note

- Leads V_1–V_6 recorded at half sensitivity
- Sinus rhythm
- Right axis deviation
- Dominant R waves in lead V_1
- T wave inversion in leads II–III, VF, V_1–V_4

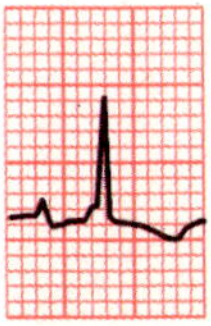

Dominant R wave in lead V_1

Fig. 5.8

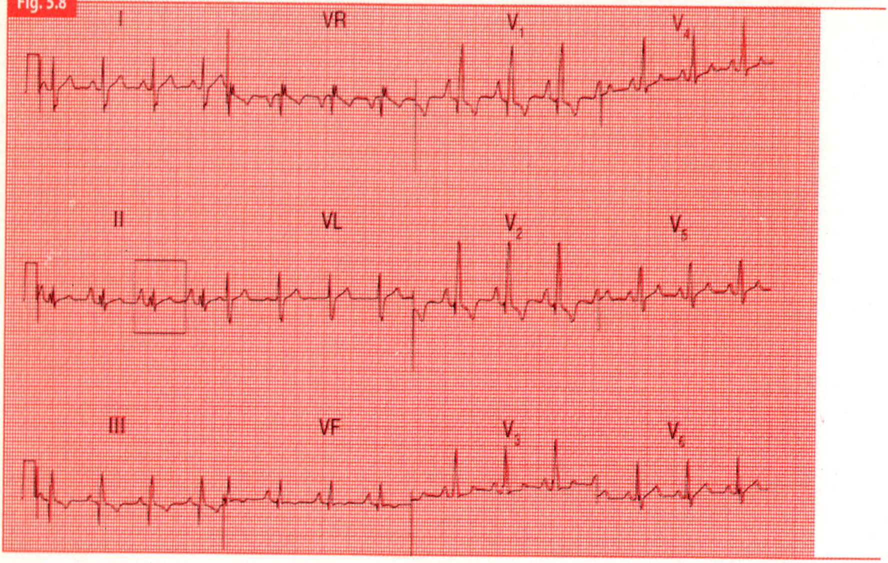

Fig. 5.9

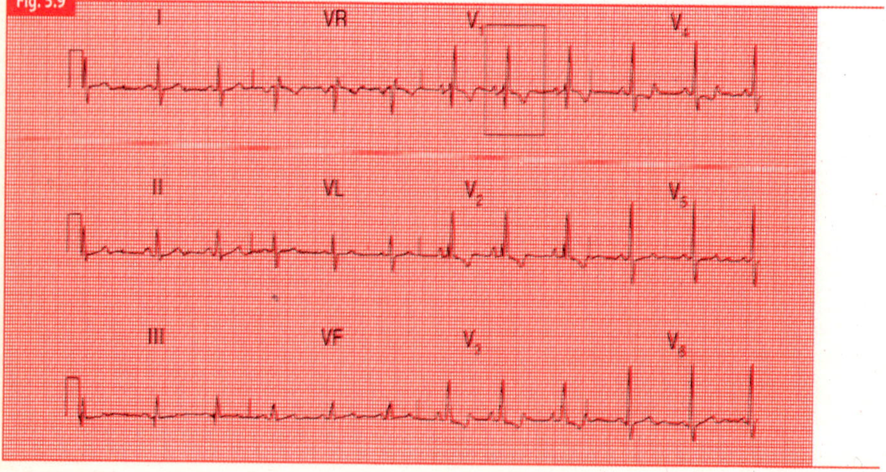

Right atrial hypertrophy and right bundle branch block, in Ebstein's anomaly

Note

- Sinus rhythm
- Peaked P waves in lead II
- Broad QRS complexes with right bundle branch block pattern

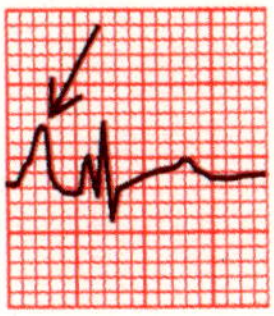

Peaked P wave in lead II

Right bundle branch block with atrial septal defect

Note

- Sinus rhythm
- Normal axis
- QRS complex duration within normal limits (108 ms)
- RBBB pattern

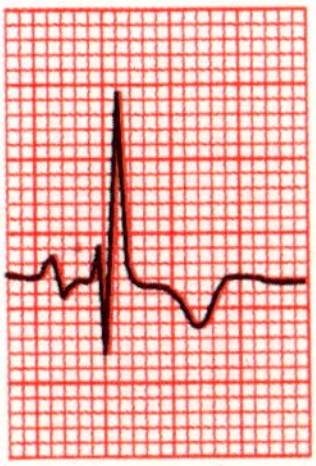

RBBB pattern in lead V_1

Fig. 5.10

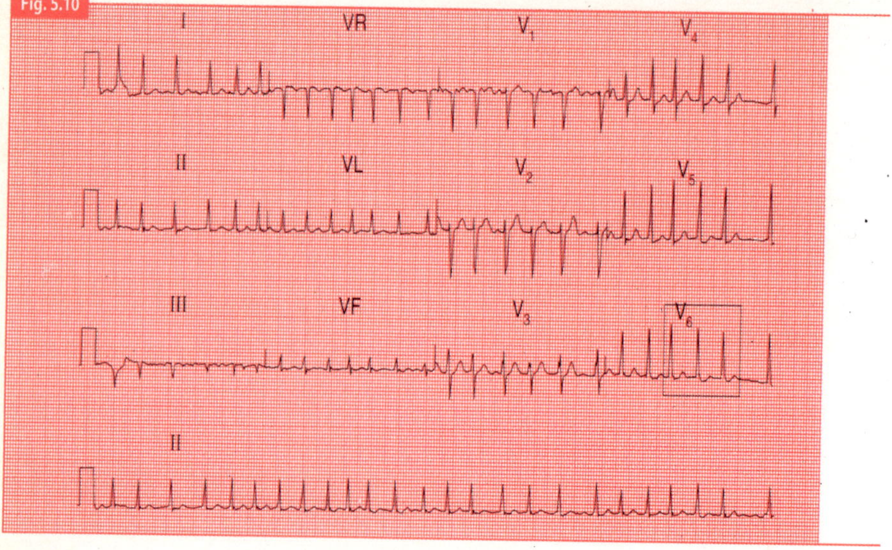

Fig. 5.11

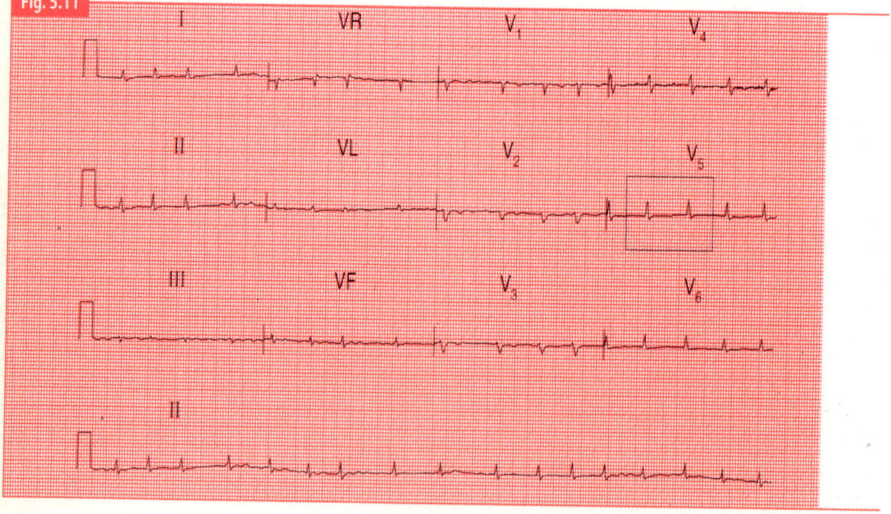

Thyrotoxicosis

Note

- Atrial fibrillation
- Ventricular rate 153/min
- Some ST segment depression in leads V_5–V_6: ?digoxin effect
- No other abnormalities

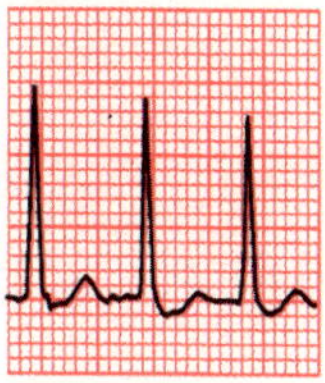

Rapid ventricular rate in lead V_6

Malignant pericardial effusion

Note

- Atrial fibrillation
- Generally small QRS complexes
- Widespread T wave flattening

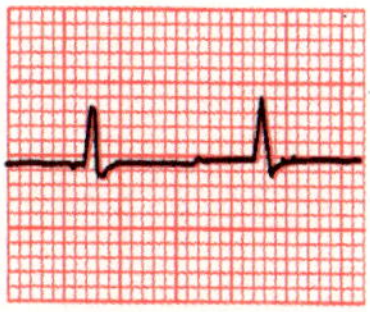

Small QRS complexes and flat T waves in lead V_5

THE ECG IN SYSTEMIC DISEASES

Cardiac involvement in a generalized disorder, particularly one that causes infiltration or the deposition of abnormal substances in the myocardium, causes arrhythmias and conduction defects.

THYROID DISEASE

Thyrotoxicosis is probably the most common non-cardiac disorder that may present as a cardiac problem. It may cause atrial fibrillation, particularly in old age. There is usually a rapid ventricular response, which is difficult to control with digoxin (Fig. 5.10). An elderly patient may complain of palpitations or the symptoms of heart failure, and arterial embolization may occur. The usual symptoms of thyrotoxicosis may be mild or even absent.

MALIGNANCY

Metastatic deposits in and around the heart can cause virtually any arrhythmia or conduction disturbance. Malignancy is the most common cause of a large pericardial effusion, and a combination of atrial fibrillation and small complexes on the ECG suggest a malignant pericardial effusion. The ECG in Figure 5.11 is from a 60-year-old man with metastatic bronchial carcinoma.

In the case of large pericardial effusions, the heart can rock with each beat within the effusion, causing alternate large and small QRS complexes. This is called 'electrical alternans'. The ECG in Figure 5.12 is from another patient with carcinoma of the bronchus, who presented with a supraventricular tachycardia. Electrical alternans suggests the presence of a pericardial effusion, though in this case the QRS complexes are of normal size.

Fig. 5.12

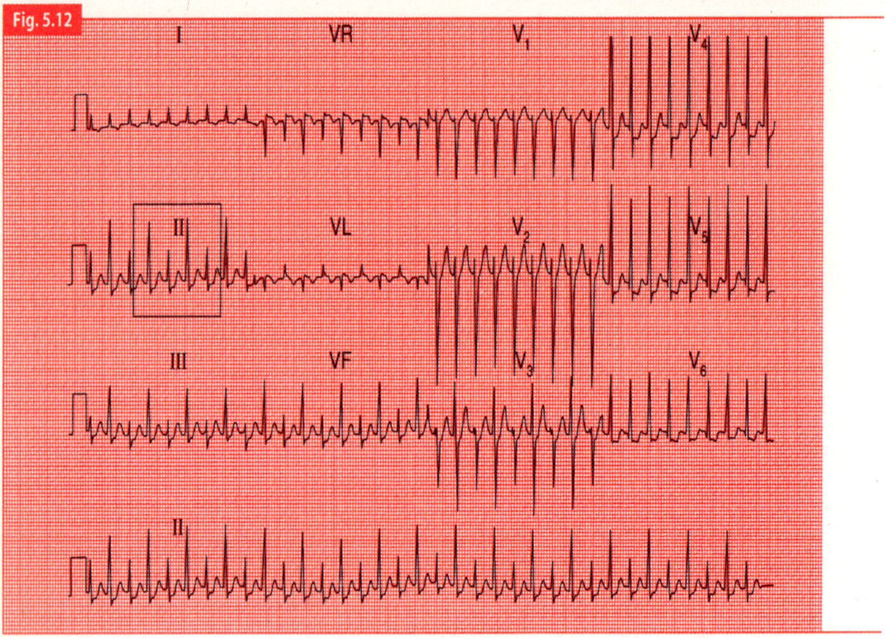

THE EFFECTS OF SERUM ELECTROLYTE ABNORMALITIES ON THE ECG

Although abnormal levels of serum potassium, magnesium and calcium can affect the ECG, the 'classical' changes are rarely seen. Occasionally an ECG may suggest that the electrolytes should be checked, but the range of normality in the ECG is so great that an ECG is an unrealistic guide to electrolyte balance. Box 5.1 lists possible causes of electrolyte imbalance, and Table 5.2 summarizes the ECG changes that may occur.

POTASSIUM

Hyperkalaemia may cause arrhythmias, including ventricular fibrillation or asystole; flattening of the P waves; widening of the QRS complexes; depression or loss of the ST segment; and, particularly, symmetrical peaking of the T waves. The ECG in Figure 5.13 is from a patient with renal failure and a potassium level of 7.4 mmol. After correction of the plasma potassium level, sinus rhythm was restored and the T waves were no longer peaked (Fig. 5.14).

Electrical alternans

Note

- Narrow complex tachycardia at 200/min (junctional tachycardia)
- Alternate large and small QRS complexes

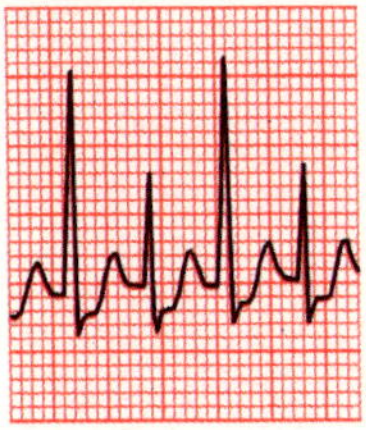

Alternate large and small QRS complexes in lead II

Box 5.1 Causes of electrolyte imbalance

Hyperkalaemia
- Renal failure
- Potassium-retaining diuretics (amiloride, spironolactone, triamterene)
- Angiotensin-converting enzyme inhibitors
- Liquorice
- Bartter's syndrome

Hypokalaemia
- Diuretic therapy
- Antidiuretic hormone secretion

Hypercalcaemia
- Hyperparathyroidism
- Renal failure
- Sarcoidosis
- Malignancy
- Myeloma
- Excess vitamin D
- Thiazide diuretics

Hypocalcaemia
- Hypoparathyroidism
- Severe diarrhoea
- Enteric fistulae
- Alkalosis
- Vitamin D deficiency

Table 5.2 The effects of electrolyte imbalance on the ECG

Electrolyte	Effect of abnormal serum electrolyte level on ECG	
	Low level	High level
Potassium or magnesium	Flat T waves Prominent U waves Depressed ST segment Prolonged QT interval First or second degree block	Flat P waves Widening of QRS complexes (nonspecific intraventricular conduction delay) Tall peaked T waves Disappearance of ST segment Arrhythmias
Calcium	Prolonged QT interval (due to long ST segment)	Short QT interval, with loss of ST segment

Fig. 5.13

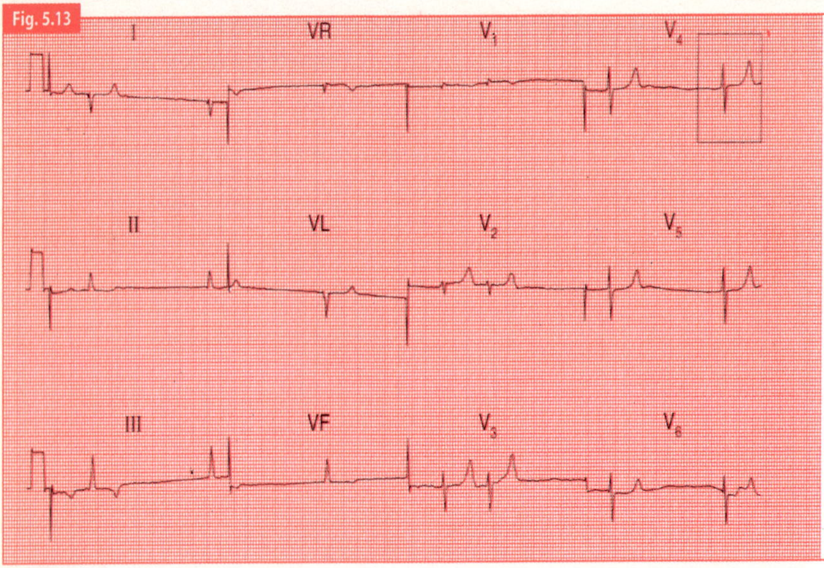

Fig. 5.14

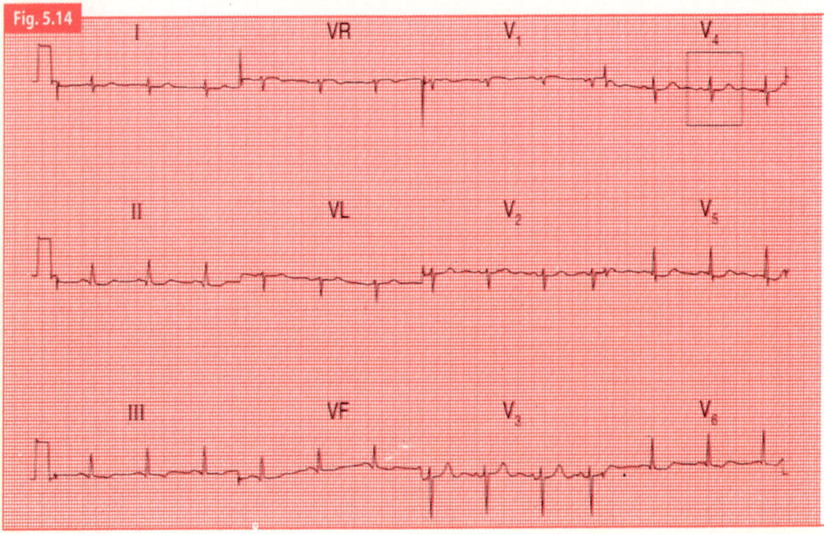

Hyperkalaemia

Note

- No P waves
- ?Atrial fibrillation
- ?Junctional escape rhythm
- Right axis deviation
- Symmetrically peaked T waves, especially in the chest leads
- Inverted T waves in leads III, VF

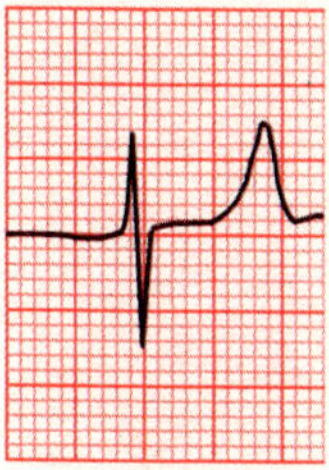

P wave absent and peaked T wave in lead V_4

Hyperkalaemia corrected

Note

- Same patient as in Figure 5.13
- Sinus rhythm
- ST segment depression in inferior lateral leads
- Normal T wave configuration

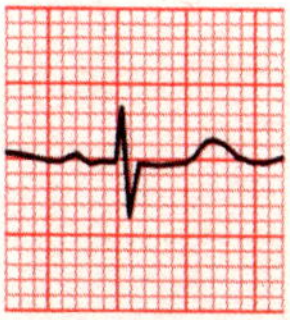

Normal P and T waves in lead V_4

Fig. 5.15

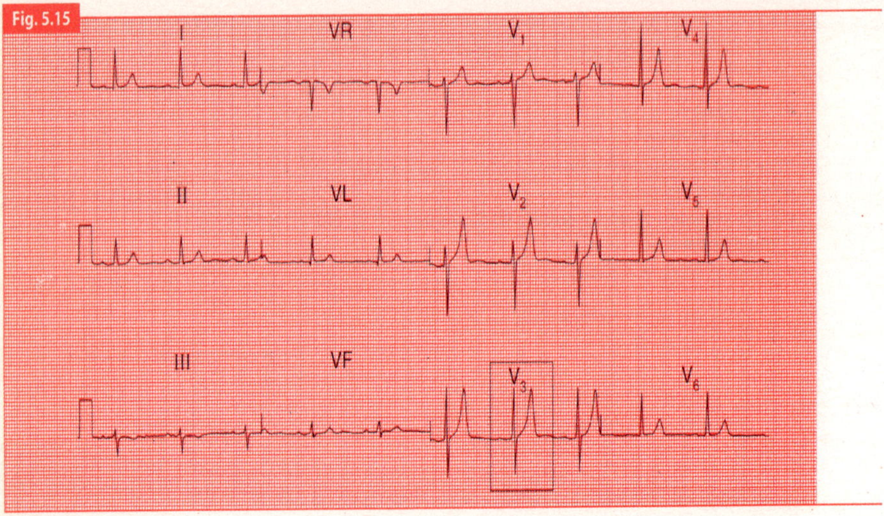

Fig. 5.16

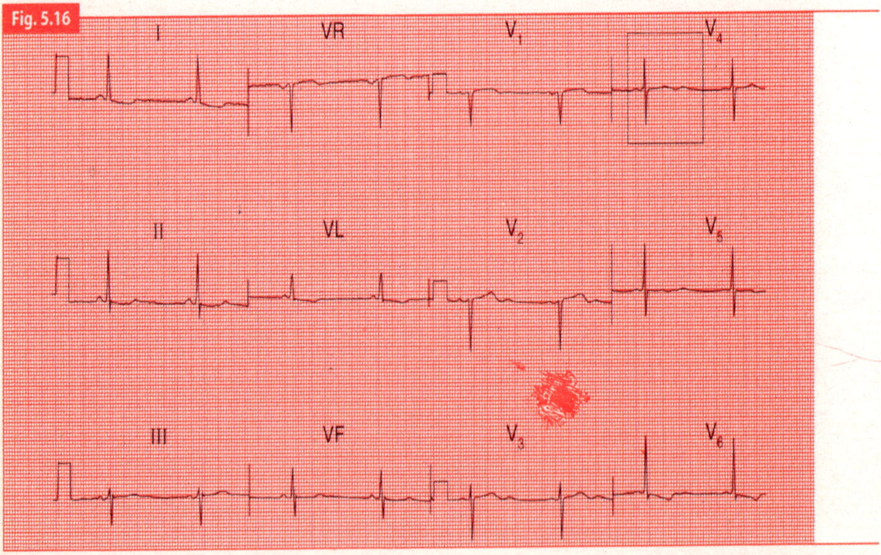

Normal ECG

Note

- Sinus rhythm
- Normal axis
- Tall peaked T waves, resembling hyperkalaemia

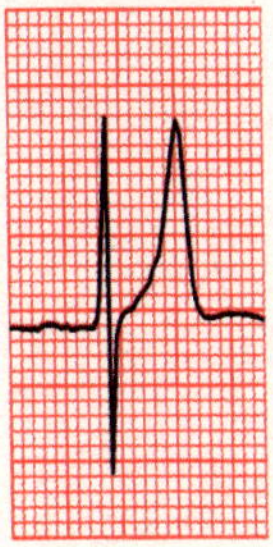

Tall, peaked T wave in lead V_3

Hypokalaemia

Note

- Leads V_1–V_6 recorded at half sensitivity
- Atrial fibrillation
- Normal axis
- Normal QRS complexes
- Flat T waves, with U waves in leads V_4–V_5

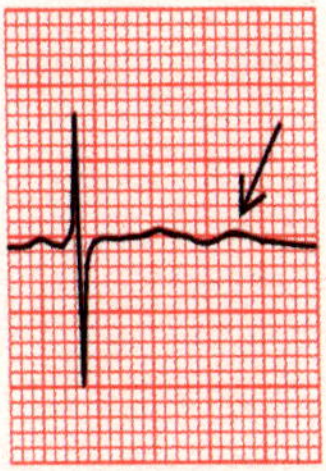

U wave in lead V_4

Remember, however, that peaked T waves are also a common finding in completely healthy patients (Fig. 5.15).

Hypokalaemia is common in patients with cardiac disease who are treated with powerful diuretics. It causes flattening of the T waves, prolongation of the QT interval, and the appearance of U waves. The ECG in Figure 5.16 was recorded from a patient with severe heart failure due to ischaemic heart disease. The serum potassium level fell to 1.9 mmol, as a result of loop diuretic treatment without either potassium supplementation or the concomitant administration of an angiotensin-converting enzyme inhibitor.

MAGNESIUM

The effects of high and low serum magnesium levels on the ECG are essentially the same as those of high and low potassium levels.

CALCIUM

Hypercalcaemia shortens, and hypocalcaemia prolongs, the QT interval. However, the ECG remains normal within a very wide range of serum calcium levels.

THE EFFECTS OF MEDICATION ON THE ECG

DIGOXIN

Atrial fibrillation is normally associated with a rapid ventricular response (sometimes inappropriately called 'fast AF'), unless conduction through the atrioventricular node is slowed by medication. Digoxin is still the best drug for controlling the ventricular rate in atrial fibrillation. The dose can be critical: the first sign of toxicity is a loss of appetite, and then the

Fig. 5.17

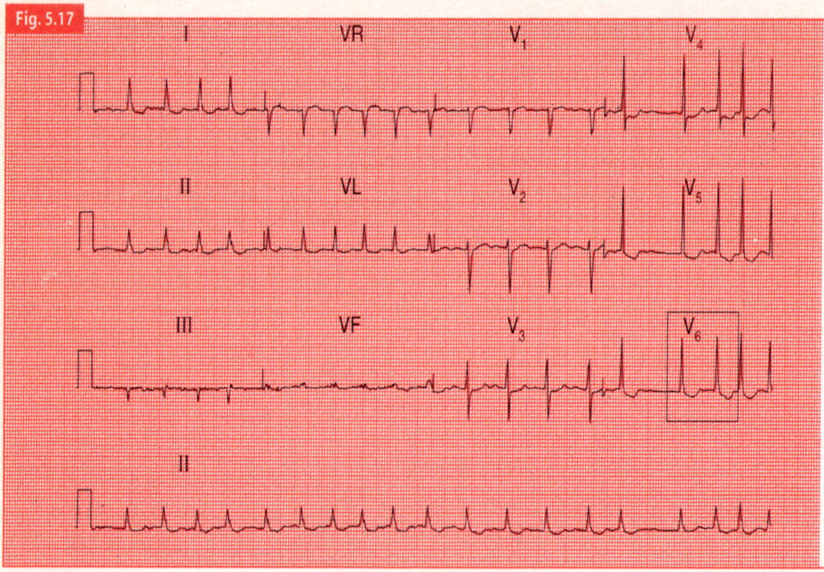

Fig. 5.18

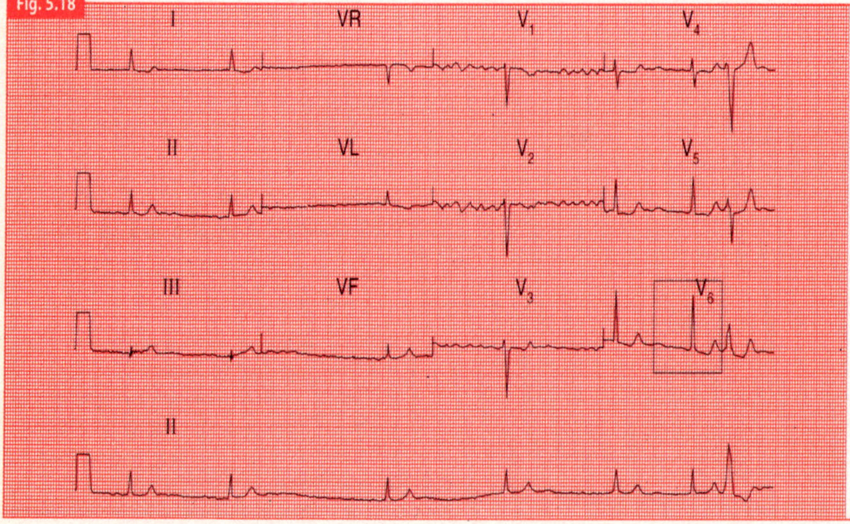

Digoxin effect

Note

- Atrial fibrillation
- Normal axis
- Normal QRS complexes
- Downward-sloping ST segments in leads V_5–V_6

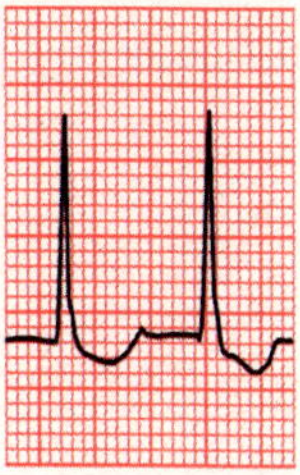

Downward-sloping ST segment in lead V_6

Digoxin toxicity

Note

- Atrial fibrillation with one ventricular extrasystole
- Ventricular rate 41/min
- Normal QRS complexes
- Digoxin effect on ST segments in lead V_6

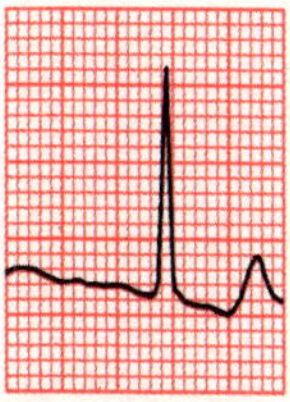

Downward-sloping ST segment in lead V_6

patient feels sick and vomits. Rarely, the patient complains of seeing yellow (xanthopsia). The main effect of digoxin on the ECG is downward sloping of the ST segments, especially in the lateral leads. The appearance is sometimes referred to as a 'reverse tick' (Fig. 5.17).

With increasing doses of digoxin the ventricular rate becomes regular and slow, and eventually complete heart block may develop. Digoxin can cause almost any arrhythmia, but especially ventricular extrasystoles and sometimes ventricular tachycardia. There is only a loose correlation between the symptoms and the ECG signs of digoxin toxicity.

The ECG in Figure 5.18 was recorded from a patient with a congestive cardiomyopathy which caused atrial fibrillation and heart failure. She was vomiting and her failure had deteriorated because her heart rate had fallen to about 40 beats/min.

The ECG in Figure 5.19 shows another example of digoxin toxicity, which caused syncopal attacks due to runs of ventricular tachycardia.

The ECG effects of digoxin are listed in Box 5.2.

Box 5.2 Effects of digoxin on the ECG

- Downward sloping ST segments
- Flattened or inverted T waves
- Short QT interval
- Almost any abnormal cardiac rhythm, but especially:
  - sinus bradycardia
  - paroxysmal atrial tachycardia with AV block
  - ventricular extrasystoles
  - ventricular tachycardia
  - any degree of AV block
- Regularization of QRS complexes in atrial fibrillation suggests toxicity

Fig. 5.19

Digoxin toxicity

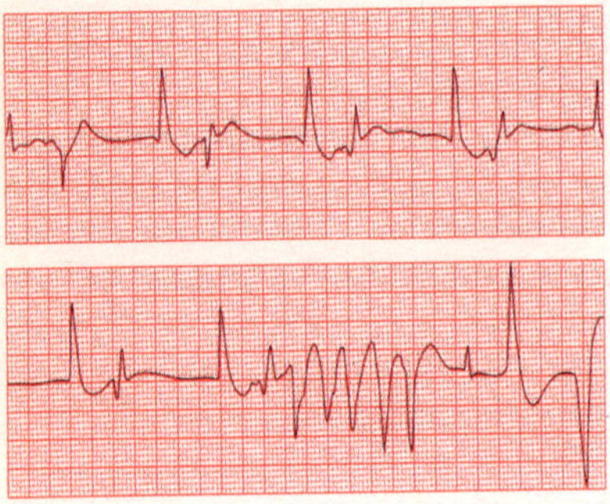

Note

- Continuous record
- Basic rhythm is atrial fibrillation: upright QRS complexes are probably the normally-conducted beats
- Each upright QRS complex is followed by a predominantly downward complex, which represents a ventricular extrasystole
- Short run of ventricular tachycardia towards the end of the recording

Fig. 5.20

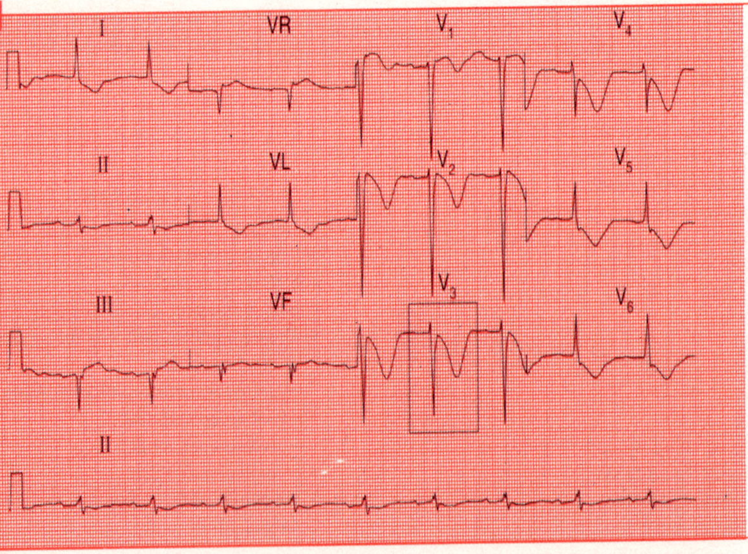

DRUGS THAT PROLONG THE QT INTERVAL

Over 200 drugs have been claimed to cause QT interval prolongation or torsade de pointes ventricular tachycardia (TdP VT). This is particularly true of the Class I and Class III antiarrhythmic drugs. It is sensible to regard all antiarrhythmic drugs as being potentially pro-arrhythmic, with the exception of the beta-blockers other than sotalol. While TdP VT is most commonly seen in patients whose ECGs have a prolonged QT interval, in some individuals the two are apparently not related. The ECG in Figure 5.20 was recorded from a patient treated with amiodarone; the T wave changes disappeared when the drug was discontinued.

Some of the more commonly used drugs which may cause QT interval prolongation and have been associated with TdP VT are listed in Box 5.3.

Several drugs that were otherwise very useful have been withdrawn because of the problems of QT interval prolongation and TdP VT. The list includes the gastric pro-motility agent cisapride, the antihistamine terfenadine, the antiplatelet agent ketanserin and the vasodilator prenylamine.

'Quinidine syncope' was recognized years before its mechanism was understood, and the ECG in Figure 5.21 is from a patient who developed TdP VT while being treated with quinidine.

Any of the drugs listed in Box 5.3 should be discontinued if the corrected QT interval exceeds 500 ms, or if the patient has symptoms suggesting an arrhythmia. It is prudent not to use drugs known to prolong the QT interval in patients with heart disease, and combinations of these drugs (e.g. erythromycin and ketoconazole) must definitely be avoided.

The appearance of T wave changes as, for example, in the patient needing lithium treatment whose ECG is shown in Figure 5.22, is not necessarily an indication to discontinue treatment.

Prolonged QT interval due to amiodarone

Note

- Sinus rhythm
- First degree block
- Normal QRS complexes
- QT interval 600 ms
- Widespread T wave inversion

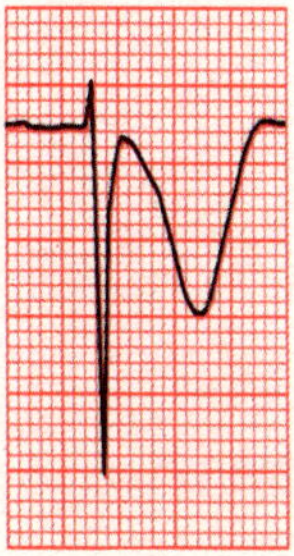

Long QT interval and inverted T wave in lead V_3

Box 5.3 Drugs associated with QT interval prolongation and TdP ventricular tachycardia

Antiarrhythmic drugs
- Amiodarone
- Bretylium
- Dofetilide
- Disopyramide
- Flecainide
- Procainamide
- Propafenone
- Quinidine
- Sotalol

Psychiatric drugs
- Amitriptyline
- Chlorpromazine
- Doxepin
- Haloperidol
- Imipramine
- Lithium
- Prochlorperazine
- Thioridazine

Antimicrobial, antifungal and antimalarial drugs
- Clarithromycin
- Chloroquine
- Co-trimoxazole (trimethoprim–sulfamethoxazole)
- Erythromycin
- Ketoconazole
- Quinine

Antihistaminic drugs
- Diphenhydramine

Others
- Alcohol
- Tacrolimus
- Tamoxifen

Fig. 5.22

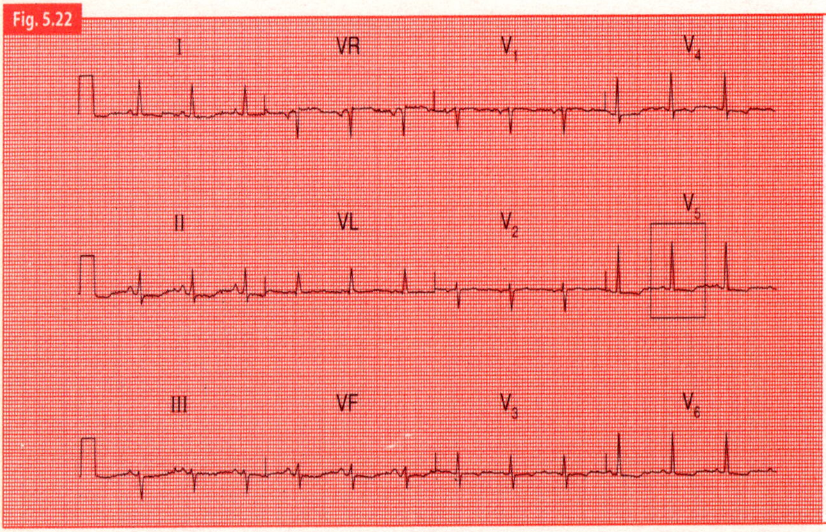

Fig. 5.21

Quinidine toxicity

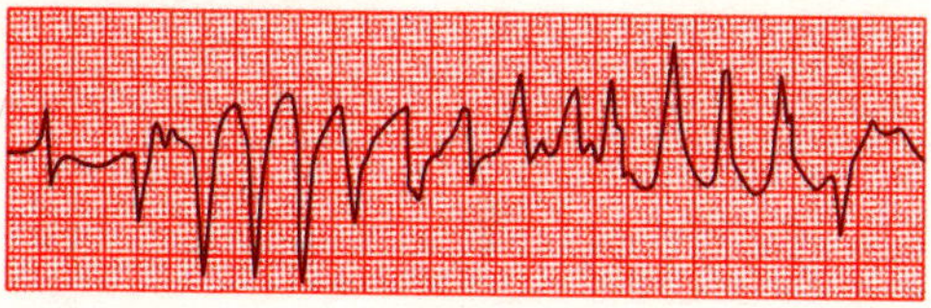

Note

- A single sinus beat is followed by a run of torsade de pointes ventricular tachycardia

Lithium treatment

Note

- Sinus rhythm
- Normal axis
- Normal QRS complexes
- Normal QT interval
- Widespread T wave inversion

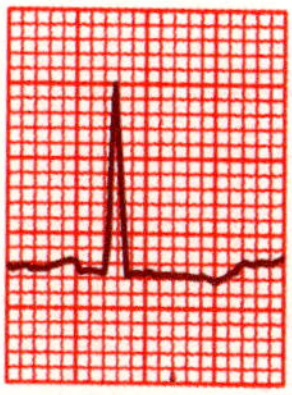

Inverted T wave in lead V_5

Fig. 5.23

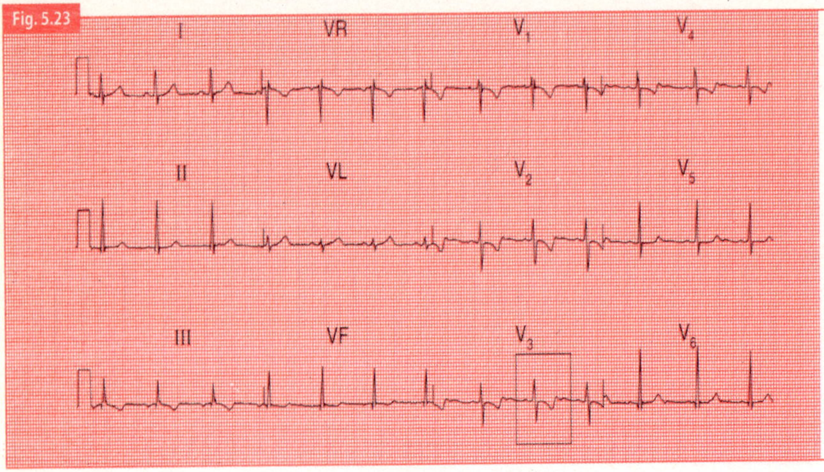

Fig. 5.24

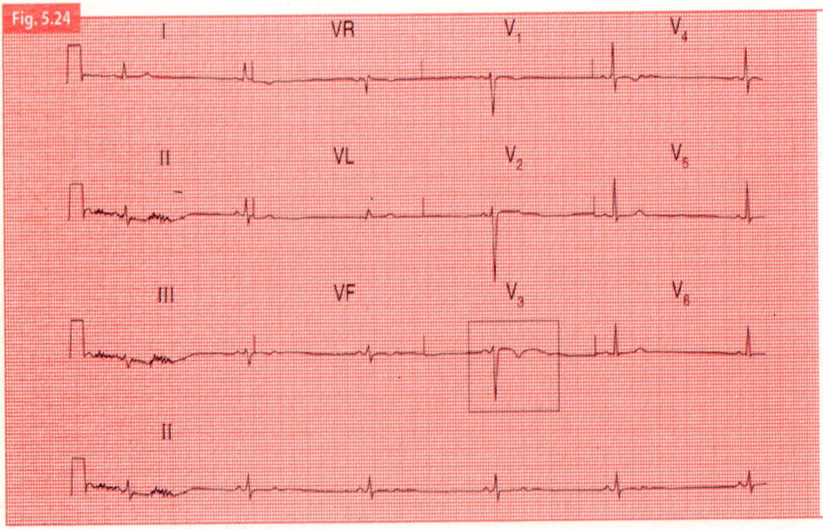

Trauma

Note

- Sinus rhythm
- Normal axis
- Partial right bundle branch block pattern
- Anterior T wave inversion

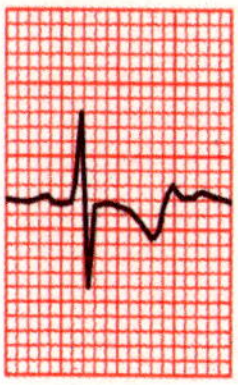

Inverted T wave in lead V_3

Anorexia nervosa

Note

- Sinus rhythm at 32/min
- Artefacts in leads II–III
- Normal axis
- Normal QRS complexes
- T wave inversion and U waves in anterior chest leads

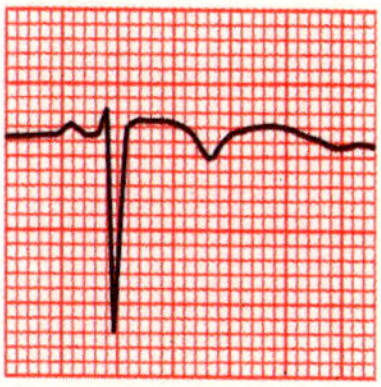

Inverted T wave and U wave in lead V_3

OTHER CAUSES OF AN ABNORMAL ECG

TRAUMA

Myocardial damage can be caused by chest injuries, either penetrating (e.g. stab wound) or closed (usually due to a steering wheel or seat belt). Direct trauma to the front of the heart can lead to occlusion of the left anterior descending coronary artery, and so to an ECG resembling that of an acute anterior myocardial infarction. However, seat belt injuries are more usually associated with myocardial contusion, as was the case in a young woman whose ECG is shown in Figure 5.23.

METABOLIC DISEASES

Most metabolic diseases, e.g. Addison's disease, are associated with nonspecific ST segment or T wave changes. There may be no apparent abnormality in the serum electrolytes. The ECG in Figure 5.24 is from a young girl with severe anorexia nervosa: her serum electrolytes and thyroid function were perfectly normal, but the ECG changes presumably reflect an intracellular electrolyte abnormality.

Fig. 5.25

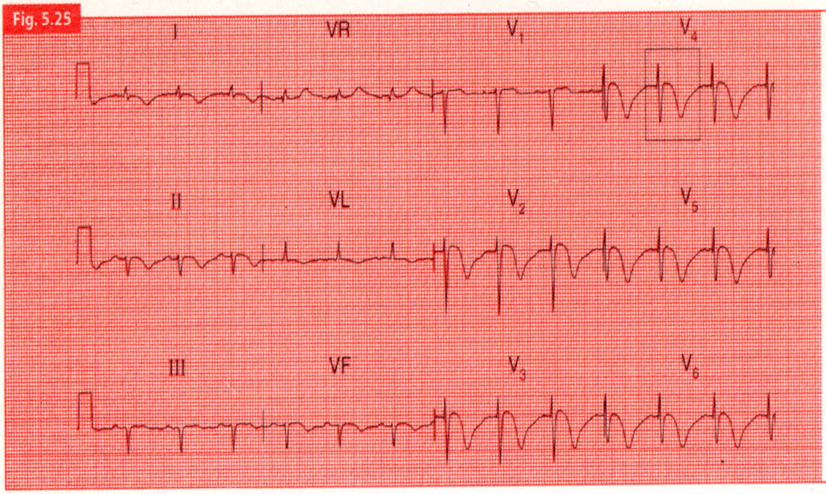

Fig. 5.26

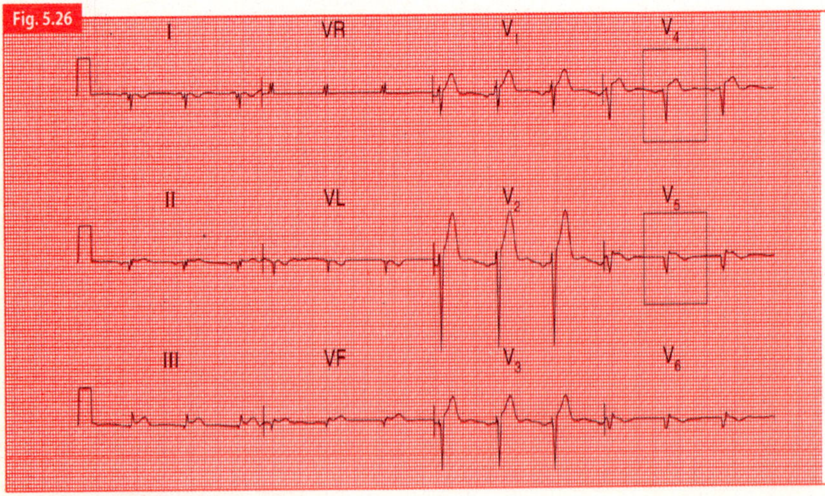

Subarachnoid haemorrhage

Note

- Sinus rhythm
- Left axis deviation
- QT interval 600 ms
- Widespread T wave inversion

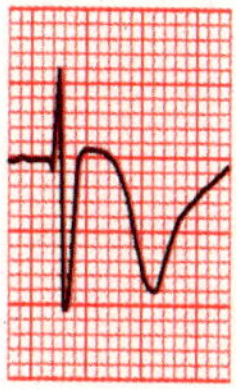

Long QT interval and inverted T wave in lead V_4

CEREBROVASCULAR ACCIDENTS

The association of a cerebrovascular accident and ECG abnormalities always suggests that the neurological problem is secondary to a cerebral embolus, which arose in the heart because of an arrhythmia or a left ventricular thrombus.

Sudden intracerebral events, particularly subarachnoid haemorrhage, can cause widespread T wave inversion. The ECG in Figure 5.25 is from a patient with subarachnoid haemorrhage.

MUSCLE DISEASE

Many of the neuromuscular disorders are associated with a cardiomyopathy. The ECG in Figure 5.26 is from a young man with no cardiovascular symptoms and a clinically normal heart, who had Friedreich's ataxia.

Friedreich's ataxia

Note

- Sinus rhythm
- Right axis deviation
- Widespread T wave abnormality
- Appearances could suggest anterolateral ischaemia

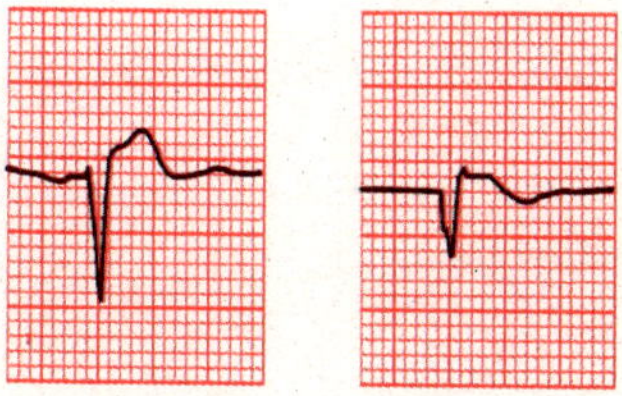

Changes in leads V_4 and V_5 suggesting an anterior infarction

6 The ECG and pacemakers, defibrillators and electrophysiology

This chapter describes the most commonly used intracardiac devices, and shows how cardiac electrophysiology can be used in the management of arrhythmias.

The 12-lead ECG is essential for the diagnosis of conduction disorders of the heart and of arrhythmias, and thus for decisions about patient management, including the need for devices such as pacemakers and implanted cardioverter defibrillators. After one of these devices has been inserted, the 12-lead ECG can be used to recognize the type of device, and to diagnose faults.

Intracardiac recordings can be made via an insulated wire with one or more exposed metal electrodes, passed percutaneously through a vein into the heart. Such recordings (endocardial ECGs) can show the spread of excitation through the heart more accurately than the surface ECG.

PACEMAKERS

Pacemakers and other cardiac devices are increasingly prevalent, especially in elderly patients. Although usually implanted and monitored by specialists, these devices are frequently encountered in a broad range of clinical contexts. The different types of pacemaker can be characterized by the number of cardiac chambers involved (see Table 6.1, p. 302). Patients often carry a card indicating the type of device implanted, but this can also be determined by its characteristic appearance on a plain chest X-ray. A chest X-ray is, therefore, a necessary part of any pacemaker assessment, and so this chapter includes a series of X-rays. It is essential that the type of device be determined before the ECG can be interpreted.

All pacemakers perform two fundamental functions: pacing and sensing. Most ECG findings in both normal and abnormal pacemaker function can be explained in terms of pacing and sensing functions.

PACING

An electrical pulse is generated between a pole at the tip of the pacing lead and either a second pole more proximally within the pacing lead (bipolar lead) or the pacemaker box itself (unipolar lead). This causes depolarization of the surrounding myocardium, the propagation of an action potential from this focus and the contraction of the paced cardiac chamber. This process is repeated at a basal rate determined when the pacemaker is programmed, although it can be suppressed as a result of device sensing (see below).

SENSING

The pacemaker continuously monitors electrical activity in the vicinity of the tip of the pacing lead.

If intrinsic cardiac depolarization is sensed in a single-chamber pacemaker, the pacemaker will inhibit pacing for a predetermined period. This prevents simultaneous pacing in the presence of spontaneous cardiac activity.

In dual-chamber pacemakers, sensing depolarization can either inhibit pacing in the same chamber or trigger pacing in a different chamber. For example, if an intrinsic ventricular beat is sensed, ventricular pacing will be inhibited for a period. If atrial depolarization is sensed, ventricular pacing will be triggered after a programmed PR interval, but only if no ventricular activity has been sensed. Thus ventricular pacing can track atrial activity in the presence of AV block, leading to appropriate coordination of atrial and ventricular systole.

PACEMAKER NOMENCLATURE

The pacing mode of most pacemaker systems can be described using the NBG pacemaker code.*

In the NBG code,

- the first character describes the chamber(s) paced (A, V or D)
- the second character describes the chamber(s) sensed (A, V, D or 0)
- the third character describes the response to a sensed event (I, D or 0)
- a fourth character (R) is used when the rate modulation is programmable.

The characters of the NBG code signify the following:

A = right atrium
V = right ventricle
D = dual
0 = none
I = inhibited

RIGHT VENTRICULAR PACEMAKERS (VVI)

One of the most commonly-used types of pacemaker, these have a single lead implanted in the right ventricle, usually at the apex (Fig. 6.1). The lead senses electrical activity in the right ventricle and, if no spontaneous cardiac activity is sensed, paces the ventricle after a predetermined interval. Note that unipolar and bipolar pacing leads cannot easily be differentiated on a routine chest X-ray. The indications for VVI pacing are listed in Box 6.1.

*NASPE/BPEG Generic, developed by the North American Society for Pacing and Electrophysiology and the British Pacing and Electrophysiology Group.

Box 6.1 Indications for VVI pacing

- Atrial fibrillation with a slow ventricular rate or pauses
- Sinoatrial disease (bradycardia–tachycardia syndrome), in which patients have atria-driven tachyarrhythmias (such as fast atrial fibrillation) but periods of relative bradycardia that prevent pharmacological rate control
- 'Backup' pacemaker, in patients with occasional pauses due to sinus node disease or atrioventricular block but a predominantly spontaneous cardiac rhythm
- In the very elderly, in whom more sophisticated devices are unlikely to improve function

ECG APPEARANCE

With bipolar right ventricular pacing, the ECG is characterized by a pacing spike followed by a broad QRS complex of left bundle branch block morphology (because cardiac depolarization originates from the lead tip in the right ventricle) (Fig. 6.2). The pacing spikes vary in size and morphology in different ECG leads and in different patients, and may not be visible in all leads.

With unipolar pacing, in which the electrical circuit is between the lead tip and the pacemaker

Fig. 6.1

Chest X-ray showing right ventricular pacemaker

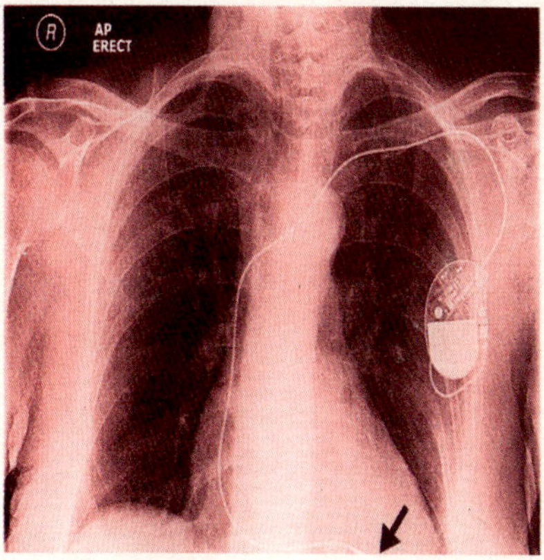

- Pacemaker unit positioned in subcutaneous pocket beneath the left shoulder
- Pacing lead passing via the subclavian vein, with the lead tip in the conventional right ventricular apical position (arrowed)

Note

box, the pacing spike is very large compared to that associated with bipolar pacing, in which the poles are close together (Fig. 6.3).

If the pacemaker senses spontaneous cardiac activity, pacing will be suppressed for a predetermined time interval. The ECG will then show intermittent pacing – varying amounts of paced ventricular rhythm and underlying ventricular rhythm (Figs 6.4 and 6.5).

The ECGs of patients with pacemakers programmed to provide a backup function for occasional slow rhythms may show no paced beats at all, if the intrinsic cardiac rate exceeds the programmed pacing rate.

The underlying atrial rhythm can be determined from the ECG, and may be important for clinical decisions, such as anticoagulation. There may be sinus rhythm, atrial fibrillation (Fig. 6.4), atrial flutter (Fig. 6.5) or complete block (Fig. 6.6).

Fig. 6.2

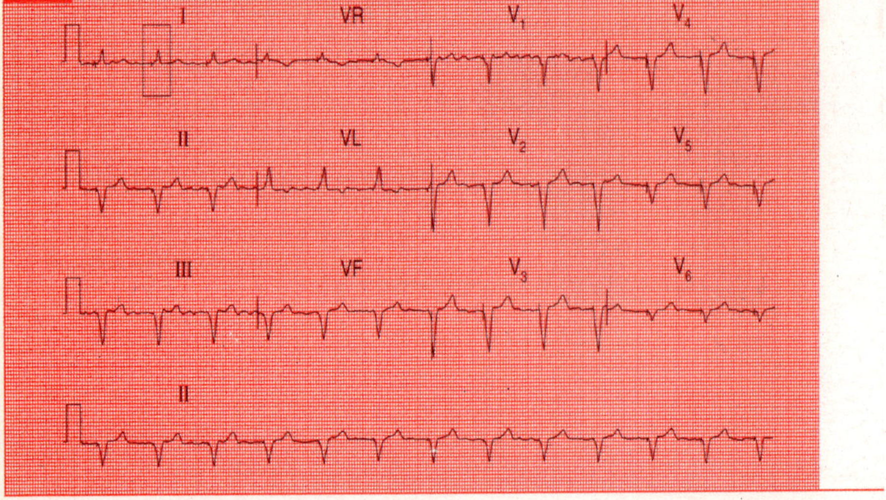
I
VR
V_1
V_4
II
VL
V_2
V_5
III
VF
V_3
V_6
II

Fig. 6.3

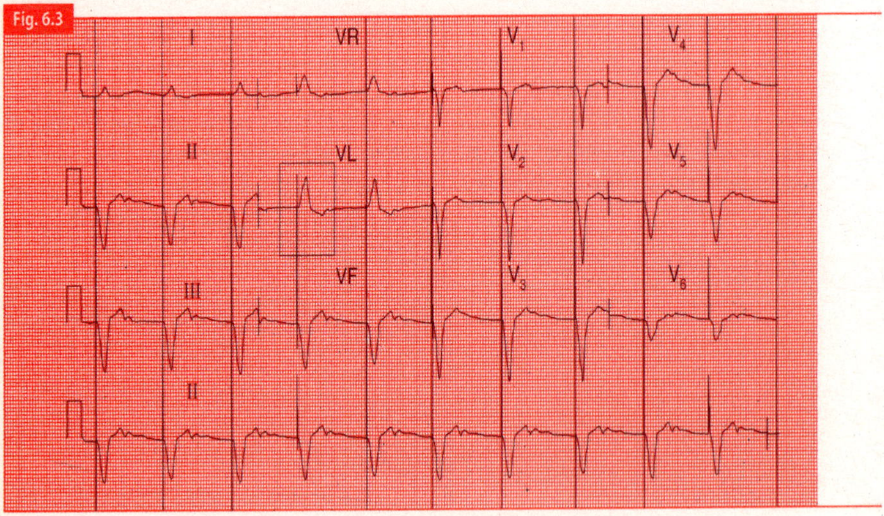
I
VR
V_1
V_4
II
VL
V_2
V_5
III
VF
V_3
V_6
II

VVI bipolar pacing

Note

- Pacing spike followed by a paced ventricular beat with a broad complex. Because the paced complex originates from the right ventricle, its morphology is similar to that seen in left bundle branch block
- The size of the pacing spike varies in different ECG leads, and may not be visible
- The unchanging morphology of the QRS complex in the rhythm strip confirms continuous right ventricular pacing
- Underlying atrial fibrillation (best seen in lead V_1)

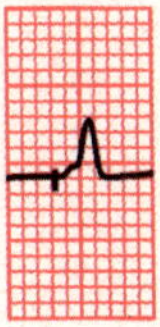

Pacing spike followed by broad QRS complex

VVI unipolar pacing

Note

- Pacing spikes much larger than with bipolar pacing

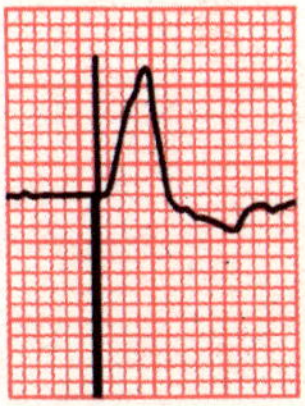

Large ventricular pacing spike

Fig. 6.4

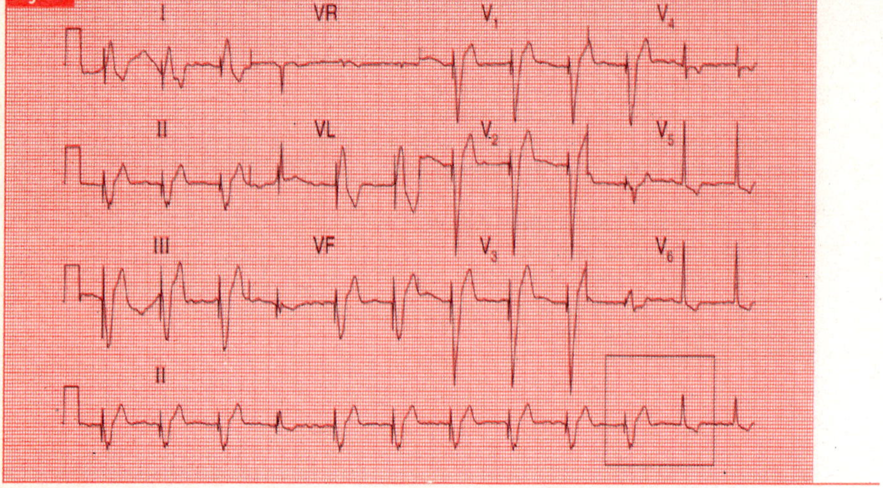
I
VR
V1
V4
II
VL
V2
V5
III
VF
V3
V6
II

Fig. 6.5

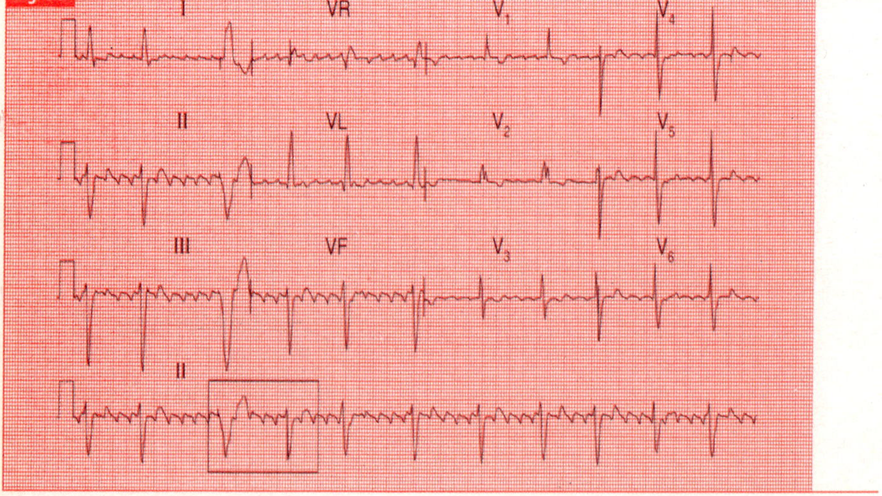
I
VR
V1
V4
II
VL
V2
V5
III
VF
V3
V6
II

Intermittent VVI pacing

Note

- Ventricular pacing
- Underlying rhythm can be seen to be atrial fibrillation
- Final two beats with narrow complexes are not paced – the intrinsic heart rate exceeds that of the pacemaker

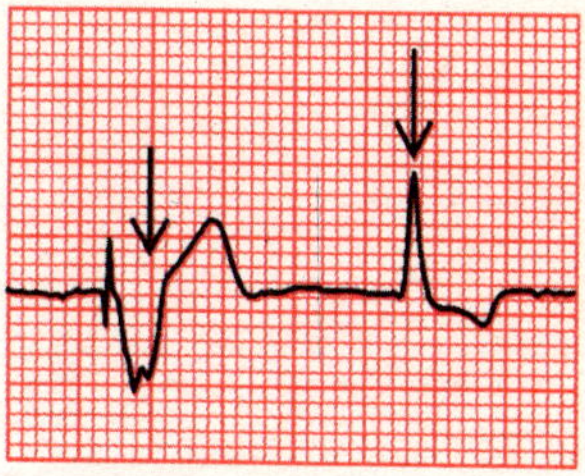

First beat paced, second beat unpaced

Atrial flutter with intermittent VVI pacing

Note

- Underlying atrial flutter with variable block
- After the second beat the subsequent pause exceeds the trigger rate for the pacemaker, and the third beat shows ventricular pacing
- All other QRS complexes are intrinsic (i.e. not paced), indicating normal ventricular sensing
- Vertical lines where the lead changes (e.g. from VL to V_2) must not be confused with pacing spikes

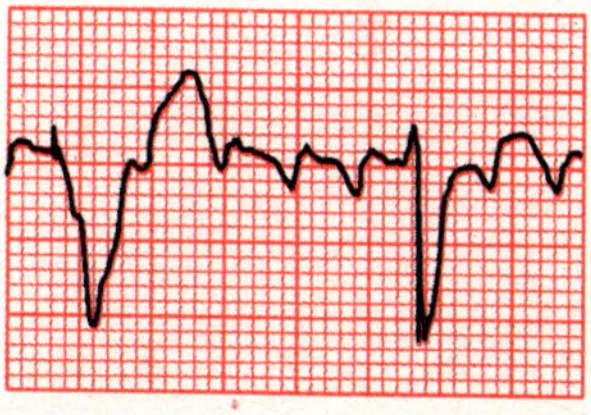

First beat paced, second beat intrinsic

Fig. 6.6

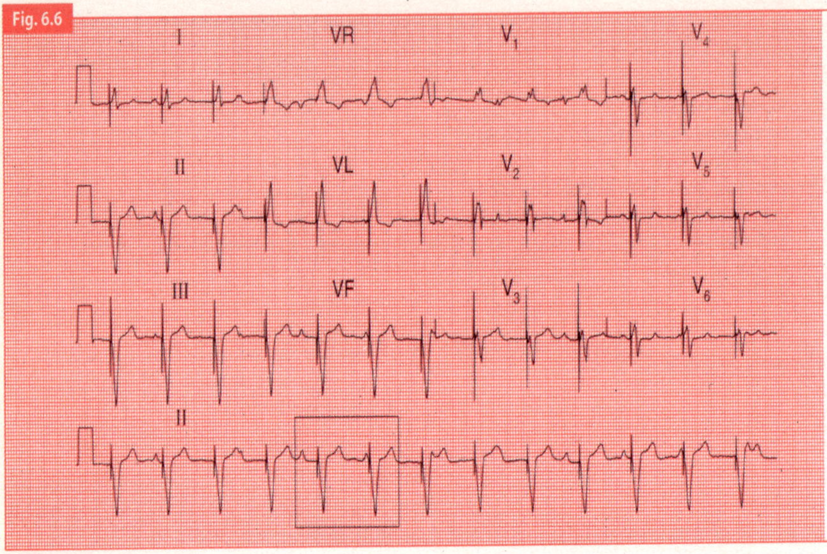

Fig. 6.7

Chest X-ray showing right atrial pacemaker

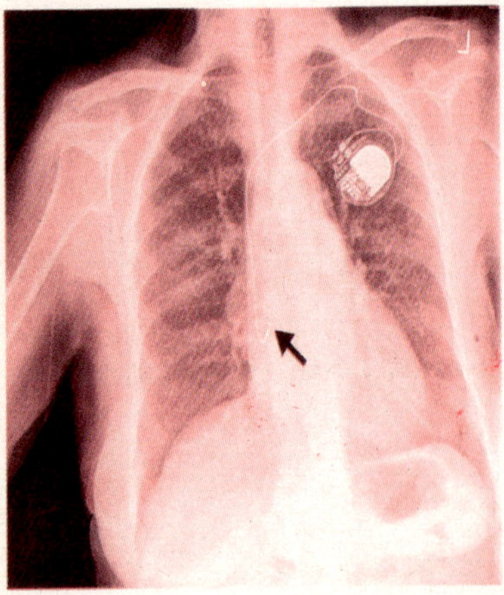

Note

- Pacemaker unit positioned in the left prepectoral position
- The single atrial lead passes via the subclavian vein to the right atrial appendage (arrowed)

VVI pacing: complete block

Note

- Ventricular pacing
- P waves can be seen, unrelated to ventricular beats
- Therefore the underlying rhythm is complete heart block

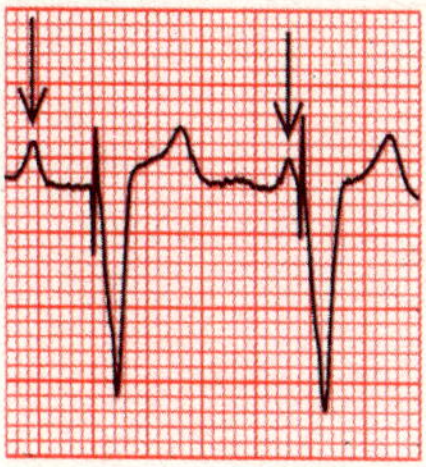

Complete block (P waves arrowed)

EXTRA FUNCTIONS

Rate response modulation (VVIR) allows an increase in pacing rate to a preset higher level in the presence of increased activity, as detected from movement. This facilitates some increase in heart rate with exercise.

RIGHT ATRIAL PACEMAKERS (AAI)

This is a rarely used mode of pacing, with a single lead implanted in the right atrium, usually in the atrial appendage (Fig. 6.7). This type of pacing senses spontaneous activity in the right atrium, and paces if the sinus node rate falls below a predetermined level.

Box 6.2 Indications for AAI pacing

- Sinus node disease with no evidence of atrioventricular node disease
- Young patients with carotid sinus syncope

The indications for AAI pacing are summarized in Box 6.2.

ECG APPEARANCE

With atrial pacing the ECG is characterized by a pacing spike followed by a paced P wave. The PR interval and QRS complex are usually normal, indicating no AV node disease (Fig. 6.8).

With intermittent pacing, if the pacemaker senses spontaneous atrial activity, atrial pacing will be suppressed for a predetermined period. Atrial pacemakers are usually implanted to provide backup during fairly rare sinus pauses. Therefore most of the time a normal ECG, with no paced beats, would be expected.

EXTRA FUNCTIONS

Rate response modulation (AAIR) allows an increase in pacing rate to a preset higher level in the presence of increased activity, as detected from movement. This allows some increase in heart rate with exercise.

'Rate drop response' allows the pacemaker to respond to sudden decreases in atrial rate by pacing at a higher rate, and is designed to try to prevent loss of consciousness during episodes of neurocardiogenic syncope.

Fig. 6.8

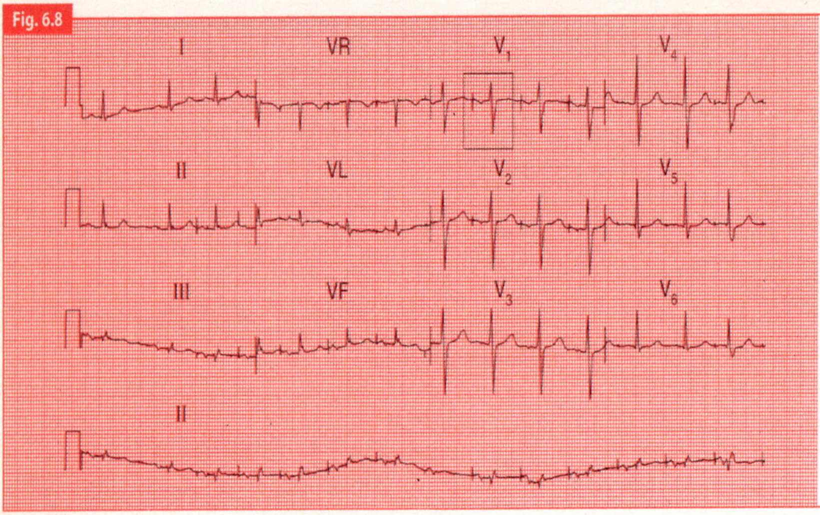

Fig. 6.9

Chest X-ray showing dual chamber pacemaker

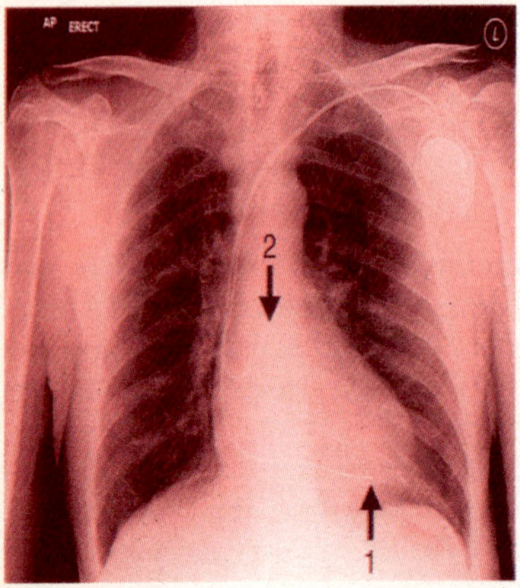

Note

- Pacemaker unit in the left prepectoral position
- Ventricular lead positioned in right ventricular apex position (arrow 1)
- Atrial lead positioned in right atrial appendage position (arrow 2)

AAI pacing

Note

- Pacing spike precedes each P wave
- The subsequent QRS complex is normal, with no evidence of AV block

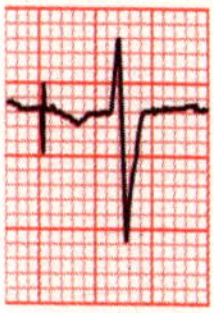

Atrial pacing spike, normal PR interval, normal QRS complex

Box 6.3 Indications for dual chamber pacing

- Atrioventricular block
- Mobitz type II second degree heart block
- Third degree heart block
- Bradycardia–tachycardia syndrome

DUAL CHAMBER PACEMAKERS (DDD)

DDD pacemakers are frequently used devices with two leads, one implanted in the right atrium and one in the right ventricle (Fig. 6.9).

The right atrial and ventricular chambers are both sensed. The atrial pacing lead will pace if no atrial activity is sensed within a predetermined interval. A maximum PR interval is also predetermined. If this is exceeded (following either a spontaneous P wave or a paced P wave) and no ventricular beat is sensed, then the ventricular paced beat is triggered.

Dual chamber pacing is appropriate with the conditions listed in Box 6.3.

ECG APPEARANCE

When both atrium and ventricle are being paced, an atrial pacing spike is followed by a paced P wave, then a ventricular pacing spike is followed by a paced ventricular beat (Fig. 6.10).

When the intrinsic atrial rate exceeds the threshold for atrial pacing, 'atrial tracking' occurs. Atrial sensing takes place, but the intrinsic PR interval is longer than the programmed AV delay – leading to ventricular pacing. The ECG shows no atrial pacing spikes, but shows spontaneous P waves followed by ventricular pacing spikes and paced ventricular beats (Fig. 6.11).

Atrial pacing with ventricular tracking would be an unusual but theoretically possible situation. It would occur if the intrinsic atrial rate was slower than the threshold for atrial pacing, but the PR interval was shorter than the programmed AV delay. Hence there would be atrial pacing and intrinsic QRS complexes. The ECG would show atrial pacing spikes, paced P waves and spontaneous conducted ventricular beats.

In intermittent pacing, spontaneous atrial or ventricular activity will be sensed – leading to the inhibition of pacing in that chamber. If the programmed maximum PR interval is not exceeded, sensed atrial contraction may be followed by an AV conducted beat and a sensed QRS complex. The ECG will then show some intrinsic rhythm and some intermittent pacing (Fig. 6.12).

Fig. 6.10

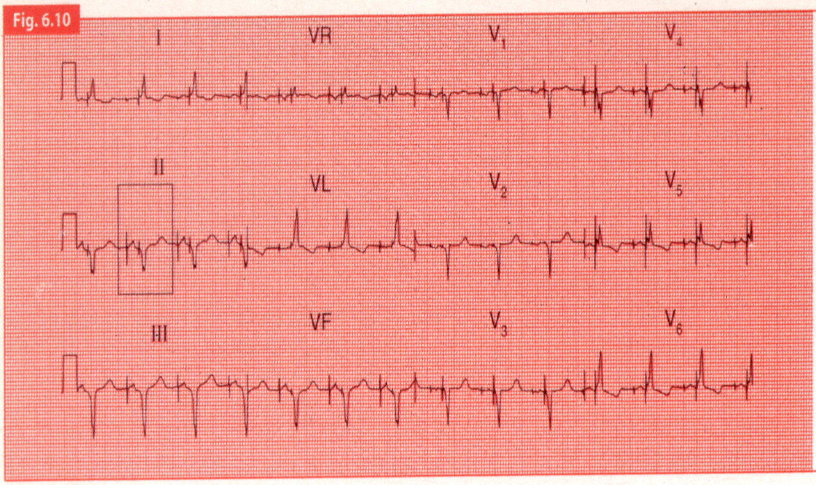

Fig. 6.11

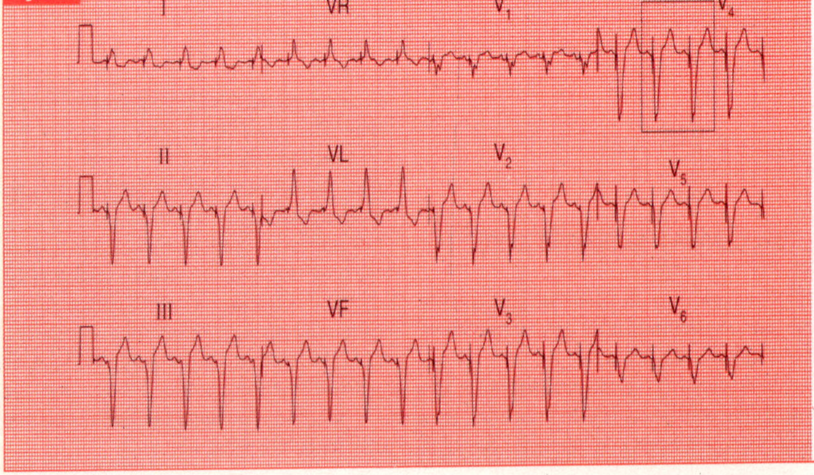

DDD pacing: atrial and ventricular pacing

Note

- Continuous atrial and ventricular pacing throughout
- Pacing spikes precede both P waves and QRS complexes

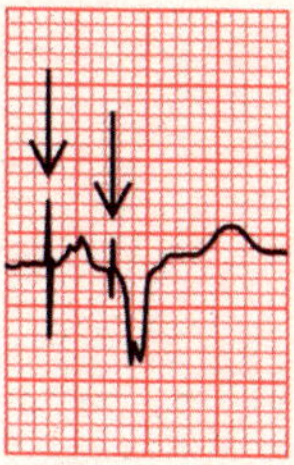

Atrial pacing followed by ventricular pacing in lead II

DDD pacing: atrial tracking

Note

- Atrial sensing and ventricular pacing
- Non-paced P waves are followed by ventricular pacing spikes and paced ventricular complexes

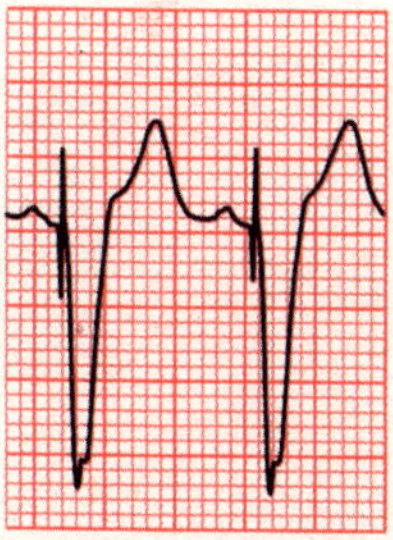

Pacing spike following P wave in lead V_4

Fig. 6.12

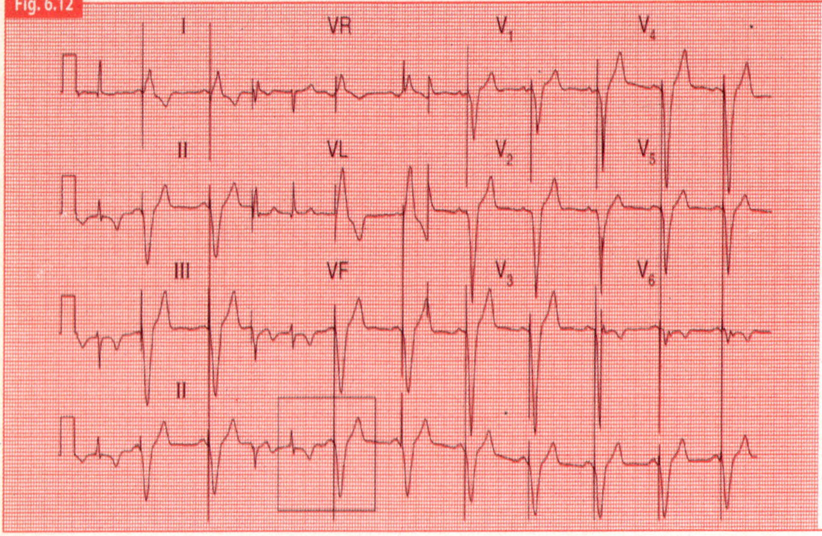

Fig. 6.13

Chest X-ray showing biventricular pacemaker

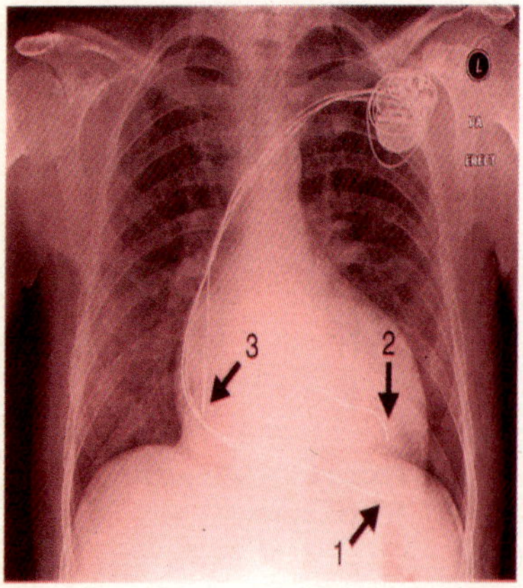

Note

- Ventricular lead in right ventricular apex position (arrow 1)
- Coronary sinus lead for left ventricular pacing (arrow 2)
- Atrial lead in right atrial appendage position (arrow 3)

DDD pacing: intermittent

Note

- Atrial tracking, with atrial sensing and ventricular pacing
- The first, fourth and fifth QRS complexes show the intrinsic underlying rhythm, with appropriate ventricular sensing
- Large pacing spikes are consistent with a unipolar ventricular lead

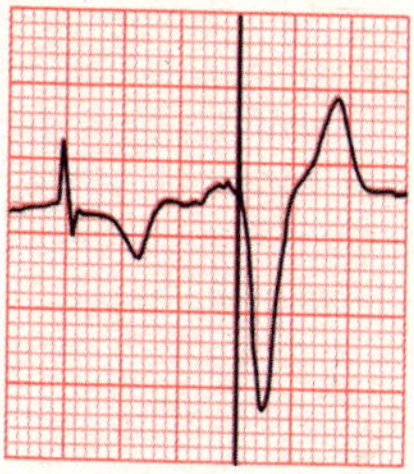

Intrinsic beat followed by a beat showing atrial sensing and ventricular pacing

SPECIALIST FUNCTIONS

Rate response (DDDR) pacing allows an increase in pacing rate to a preset higher level in the presence of increased activity, allowing some increase in heart rate with exercise.

Anti-AF algorithms trigger atrial pacing if atrial activity is sensed at a high rate, suggesting the onset of atrial arrhythmia. The aim is to control the atria at a lower rate.

CARDIAC RESYNCHRONIZATION THERAPY (CRT)

This technique is also known as biventricular pacing, or simply 'bivent'.

Patients with severe heart failure, especially those whose ECG shows left bundle branch block with a broad QRS complex, may have dyssynchronous cardiac contraction. Instead of both sides of the left ventricle contracting simultaneously in systole, there is a substantial delay between contraction of the left ventricular septum and the free wall. This reduces the stroke volume and exacerbates the heart failure. Contraction can be resynchronized by pacing the left ventricular free wall and the septum simultaneously. This is achieved by two pacing leads – one placed in a branch of the coronary sinus (the venous side of the coronary circulation, which drains into the right atrium), with a second, right ventricular lead, to pace the septum. Resynchronization improves both cardiac output and symptomatic heart failure. In addition to right ventricular and coronary sinus leads, there will usually be an atrial lead if sinus rhythm is present, as atrial systole may make an important contribution to cardiac output (Fig. 6.13).

INDICATIONS FOR CRT

Numerous clinical studies have shown that in appropriate patients, CRT can improve left ventricular function and ejection fraction, and can improve exercise capacity. In patients still symptomatic from heart failure despite optimal medical therapy, CRT has been shown to reduce morbidity and all-cause mortality. CRT is therefore now considered a standard therapy (see Box 6.4), but its role in patients with less severe symptoms, atrial fibrillation or pacemaker dependence, has not been established. Since it is an invasive and costly procedure, patient selection is clearly extremely important.

Box 6.4 Indications for cardiac resynchronization therapy

These remain uncertain, but it is currently recommended for patients:

- on optimal pharmacotherapy *and*
- with an ejection fraction of less than 35% *and*
- left bundle branch block with a QRS complex longer than 150 ms (or 120–149 ms and with echocardiographic evidence of dyssynchrony) *and*
- heart failure symptoms in NYHA Class III or IV

Fig. 6.14

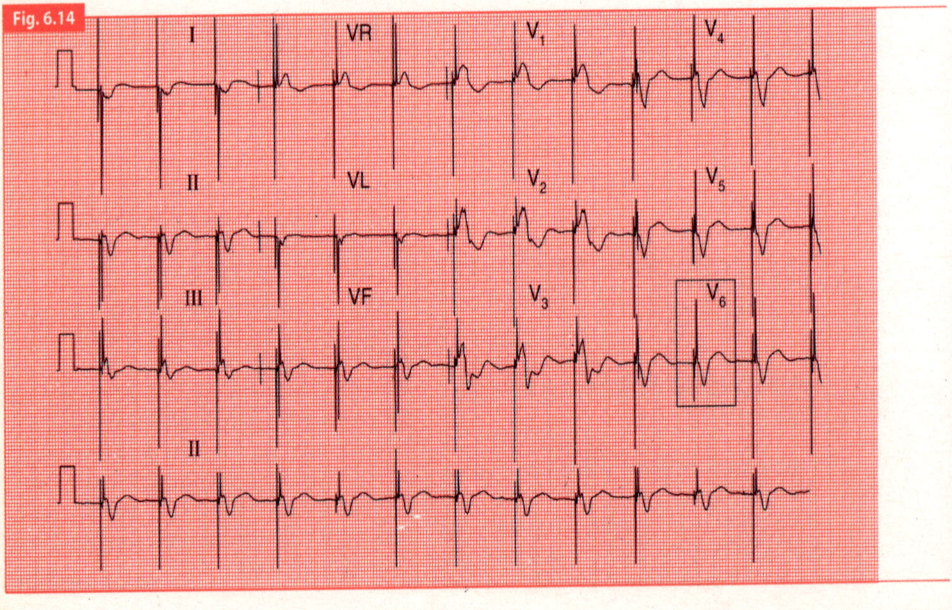

ECG APPEARANCE

Biventricular pacing is 'obligate', because resynchronization cannot be achieved unless the heart is in a paced rhythm. If necessary, pacing is ensured careful programming of the AV delay or by pharmacological suppression of the intrinsic rhythm.

The pacing spike may be complex and may have two components. The QRS complex of the paced beat may have either a narrowed left bundle branch block morphology or a right bundle branch block morphology (Fig. 6.14).

Patients without an atrial lead will usually have atrial fibrillation or atrial flutter.

SPECIALIST FUNCTIONS

Patients with severe left ventricular dysfunction are at increased risk of ventricular arrhythmias, so some CRT devices incorporate a ventricular implanted cardioverter defibrillation element (CRTD). This device will function in the same way as a conventional biventricular pacing device, but with the additional function of an ICD (see below).

Biventricular pacing

Note

- Complex ventricular pacing spike, sometimes with two distinct elements derived from the right ventricular and coronary sinus leads
- Right bundle branch block morphology in the QRS complexes
- Obligate pacing throughout

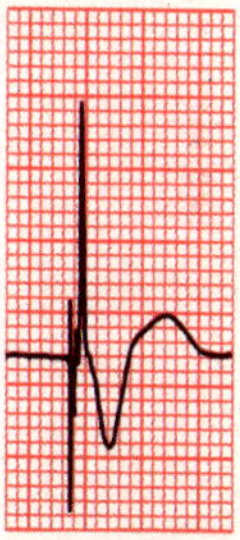

Two juxtaposed pacing spikes

Fig. 6.15

Chest X-ray showing single chamber ICD

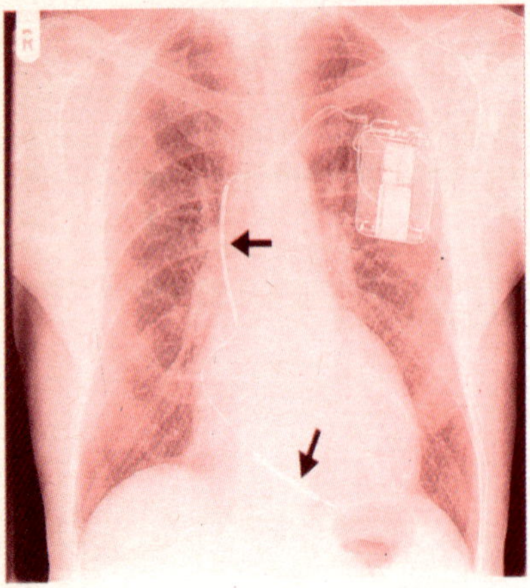

Note

- Single right ventricular lead, with thicker areas indicating the poles of the shocking coils (arrowed)

Fig. 6.16

ICD cardioversion of ventricular fibrillation

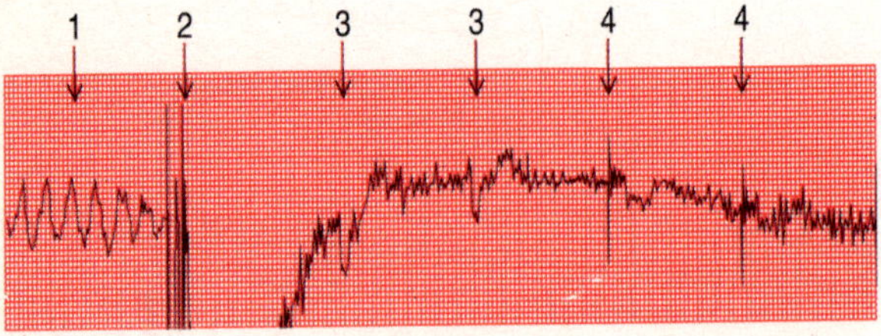

Note

- Ventricular fibrillation (1) followed by ICD-mediated cardioversion (2)
- Intrinsic QRS complexes (3)
- Paced ventricular responses (4)

IMPLANTED CARDIOVERTER DEFIBRILLATOR (ICD) DEVICES

These devices are designed for patients at increased risk of ventricular arrhythmia or sudden cardiac death. They have the following functions:

- pacemaker
- defibrillator
- control of ventricular tachycardia.

PACEMAKER FUNCTION

ICD devices have the same functions as a conventional pacemaker. They can be single or dual chamber, or biventricular (CRTD). In patients who do not require the pacing function, the ICD will usually be a single chamber system, programmed as a backup VVI. The device will then be in continuous sensing mode.

DEFIBRILLATOR FUNCTION

The chest X-ray appearances of ICD devices are similar to those of conventional pacemakers. However, devices with a defibrillating function are bigger, incorporating more battery power for the delivery of shocks. In addition, the right ventricular lead contains the two poles of the shocking coil and so is thicker than a conventional lead (Fig. 6.15).

In addition to the normal sensing functions of a pacemaker, an ICD can sense high rates of ventricular activity. If a predetermined ventricular rate is exceeded, an electrical shock discharges between the two poles of the defibrillator coil in the ventricular lead, with the aim of cardioverting a life-threatening ventricular arrhythmia (Fig. 6.16). If the ventricular rate does not fall below the threshold following one shock, then further shocks may be delivered.

ANTI-TACHYCARDIA PACING

The device may also attempt to control ventricular tachycardia by 'overdrive pacing'. If ventricular activity is detected within a certain range (usually significantly above normal cardiac rates but below the threshold set for defibrillation), the ICD will attempt to pace the ventricle at a high rate before reducing the rate of pacing. Ventricular capture with rapid pacing can sometimes terminate ventricular tachycardia. If anti-tachycardia pacing in this way is unsuccessful after a set number of attempts, the ICD will then usually default to defibrillation.

INDICATIONS FOR ICD DEVICES

These are summarized in Box 6.5.

Box 6.5 Indications for ICD insertion

These remain subject to ongoing clinical trials. Current recommendations are for the following patient groups:

- Survived cardiac arrest due to ventricular fibrillation or ventricular tachycardia
- Spontaneous sustained ventricular tachycardia, causing syncope or haemodynamic compromise
- Sustained ventricular tachycardia or cardiac arrest, and ejection fraction < 35% (but symptoms no worse than NYHA Class III)
- Familial risk of sudden cardiac death due to hypertrophic cardiomyopathy, long QT syndrome, Brugada syndrome, or ARVD (arrhythmogenic right ventricular dysplasia)
- Surgical repair of congenital heart disease
- Non-sustained ventricular tachycardia and ejection fraction < 35% (but symptoms no worse than NYHA Class III), plus a history of myocardial infarction (> 4 weeks old), plus inducible ventricular tachycardia at electrophysiology
- Ejection fraction < 35% and QRS complexes >120 ms and no myocardial infarction in the previous 4 weeks

Types of device and clinical indications

Device function	Chamber(s) with implanted electrode	Clinical indications
Single chamber		
VVI	Right ventricle	Slow atrial fibrillation, or atrial fibrillation with pauses 'Backup' with sinus node disease or atrioventricular block Bradycardia–tachycardia syndrome Very elderly patients
AAI	Right atrium	Sinus node disease without atrioventricular block Carotid sinus syncope
VVI/ICD	Right ventricle	Survived cardiac arrest due to ventricular fibrillation or ventricular tachycardia Spontaneous sustained ventricular tachycardia causing syncope or haemodynamic compromise Sustained ventricular tachycardia or cardiac arrest and ejection fraction < 35% with no worse than NYHA Class III* Familial risk of sudden cardiac death (HCM (hypertrophic cardiomyopathy), long QT syndrome, Brugada syndrome, ARVD (arrhythmogenic right ventricular dysplasia)) Surgical repair of congenital heart disease Non-sustained ventricular tachycardia and ejection fraction < 35% with no worse than NYHA Class III*, plus a history of myocardial infarction (> 4 weeks old) and inducible ventricular tachycardia at electrophysiology Ejection fraction < 30% and QRS complex >120 ms and no myocardial infarction in the previous 4 weeks

Table 6.1 Contd

Device function	Chamber(s) with implanted electrode	Clinical indications
Dual chamber		
DDD	Right ventricle Right atrium	Atrioventricular block, usually third degree block or Mobitz type II second degree block Bradycardia–tachycardia syndrome
DDD/ICD	Right ventricle – shocking lead Right atrium – pacing lead	Indications as for VVI/ICD but in patient requiring DDD pacemaker function
Biventricular		
CRT	Right ventricle Left ventricle via coronary sinus ± Right atrium	NYHA Class III* or IV* heart failure and ejection fraction < 35%, plus either left bundle branch block with QRS complexes > 150 ms, or QRS complexes 120–150 ms with echocardiographic dyssynchrony
CRTD	Right ventricle – shocking lead Coronary sinus left ventricular pacing lead ± Right atrial pacing lead	Indications as for CRT and ICD Patient groups benefiting from combined device not yet clearly defined

*New York Heart Association Class III/IV – moderate/severe heart failure

ECG APPEARANCE

ECGs from patients with ICDs are the same as those from patients with conventional pacemakers, except when ventricular arrhythmia is detected.

ABNORMAL PACEMAKER FUNCTION

Pacemaker failure is rare. Most failures are due to problems with the pacing and/or sensing functions of the device. Complete diagnosis will usually require remote interrogation of the pacemaker, by placing over the implanted device a wand or header connected to a specialist programmer. This reveals information about how the device has been performing, as well as assessment of the leads and pacemaker function. There are various potential causes of device failure. Early after implantation, lead displacement may occur (Fig. 6.17). Rarer causes include lead insulation failure or lead fracture (Fig. 6.18). Unexpected battery depletion is rare, because devices are usually monitored regularly.

The investigation of pacemaker malfunction requires specialist techniques and expertise, and the

Fig. 6.17

Chest X-ray showing right atrial and ventricular lead displacement

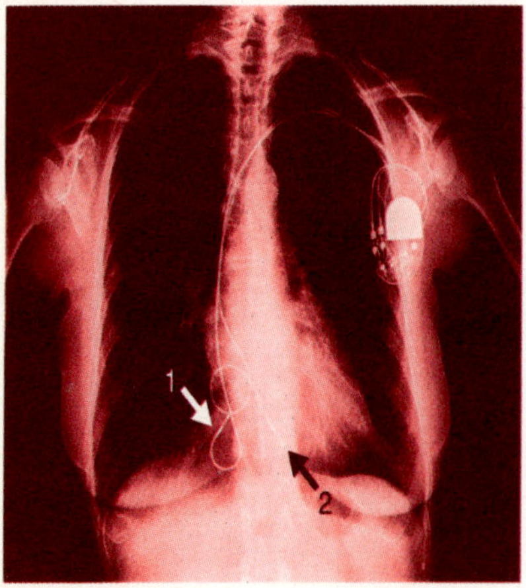

Note

- Compare with Figure 6.9
- The right atrial lead has been displaced from the atrial appendage, to a position much lower in the right atrium (arrow 1)
- The right ventricular lead is looped in the right atrium, with the tip displaced from the apex of the right ventricle (arrow 2)
- Atrial and ventricular pacing and sensing were lost in this patient

Fig. 6.18

Chest X-ray showing fractured pacing lead

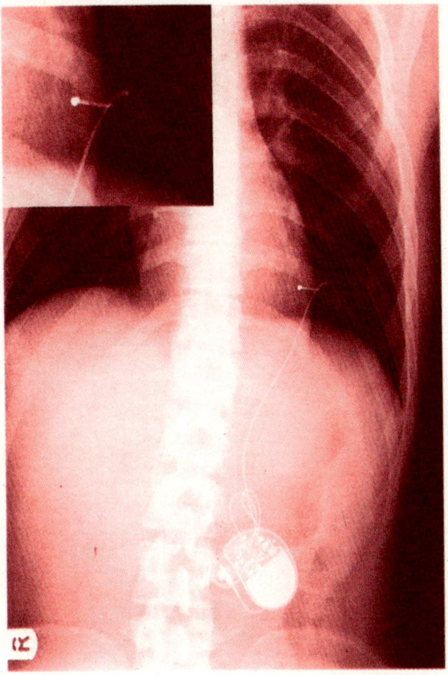

Note

- Abdominally placed pacemaker unit (in a child)
- Epicardial lead placed on the epicardial surface of the heart rather than within the right ventricle (endocardial)
- Fracture of the lead just proximal to the lead tip (enlarged inset)

12-lead ECG can be extremely helpful in showing what has gone wrong.

FAILED PACING CAPTURE

This occurs when the voltage delivered to the pacemaker lead fails to trigger myocardial depolarization. It is characterized by the presence of pacing spikes but no subsequent atrial or ventricular depolarization (Figs 6.19 and 6.20).

UNDER-SENSING

'Under-sensing' occurs when the device develops an inability to detect intrinsic cardiac activity, and therefore fails to suppress pacing in response to an intrinsic beat. The ECG is characterized by the presence of paced and normal beats closer together than would be expected from the programmed interval (Figs 6.21 and 6.22).

Fig. 6.19

Failed pacemaker capture

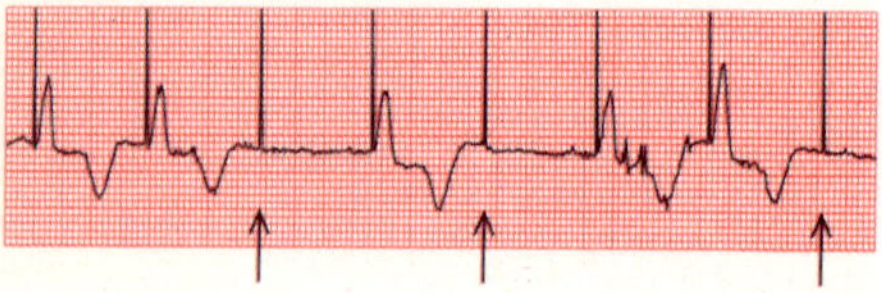

Note

- Intermittent failed right ventricular capture – pacing spikes (arrowed) not followed by a QRS complex (VVI pacemaker; no underlying cardiac rhythm)

Fig. 6.20

Failed pacemaker capture. Redrawn by permission of Medtronic

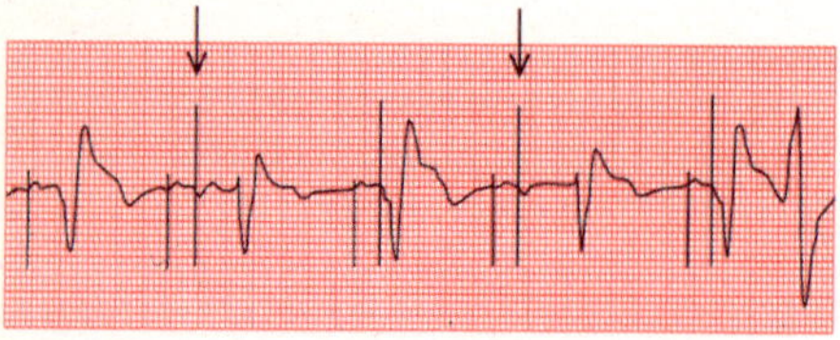

Note

- Intermittent failed right ventricular capture (arrowed)
- Ventricular sensing and atrial function appear normal (DDD pacemaker)

Fig. 6.21

Pacemaker under-sensing

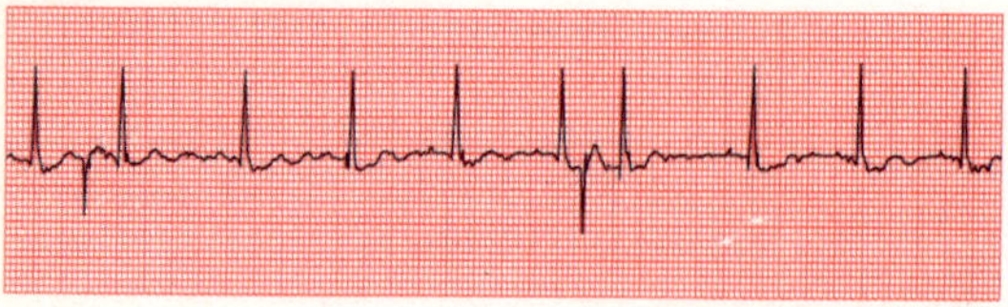

Note

- Atrial under-sensing (AAI pacemaker)
- Inappropriate atrial pacing spikes, which capture and conduct from atria to ventricles despite an adequate rate of intrinsic atrial activity – indicating failed atrial sensing

Fig. 6.22

Pacemaker under-sensing. Redrawn by permission of Medtronic

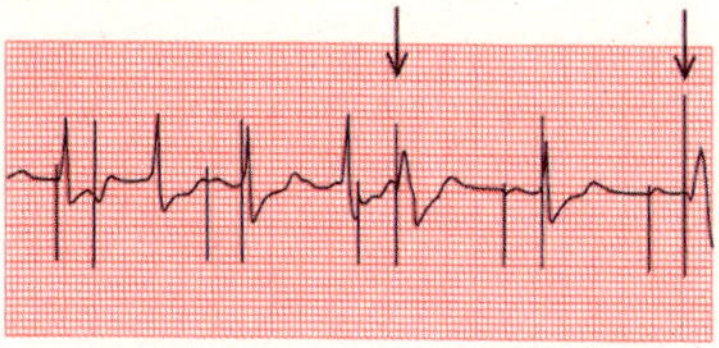

Note

- Ventricular under-sensing (DDD pacemaker)
- Atrial and ventricular pacing spikes occur despite an underlying rhythm, indicating failed sensing
- The third and fifth ventricular pacing spikes are normally conducted (arrowed). The remainder form fusion complexes, between the paced and intrinsic QRS complexes

Fig. 6.23

Pacemaker over-sensing. Redrawn by permission of Medtronic

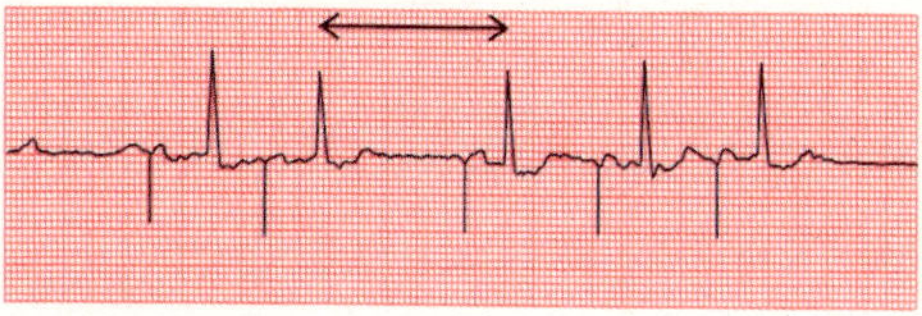

Note

- There is an inappropriate gap between the paced atrial and tracked ventricular complexes (arrowed). This could be due to atrial or ventricular over-sensing. In this case the ventricular lead was at fault.

OVER-SENSING OR FAR-FIELD SENSING

This arises when sensing occurs in the absence of real intrinsic cardiac activity, triggering the inappropriate suppression of pacing. The ECG is characterized by inappropriately long intervals between beats, when pacing would be expected (Fig. 6.23).

PACEMAKER-MEDIATED TACHYCARDIA

A rare problem occurs when ventricular pacing triggers retrogradely conducted atrial depolarization, which is then sensed and triggers further ventricular pacing at an inappropriately short interval (Fig. 6.24). Pacemakers have a function for

Fig. 6.24

Pacemaker-mediated tachycardia. Redrawn by permission of Medtronic

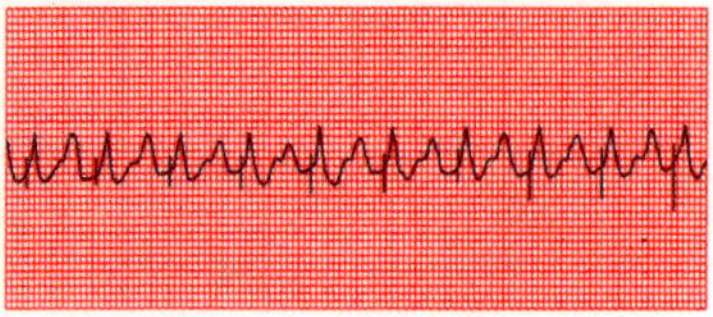

Note

- Tachyarrhythmia with pacing spike preceding each QRS complex

preventing this, called PVARP (post-ventricular atrial refractory period). This is a refractory period after ventricular pacing, in which atrial activity cannot be sensed. Inappropriately rapid pacing will require specialist assessment.

MAGNET RATE

A simple check of pacemaker function can be made by applying a magnet to the skin over the device. This will trigger obligate pacing at the 'magnet rate' (Fig. 6.25). Pacing spikes will be delivered at this fixed preset rate regardless of the intrinsic rhythm, and should cause depolarization unless delivered at the time of an intrinsic beat, when fusion may occur. The pacemaker will return to normal programmed function when the magnet is removed.

ABNORMAL ICD FUNCTION

Either the pacing function or the defibrillator function of an ICD device may fail. The defibrillator function may either fail to appropriately initiate ventricular arrhythmia therapy, or may deliver inappropriate shocks. This will require specialist input and analysis. In the event of inappropriate repeated shock delivery, an ICD can be inactivated in a monitored patient by the application of a magnet.

ICDs should always be interrogated shortly after shock delivery, even if this was appropriate, to check device function and battery life. The presence of pacemakers or ICDs in no way precludes external defibrillation, provided that the paddles are not applied directly over the device.

CARDIAC ELECTROPHYSIOLOGY AND THE ECG

Electrophysiology is the process of recording the ECG from inside the heart, using electrodes inserted via a peripheral vein. This is a highly specialized area, and yields additional information to that obtained from a conventional 12-lead ECG.

The main purpose of electrophysiological studies is to identify the site of origin of arrhythmia. If the origin can be localized, the arrhythmia may be prevented permanently by ablation. This technique uses local endocardial (or more rarely epicardial) cautery burns to abolish areas of abnormal cardiac electrical activity, or to interrupt re-entry circuits causing arrhythmia.

Fig. 6.25

Magnet pacing – DDD pacemaker

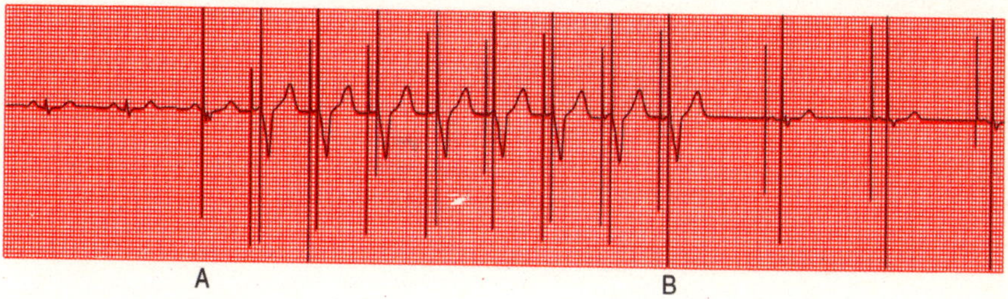

Note

- Sinus rhythm before magnet application (A)
- Magnet triggers D00 pacing
- Following magnet removal (B), pacing continues until underlying rhythm returns

Arrhythmias occur either because of an abnormality of focal depolarization of the heart, or because of re-entry circuits. Before the advent of electrical (ablation) therapy (see below), the cause of arrhythmias was a fairly esoteric subject. Now, however, it is essential to understand the electrical mechanisms that can underlie arrhythmias, because they form the focus of ablation therapy.

ENHANCED AUTOMATICITY AND TRIGGERED ACTIVITY

If the intrinsic frequency of depolarization of the atrial, junctional or ventricular conducting tissue is increased, an abnormal rhythm may occur. This phenomenon is called 'enhanced automaticity'. Single early beats, or extrasystoles, may be due to enhanced automaticity arising from a myocardial focus. The most common example of a sustained rhythm due to enhanced automaticity is 'accelerated idioventricular rhythm', which is common after acute myocardial infarction. The ECG appearance (Fig. 6.26) resembles that of a slow ventricular tachycardia, and that is the old-fashioned name for this condition. This rhythm causes no symptoms, and should not be treated.

If the junctional intrinsic frequency is enhanced to a point at which it approximates to that of the SA node, an 'accelerated idionodal rhythm' results. This may appear to 'overtake' the P waves (Fig. 6.27). This rhythm used to be called a 'wandering pacemaker'.

Enhanced automaticity is also thought to be the mechanism causing some non-paroxysmal

Fig. 6.26

Accelerated idioventricular rhythm

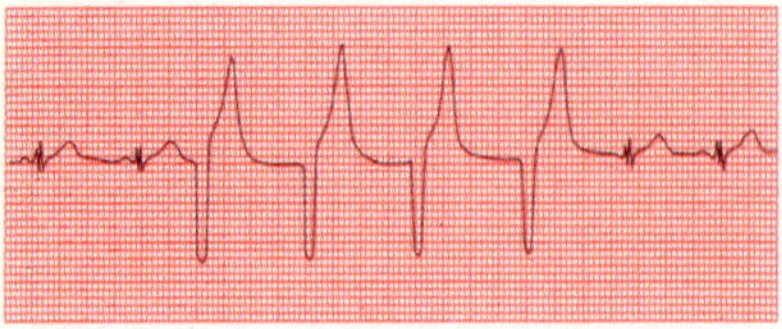

Note

- After two sinus beats, there are four beats of ventricular origin with a rate of 75/min
- Sinus rhythm is then restored

Fig. 6.28

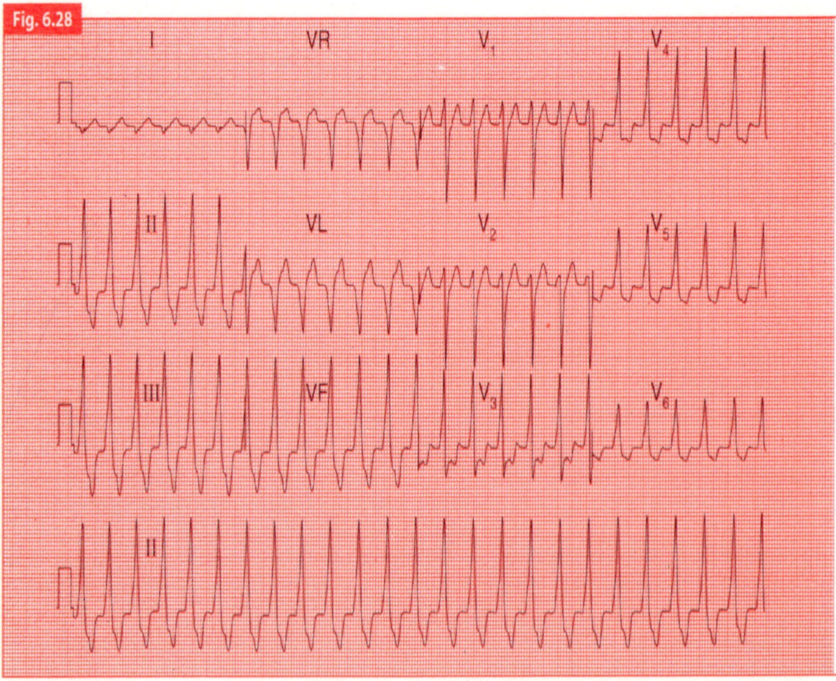

Fig. 6.27

Accelerated idionodal rhythm

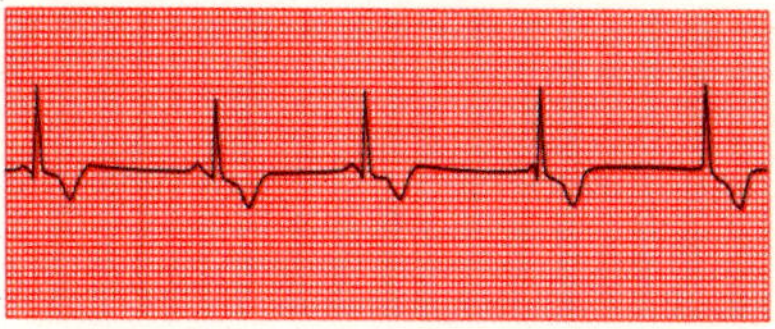

Note

- After three sinus beats, the sinus rate slows slightly
- A nodal rhythm appears and 'overtakes' the P waves

Right ventricular outflow tract ventricular tachycardia (RVOT-VT)

Note

- Broad complex tachycardia
- Left bundle branch block and right axis deviation, typical of RVOT-VT

tachycardias, particularly those due to digoxin intoxication.

'Triggered activity' results from late depolarizations which occur after normal depolarization, during what would normally be a period of repolarization. Like enhanced automaticity, this can cause extrasystoles or sustained arrhythmia, such as right ventricular outflow tract ventricular tachycardia (RVOT-VT) (Fig. 6.28).

ABNORMALITIES OF CARDIAC RHYTHM DUE TO RE-ENTRY

Normal conduction results in the uniform spread of the depolarization wave front in a constant direction. Should the direction of depolarization be reversed in some part of the heart, it becomes possible for a circular or 're-entry' pathway to be set up. This has been discussed in the context of the Wolff–Parkinson–White syndrome, an example of atrioventricular re-entry (AVRE) tachycardia (see p. 67).

Atrial tachycardia and atrial flutter

Re-entry within the atrial muscle causes a tachycardia characterized by P waves with a shape different from that of those related to sinus rhythm. The PR interval is usually short (Fig. 6.29). Atrial tachycardia can also result from enhanced automaticity. Atrial flutter is an organized atrial tachycardia, due to re-entry through a small circuit within the atrial muscle.

Fig. 6.29

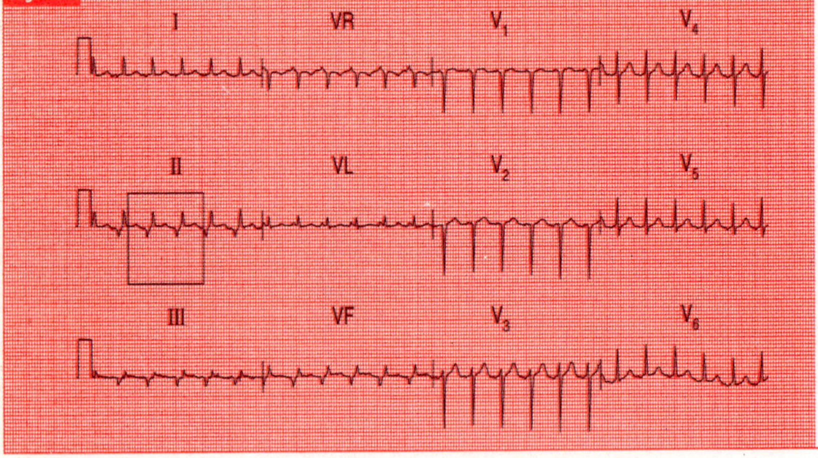

Fig. 6.30

AV nodal re-entry tachycardia

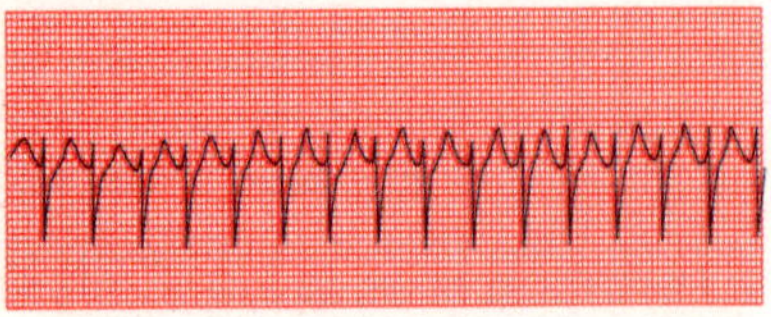

Note

- No P waves can be seen
- QRS complexes are narrow, and completely regular at 165/min

AV nodal re-entry (AVNRE) tachycardia

This occurs because of a congenital abnormality of the AV node, which allows re-entry to start and be sustained within the node itself. The resting ECG has no distinguishing features. During tachycardia, atrial and ventricular activation are virtually simultaneous, so the P wave is hidden within the QRS complex (Fig. 6.30). AVNRE used to be called 'junctional tachycardia'.

Ventricular tachycardia

Ventricular tachycardia may be due to re-entry through circuits within the ventricles (for example around areas of scar tissue following myocardial infarction), or may result from enhanced automaticity or triggered activity. The broad QRS complexes are of a constant configuration and are fairly regular if the re-entry pathway is constant (Fig. 6.31).

DIFFERENTIATION BETWEEN RE-ENTRY AND ENHANCED AUTOMATICITY

Except in the case of the pre-excitation syndromes, there is no certain way of distinguishing from the surface ECG between a tachycardia due to enhanced automaticity and one due to re-entry. In general, however, tachycardias that follow or are terminated by extrasystoles, and those that can be initiated or

Atrial tachycardia

Note

- P waves visible, but they are inverted in several leads
- Rate 140/min
- Normal QRS complexes

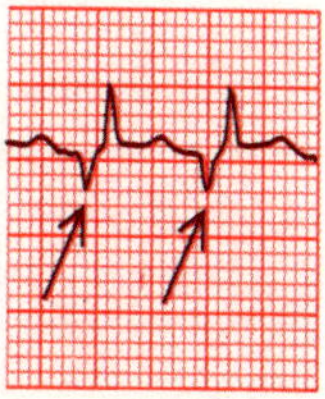

Inverted P waves in lead II

Fig. 6.31

Ventricular tachycardia

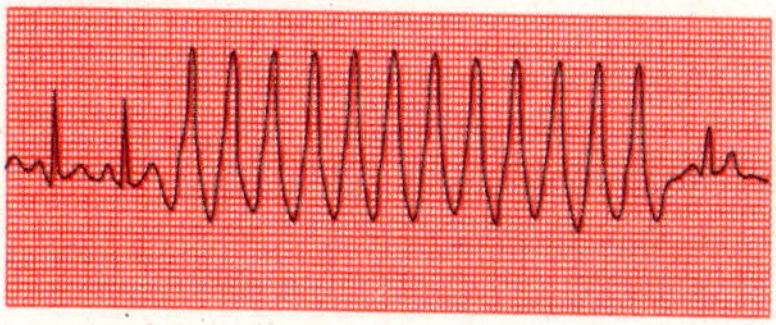

Note

- Two sinus beats are followed by ventricular tachycardia at 200/min
- The complexes are regular, with little variation in shape
- Sinus rhythm is then restored

inhibited by appropriately timed intracardiac pacing impulses, are likely to be due to re-entry (Figs 6.32 and 6.33).

The differentiation between tachycardias caused by enhanced automaticity and those caused by re-entry does not affect the choice of drug treatment, and both can be treated by ablation.

ELECTROPHYSIOLOGY AND CATHETER ABLATION

THE ENDOCARDIAL ECG

Electrical mapping catheters introduced via a transvenous route into the heart can be used to measure the pattern of electrical activation in the heart. Usually catheters are placed in the right atrium; the right ventricle; across the tricuspid valve (close to the His bundle); and in the coronary sinus (to measure the pattern of left ventricular depolarization). Figure 6.34 shows an X-ray taken during a fairly typical investigation, with exploring electrodes in different cardial chambers. More sophisticated mapping catheters, including looped catheters and balloon catheters, may be employed in more complex cases.

The endocardial ECG used during electrophysiological studies simultaneously displays depolarizations recorded from several catheters, each with multiple electrodes. The ECG is used to show the relative timing of depolarization as it moves through the heart. The component elements of this wave of depolarization are best illustrated from recordings taken by the His catheter. The 'A' wave of atrial depolarization (the P wave of the surface ECG) is normally followed by the sharp deflection of the 'H spike', caused by the depolarization of the His bundle (Fig. 6.35). The AH interval is 55–120 ms in normal subjects, with most of this period being due to delay within the AV node. The 'V' wave normally follows, representing ventricular depolarization (the QRS complex of the surface ECG). The HV interval (normal range 33–35 ms) measures the time taken for depolarization to spread from the His bundle to the first part of the interventricular septum.

Fig. 6.32

Atrial tachycardia

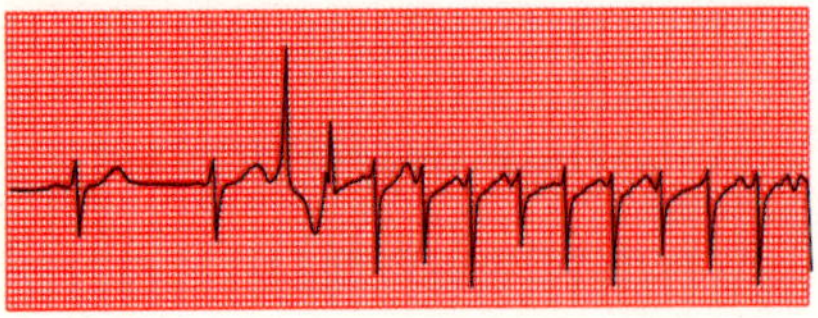

Note

- After two sinus beats there is one ventricular extrasystole, and then a narrow complex that is probably supraventricular
- Atrial tachycardia is induced
- P waves are visible at the end of the T wave of the preceding beat

Fig. 6.33

AV nodal re-entry (AVNRE) tachycardia

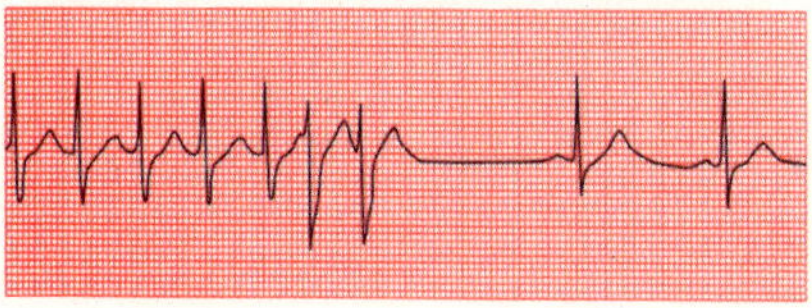

Note

- Five beats of AVNRE tachycardia at 143/min are followed by two ventricular extrasystoles
- These interrupt the tachycardia, and sinus rhythm is restored

Fig. 6.34

Still fluoroscopic image of transvenous catheters during electrophysiology. Redrawn by permission of P. Stafford and G. A. Ng, Glenfield Hospital, Leicester

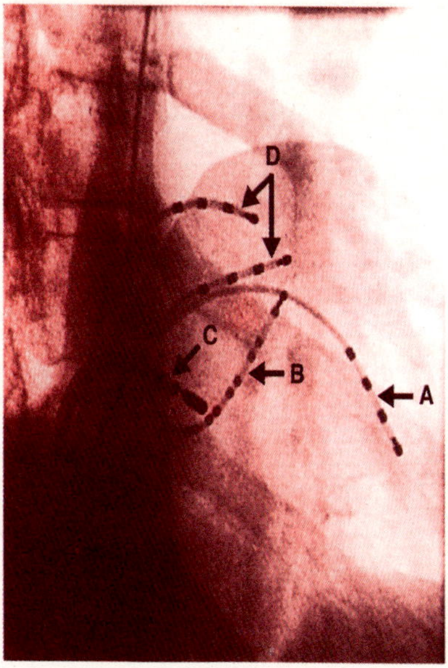

Note

- Catheters have multiple electrodes (dark bands) to enable mapping of the propagation of endocardial electrical activity
- Catheters shown are: right ventricular (A), coronary sinus (B), His bundle (C) and atrial (D)

Figure 6.36 shows an endocardial ECG from a patient with first degree heart block, in this case due to prolongation of the AH interval.

A His bundle electrogram also demonstrates the site of second degree block. In the case of 2:1 block, this is usually in the His bundle rather than the AV

Fig. 6.35

Normal His bundle electrogram

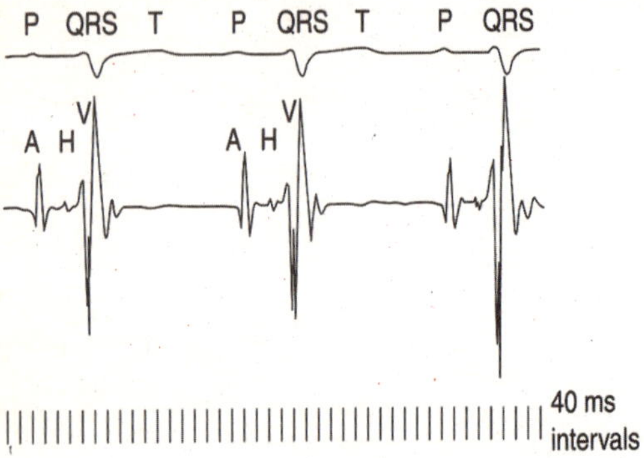

Note

- Upper trace shows the usual ECG recorded from the body surface
- The P waves, QRS complexes and T waves are broad and flat because the record was made with a fast paper speed
- The lower trace shows the intracardiac recording. The A and V waves correspond to the P waves and QRS complexes, but have a totally different appearance
- His bundle depolarization is shown as a small spike labelled 'H'

Fig. 6.36

His electrogram: first degree block

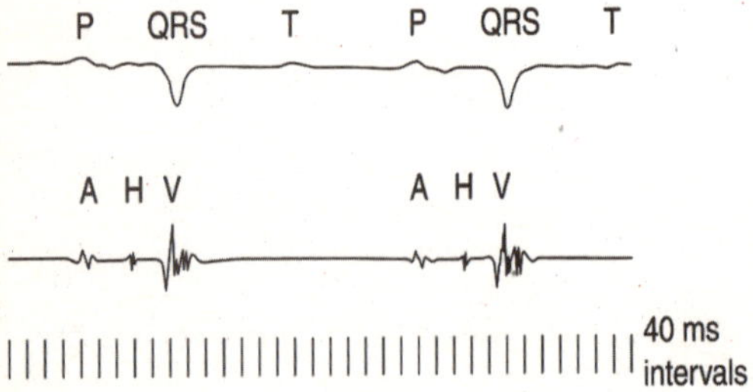

Note

- Upper record shows surface ECG
- PR interval 200 ms
- Lower record shows His electrogram
- AH interval is prolonged (150 ms), but the HV interval is normal (70 ms)

node. Therefore a normal H (or His) spike will be seen, but in the non-conducted beats the H spike will not be followed by a V wave (Figs 6.37 and 6.38).

The ordinary surface ECG provides all the information necessary for pacemaker insertion or for the identification of heart block. However, records of His bundle conduction provide a simple example of an electrophysiological record. The studies required for ablation are a good deal more complex.

Fig. 6.37

Second degree block (2:1)

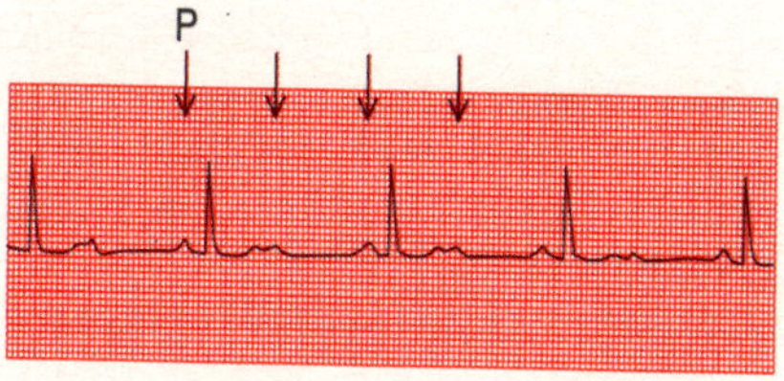

Note

- The conducted beats have a normal PR interval
- Alternate P waves are not followed by a QRS complex

Fig. 6.38

His electrogram: second degree block

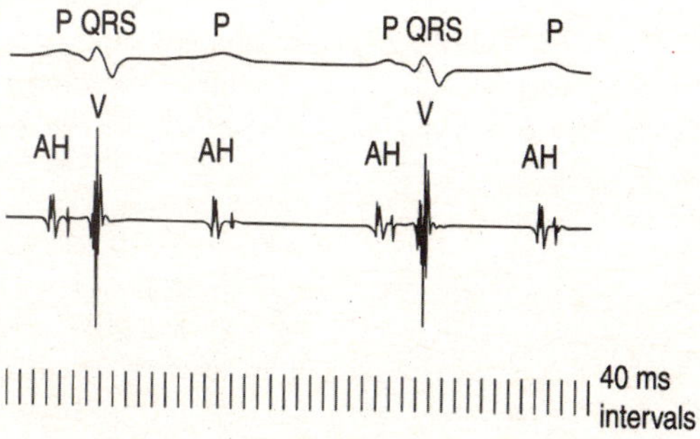

Note

- Upper trace shows the surface ECG
- As in the case of other His electrograms, the paper speed is fast – so the P–QRS–T complexes are flattened and spread out
- Lower trace shows first a normal A wave, H spike and V wave, but then an A wave and an H spike with no V wave
- The sequence is then repeated

ELECTROPHYSIOLOGICAL MAPPING AND CATHETER ABLATION

If an abnormal conduction pathway, e.g. in the Wolff–Parkinson–White syndrome, can be located (mapped) and permanently interrupted, a paroxysmal re-entry tachycardia can be prevented. In other words, the patient can be cured without the need for further drug therapy. This used to be done surgically, but now abnormal re-entry pathways are ablated (cauterized) by burning with radiofrequency energy applied through an intra-cardiac catheter. Ablation can also be used to destroy a focus of enhanced automaticity or triggered activity that is the cause of an arrhythmia.

The endocardial ECG is used to identify both the mechanism of an arrhythmia and the optimal position for the administration of a catheter-mediated radiofrequency ablation burn. The resting pattern of the cardiac electrical activity, as well as the pattern of activity in response to atrial or ventricular pacing and attempted pharmacological stimulation of the arrhythmia, may be recorded during electrophysiological studies. Real-time analysis of the endocardial ECG allows the precise assessment of the relative timing of atrial and ventricular depolarization in different anatomical positions within the heart. This in turn provides information on the propagation of depolarization. Abnormal sources or routes of depolarization can then be mapped, and a position identified for radiofrequency ablation.

An example of the use of the endocardial ECG in catheter ablation is shown in Figure 6.39.

It is important to recognize that the paper speed used in electrophysiology is usually greater than that used for 12-lead ECGs, and so the scale of the trace differs. Figure 6.39 shows continuous traces from surface ECG leads I and V_1. Intracardiac electrograms are recorded at the proximal (CS-prox) and distal (CS-dist) poles of a multipolar catheter placed in the coronary sinus (CS) (Fig. 6.34). The coronary sinus runs in the groove of the left atrioventricular sulcus, so both atrial (A) and ventricular (V) electrograms are recorded. The atrial electrograms from the CS arise from atrial tissue close to the AV junction. These areas depolarize late in atrial systole, so coincide with the end of the P wave seen in the surface ECG leads. The final electrogram shown in Figure 6.39 was recorded from the tip of the mapping/ablation catheter (MAP). This single-tip catheter is used as a mapping electrode, to probe for the optimal site for ablation, and is also used to deliver the radiofrequency ablation burn once this position is found.

The first three beats recorded in Figure 6.39 show sinus rhythm, conducted with pre-excitation via a left-sided accessory pathway – with a negative delta wave in lead I, positive delta wave in lead V_1, and closely spaced atrial (A) and ventricular (V) electrograms recorded by the CS catheter. On applying radiofrequency energy for ablation (RF on), there was an almost immediate loss of pre-excitation, with the disappearance of delta waves in the ECG leads in the following beats. The interval between atrial and ventricular electrograms within each beat increased at the CS catheter, indicating normal conduction via the atrioventricular node and no conduction via the accessory pathway. The PR interval also increased, from less than 120 ms in the first three beats to 180 ms following successful radiofrequency ablation of the accessory pathway.

Fig. 6.39

Endocardial ECG: ablation of left-sided accessory pathway. Redrawn by permission of P. Stafford and G. A. Ng, Glenfield Hospital, Leicester

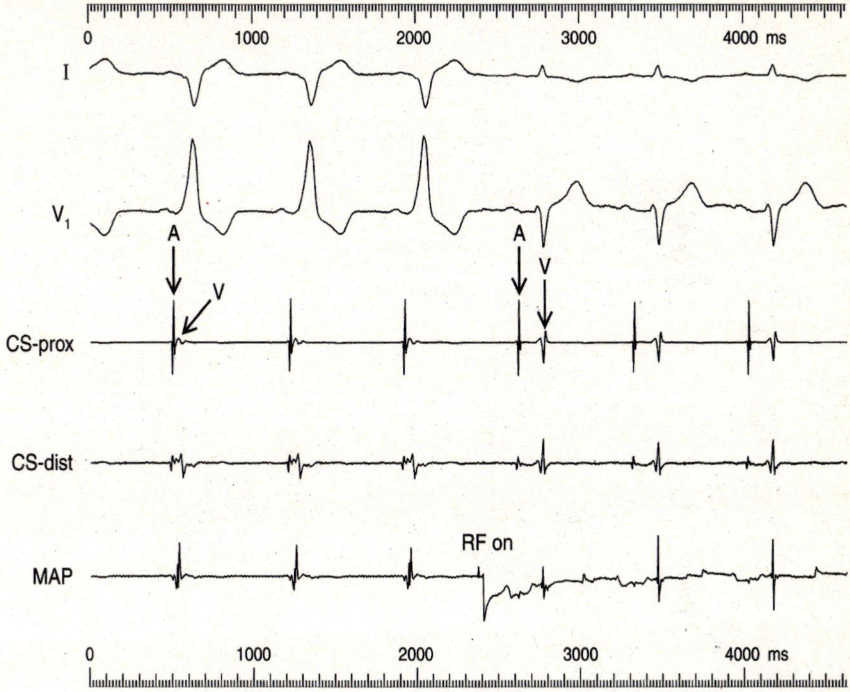

Note

- Increased paper speed compared to 12-lead ECG
- Delta wave in first three beats: positive in lead V_1, negative in lead I, PR interval < 120 ms
- Atrial (A) and ventricular (V) depolarization are almost superimposed before ablation, indicating conduction via an accessory pathway
- After ablation (RF on): delta wave in leads I and V_1 is lost; increased PR interval (180 ms); increased separation of atrial and ventricular depolarization recorded in the coronary sinus. These changes indicate AV nodal conduction

ARRHYTHMIAS AMENABLE TO ABLATION

Atrial flutter

Typical atrial flutter results from a re-entry circuit within the atria. This can be abolished by ablating an area known as the right atrial isthmus, which prevents re-entry from occurring (Fig. 6.40).

Atrial fibrillation

There is increasing evidence that in a high proportion of patients, atrial fibrillation is initiated either by enhanced atrial automaticity or by triggered activity arising in the vicinity of the pulmonary veins, probably in atrial tissue within the pulmonary vein ostia. Pulmonary vein isolation by ablation (Fig. 6.41) can

Fig. 6.40

Typical atrial flutter ablation

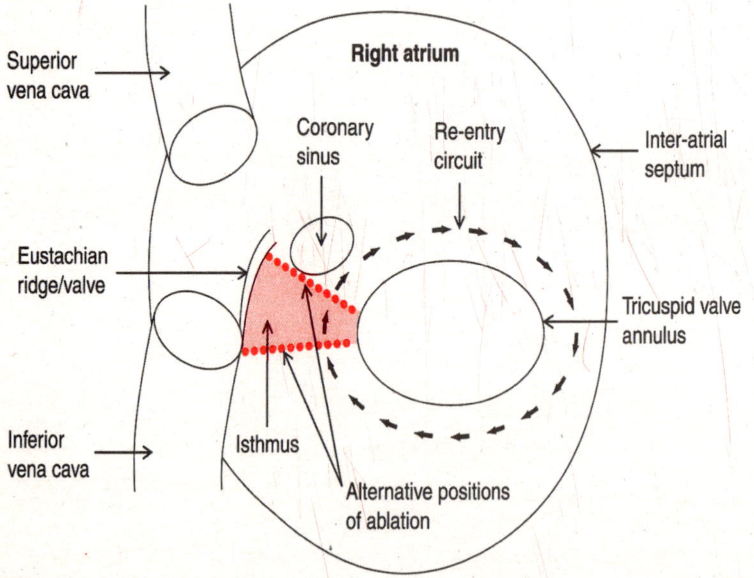

Note

- Arrhythmia occurs due to a re-entry circuit around the tricuspid valve annulus
- The re-entry circuit requires conduction through a narrow 'isthmus' of conducting tissue between the tricuspid valve annulus, the inferior vena cava, the coronary sinus and Eustachian ridge/valve
- Radiofrequency ablation of this isthmus interrupts and prevents re-entry

Fig. 6.41

Pulmonary vein isolation by ablation

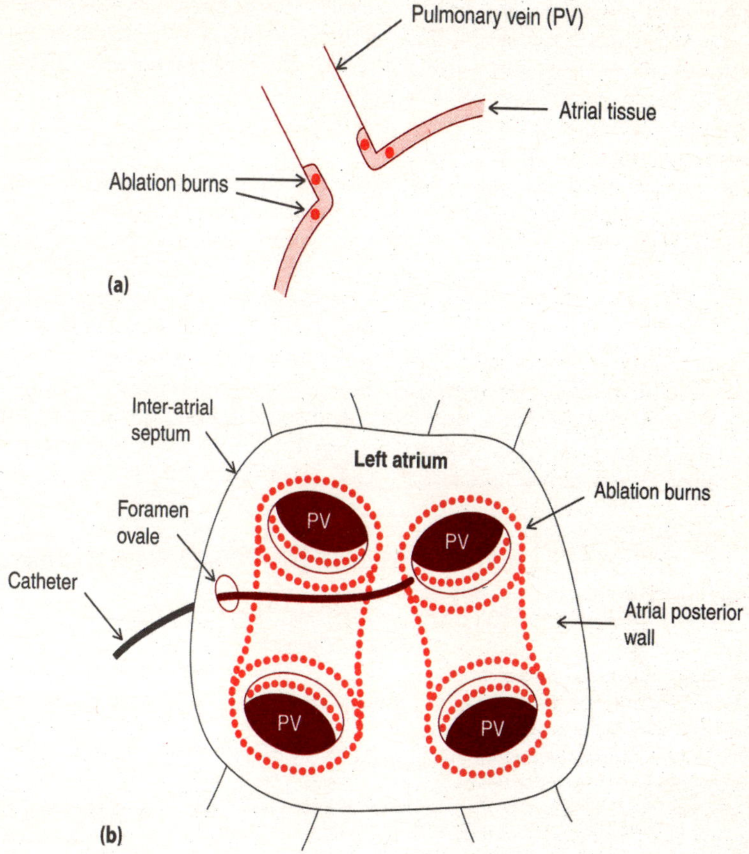

Note

- Atrial tissue extending into the pulmonary venous ostia acts as the substrate for the initiation of atrial fibrillation
- The aim of ablation is to isolate atrial tissue within the pulmonary veins from the rest of the atrium (a)
- Anatomy of pulmonary venous drainage is variable. Most commonly four veins drain into the posterior left atrium
- Ablation requires trans-septal puncture (through the foramen ovale), to allow trans-venous catheters to access the left atrium (b)

suppress the initiation of paroxysmal atrial fibrillation and also reduce relapse after the cardioversion of permanent atrial fibrillation. The ablation treatment of atrial fibrillation is more difficult than that of atrial flutter, because the left atrium has to be entered through the inter-atrial septum, and more burns are needed. At present this technique is usually regarded as a second-line option, limited to patients with symptoms refractory to conventional medical therapy, although its wider application is the subject of ongoing study.

Pathway ablation

Atrioventricular re-entry tachycardias, such as in the Wolff–Parkinson–White syndrome, can be treated by ablation of the accessory pathway, as described above. This prevents re-entry and eliminates both pre-excitation and episodes of supraventricular tachycardia. The ablation of pathways close to the AV node, including those involved in atrioventricular nodal re-entry tachycardia, can be attempted. However, there is a risk of AV block, with the associated necessity for a permanent pacemaker (see below).

Ventricular tachycardia

Some forms of ventricular tachycardia are amenable to catheter radiofrequency ablation treatment. These include right ventricular outflow tract VT, where triggered activity is the cause, and also VT in some patients with surgically corrected congenital heart disease, if a simple ventricular re-entry circuit can be demonstrated. Ischaemic VT is not usually amenable to electrophysiological ablation, because often there are multiple potential foci of increased automaticity and potential re-entry circuits, due to areas of myocardial scarring. More sophisticated

Box 6.6 Indications and complications of electrophysiology

Indications

- Atrioventricular re-entry tachycardias, including the Wolff–Parkinson–White syndrome
- Atrial fibrillation or atrial flutter, either paroxysmal or permanent, where the symptoms are refractory to conventional therapy or where medical therapy is contraindicated or poorly tolerated
- Ventricular tachycardias outside the context of ischaemic heart disease, including those associated with congenital heart disease and right ventricular outflow tract ventricular tachycardia
- Non-sustained ventricular tachycardia, as part of preparation for an ICD device (see indications for ICD devices): a ventricular tachycardia stimulation study
- AV node ablation, for atrial arrhythmias and AVNRE refractory to conventional medical therapies

Complications

- Peri-procedural stroke or TIA (transient ischaemic attack) (1%)
- Groin haematoma (7%)
- Pericardial tamponade (1%)
- Arteriovenous fistula (< 1%)
- Higher degree AV block (with pathways close to the AV node)
- Pulmonary vein stenosis (1%) (pulmonary vein isolation only)
- Repeated procedures (complex studies may require repeat procedures)

ventricular mapping tools are becoming available which allow potential ablation treatment even for ischaemic VT.

AV node ablation

Patients with atrially driven tachyarrhythmias, AVNRE tachycardia or atrial fibrillation, which cannot be controlled by pharmacological means, may undergo catheter ablation of the AV node. This leads to complete AV block, and bradycardia is prevented by the implantation of a permanent pacemaker ('ablate and pace').

INDICATIONS FOR ELECTROPHYSIOLOGY

The indications for electrophysiology, and the associated hazards, are summarized in Box 6.6.

7 Conclusions: four steps to making the most of the ECG

The theme of this book has been that the ECG is just one way of helping with the management of patients. The ECG is not an end in itself, and must always be seen in the context of the patient from whom it was recorded. To make the most of an ECG you need to think in four steps:

1. Describe it.
2. Interpret it.
3. See how it helps with the diagnosis.
4. Ask how it helps with treatment.

DESCRIPTION

An ECG can be described by anyone with the most basic knowledge, but an accurate description is needed as a basis for the later steps. The description starts with the rate of the heartbeat and its regularity, as measured by the intervals between the QRS complexes. The P waves must be identified; and if there are none, a clear statement of their absence is necessary. The relationship of the P waves to the QRS complexes is the next logical step, and the PR interval must be measured. The shape of the P wave needs to be recorded if it is abnormally peaked or bifid.

The QRS complexes need to be described in terms of their width and height, and also their shape: whether Q waves are present; whether there is more than one R wave in the QRS complex; and whether there are S waves in the leads where they would be expected. If there are Q waves, are they small and narrow, and are they only seen in the lateral leads, where they may be due to septal depolarization? If there are pathological Q waves, in which leads are they present and do they suggest a possible inferior or anterior myocardial infarction? The cardiac axis should be defined.

Elevation or depression of the ST segment must be noted. If the ST segment is elevated, does it follow an S wave, so indicating 'high take-off'? The T waves must be inspected in each lead, and while inversion in VR and V_1 is always normal, inversion in any other leads should be recorded. The QT interval should be measured and if it appears long, should be corrected for heart rate.

All these features can be identified without any knowledge of the patient, or indeed much knowledge of cardiology. The description of an ECG is reasonably well done by the automatic 'interpretation' function built into most modern ECG recorders, but it is important to remember that these are far from perfect. Automatic recorders tend to over-interpret ECGs (so that nothing of importance is missed), and their descriptions are not always totally accurate. They can be poor at identifying P waves and they often miss ST segment changes, and sometimes T wave inversion. Therefore you should never depend solely on a description provided by the ECG recorder itself.

INTERPRETATION

Once you have described the ECG you can interpret it, but a proper interpretation requires knowledge of the patient.

Always establish the cardiac rhythm first, because it may influence your interpretation of the rest of the ECG. For example, ventricular tachycardia, with its broad QRS complexes, will prevent any further interpretation – as will the broad complexes of complete heart block. The rhythm is established from the presence or absence of P waves and their relationship to the QRS complexes, from which arrhythmias and conduction defects can be accurately identified. On the whole, this part of ECG interpretation can be independent of the patient.

Otherwise, the accurate interpretation of an ECG will depend on the characteristics of the patient. If the ECG has been recorded from a healthy subject, or a patient with no clinical suggestion of cardiac disease, then it is essential to remember the range of normality of the ECG. First degree block, and supraventricular or ventricular extrasystoles, are commonly seen in healthy people. P waves can be bifid in healthy people; right axis deviation can be normal in tall thin people; and minor degrees of left axis deviation (especially with a narrow QRS complex) are normal in fat people and in pregnancy. An RSR^1 pattern with a normal QRS complex duration in lead V_1 is perfectly normal; and in some perfectly normal people there can be a small dominant R wave in lead V_1. Tall QRS complexes are frequently seen in healthy young people, and do not in themselves indicate left ventricular hypertrophy. 'Septal' Q waves may be present in leads VL and V_5–V_6. Inverted T waves in the anterior chest leads can be normal in black people, while in white people they may be due to hypertrophic cardiomyopathy. Peaked T waves are often of no significance at all, though they can be due to hyperkalaemia.

In a patient with chest pain, however, the interpretation of the same ECG abnormalities can be quite different. T wave inversion in the anterior chest leads may indicate a non-ST segment elevation myocardial infarction. Left bundle branch block may be the result of an old or new infarction. A change of cardiac axis to the right may be due to a pulmonary embolism. A dominant R wave in lead V_1 might be due to a posterior myocardial infarction.

In a patient with breathlessness, right axis deviation, a dominant R wave in lead V_1 or T wave inversion in leads V_1–V_3 may indicate multiple pulmonary emboli or idiopathic pulmonary hypertension. A deep S wave in lead V_6 may be due to chronic lung disease or to a pulmonary embolus. In patients complaining of attacks of dizziness, a finding such as first degree block, of little significance in a healthy subject, might indicate transient episodes of higher degrees of block causing a symptomatic bradycardia. A prolonged QT interval might point to episodes of torsade de pointes ventricular tachycardia.

Any described abnormality in an ECG must therefore be interpreted in the context of a knowledge of the patient's condition; otherwise, ECG changes will support a less focused differential diagnosis.

DIAGNOSIS

The ECG is essential for the diagnosis of problems involving rhythm and conduction, and here the interpretation and the diagnosis are clearly strongly linked. But it is necessary to remember that the identification of a specific arrhythmia does not complete the diagnosis, which should include the cause of the arrhythmia. For example, the cause of atrial fibrillation may be ischaemic or rheumatic heart disease, or alcoholism, or thyrotoxicosis, or a cardiomyopathy, and so on. Heart block may be due to idiopathic His bundle fibrosis, but it also raises the possibility of ischaemic or hypertensive heart disease. Left bundle branch block may be due to aortic stenosis, and right bundle branch block may be associated with an atrial septal defect.

ECG appearances that suggest faults in the recording technique may sometimes point to a clinical diagnosis. For example, artefacts due to movement may suggest a neurological disorder such as Parkinson's disease. Low-voltage QRS complexes may be due not to poor standardization, but to obesity, emphysema, myxoedema or a pericardial effusion.

An ECG cannot diagnose the presence of heart failure, though with a totally normal ECG, heart failure is unlikely. The ECG may, however, help in diagnosing the cause of heart failure, which is often the key to treatment – atrial fibrillation and ventricular hypertrophy may suggest valve disease, as may left bundle branch block, or there may be evidence of an old myocardial infarction. Similarly, the ECG is not a good way of identifying electrolyte abnormalities, but flat T waves, U waves, and long QT intervals should at least suggest the possibility that there may be an electrolyte problem. A long QT interval, on the other hand, may be due to one of the congenital syndromes or to one of a wide variety of drugs.

The accurate identification of an ECG abnormality is thus only part of the diagnostic process: we still need to determine the underlying cause. The ECG often points the way to appropriate further investigations, such as chest X-rays, echocardiography, blood tests for electrolyte abnormalities, or cardiac catheterization, and the ECG is simply part of the diagnostic process.

TREATMENT

The ECG is obviously paramount in determining the treatment of an arrhythmia or conduction defects. It is also crucial for the proper use of acute interventions in both ST segment elevation and non-ST segment elevation myocardial infarction. But its limitations must also be understood: in particular, it must be remembered that the ECG can be normal in the early stages of a myocardial infarction, and a normal, or near-normal, ECG is not an adequate reason for sending a patient with chest pain home from an A & E department.

Without an understanding of the ECG, devices such as pacemakers and implanted cardioverter defibrillators (ICDs) could not have been invented. These devices, and the techniques that use them, such as dual chamber pacing and cardiac resynchronization therapy, are the province of the specialist. But as these devices and techniques become increasingly prevalent, they will be encountered more and more by general practitioners and specialists in non-cardiac disciplines. For example, patients with these devices tend to be elderly, and it is the elderly who most frequently experience multiple medical problems – so non-cardiac specialists are bound to come across patients who have problems, but who also have a modern electrical device that is working perfectly normally. A basic understanding of these devices and techniques is therefore needed by a wide range of clinicians, and it is to them that Chapter 6 of this book was addressed.

CONCLUSION

The ECG is easy to describe and interpret, but it is often more difficult to appreciate the range of normality, and to remember that a full diagnosis encompasses the cause of any abnormality that may have been identified. The ECG is an essential part of the overall diagnostic process in a wide variety of patients, and in some it influences treatment. The most important thing to remember is that diagnosis and management depend on a full consideration of the individual patient, not just of the ECG.

Now test yourself

150 ECG Problems, a companion to this volume, gives 150 clinical scenarios with full related ECGs, and poses questions about ECG interpretation and the diagnosis and management of patients.

Index

Note: Page numbers in **bold** refer to figures and tables.
Abbreviations used in subentries: LBBB, left bundle branch block; RBBB, right bundle branch block.

A

B

C

D

E

F

G

H

M

N

O

P

S

T

U

V

W

X